Spinal Diseases

Guest Editor

RONALDO C. da COSTA, DMV, MSc, PhD

VETERINARY CLINICS
OF NORTH AMERICA:
SMALL ANIMAL PRACTICE

www.vetsmall.theclinics.com

September 2010 • Volume 40 • Number 5

SAUNDERS an imprint of ELSEVIER, Inc.

W.B. SAUNDERS COMPANY
A Division of Elsevier Inc.

1600 John F. Kennedy Blvd. • Suite 1800 • Philadelphia, PA 19103-2899
http://www.vetsmall.theclinics.com

VETERINARY CLINICS OF NORTH AMERICA: SMALL ANIMAL PRACTICE Volume 40, Number 5 September 2010 ISSN 0195-5616, ISBN-13: 978-1-4377-2507-0

Editor: John Vassallo; j.vassallo@elsevier.com
Developmental Editor: Donald Mumford

Veterinary Clinics of North America: Small Animal Practice (ISSN 0195-5616) is published bimonthly (For Post Office use only: volume 40 issue 5 of 6) by Elsevier Inc., 360 Park Avenue South, New York, NY 10010-1710. Months of issue are January, March, May, July, September, and November. Business and Editorial Offices: 1600 John F. Kennedy Blvd., Ste. 1800, Philadelphia, PA 19103-2899. Customer Service Office: 3251 Riverport Lane, Maryland Heights, MO 63043. Periodicals postage paid at New York, NY and additional mailing offices. Subscription prices are $245.00 per year (domestic individuals), $388.00 per year (domestic institutions), $122.00 per year (domestic students/residents), $324.00 per year (Canadian individuals), $477.00 per year (Canadian institutions), $360.00 per year (international individuals), $477.00 per year (international institutions), and $177.00 per year (international and Canadian students/residents). To receive student/resident rate, orders must be accompained by name of affiliated institution, date of term, and the *signature* of program/residency coordinator on institution letterhead. Orders will be billed at individual rate until proof of status is received. Foreign air speed delivery is included in all *Clinics* subscription prices. All prices are subject to change without notice. **POSTMASTER:** Send address changes to *Veterinary Clinics of North America: Small Animal Practice*, Elsevier Health Sciences Division, Subscription Customer Service, 3251 Riverport Lane, Maryland Heights, MO 63043. Customer Service (orders, claims, online, change of address): Elsevier Periodicals Customer Service, Elsevier Health Sciences Division Subscription Customer Service 3251 Riverport Lane Maryland Heights, MO 63043. Tel: 1-800-654-2452 (U.S. and Canada); 314-447-8871 (outside U.S. and Canada). Fax: 314-447-8029. E-mail: journalscustomerservice-usa@elsevier.com (for print support); journalsonlinesupport-usa@elsevier.com (for online support).

Reprints. For copies of 100 or more of articles in this publication, please contact the Commercial Reprints Department, Elsevier Inc., 360 Park Avenue South, New York, NY 10010-1710. Tel.: 212-633-3812; Fax: 212-462-1935; E-mail: reprints@elsevier.com.

Veterinary Clinics of North America: Small Animal Practice is also published in Japanese by Inter Zoo Publishing Co., Ltd., Aoyama Crystal-Bldg 5F, 3-5-12 Kitaaoyama, Minato-ku, Tokyo 107-0061, Japan.

Veterinary Clinics of North America: Small Animal Practice is covered in *Current Contents/Agriculture, Biology and Environmental Sciences, Science Citation Index, ASCA, MEDLINE/PubMed (Index Medicus), Excerpta Medica, and BIOSIS.*

Printed and bound by CPI Group (UK) Ltd, Croydon, CR0 4YY
Transferred to Digital Print 2011

Contributors

GUEST EDITOR

RONALDO C. da COSTA, DMV, MSc, PhD
Diplomate, American College of Veterinary Internal Medicine (Neurology); Assistant Professor and Service Head, Neurology and Neurosurgery, Department of Veterinary Clinical Sciences, College of Veterinary Medicine, The Ohio State University, Columbus, Ohio

AUTHORS

RODNEY S. BAGLEY, DVM
Diplomate, American College of Veterinary Internal Medicine (Neurology, Internal Medicine); Professor of Neurology and Neurosurgery; Chair, Department of Clinical Sciences, Iowa State University, College of Veterinary Medicine, Ames, Iowa

NIKLAS BERGKNUT, DVM, MS
Department of Clinical Sciences of Companion Animals, Faculty of Veterinary Medicine, Utrecht University, Utrecht, The Netherlands; Division of Small Animals, Department of Clinical Sciences, Faculty of Veterinary Medicine and Animal Sciences, Swedish University of Agricultural Sciences, Uppsala, Sweden

BRIGITTE A. BRISSON, DMV, DVSc
Diplomate, American College of Veterinary Surgeons; Associate Professor and Chief of Small Animal Surgery, Department of Clinical Studies, Ontario Veterinary College, University of Guelph, Guelph, Ontario, Canada

JOAN R. COATES, DVM, MS
Diplomate, American College of Veterinary Internal Medicine (Neurology); Associate Professor of Veterinary Neurology and Neurosurgery, Department of Veterinary Medicine and Surgery, College of Veterinary Medicine, University of Missouri Columbia, Columbia, Missouri

RONALDO C. da COSTA, DMV, MSc, PhD
Diplomate, American College of Veterinary Internal Medicine (Neurology); Assistant Professor and Service Head, Neurology and Neurosurgery, Department of Veterinary Clinical Sciences, College of Veterinary Medicine, The Ohio State University, Columbus, Ohio

LUISA DE RISIO, DVM, MRCVS, PhD
Diplomate, European College of Veterinary Neurology; European and RCVS Specialist in Veterinary Neurology; Head of Neurology/Neurosurgery Unit, Centre for Small Animal Studies, Animal Health Trust, Kentford, Newmarket, Suffolk, United Kingdom

NICK D. JEFFERY, BVSc, PhD, FRCVS
Diplomate, European College of Veterinary Surgeons; Diplomate, European College of Veterinary Neurology; Professor of Veterinary Clinical Studies, Department of Veterinary Medicine, University of Cambridge, Cambridge, United Kingdom

KATIA MARIONI-HENRY, DVM, MRCVS, PhD
Diplomate, American College of Veterinary Internal Medicine (Neurology); Diplomate, European College of Veterinary Neurology; Southern Counties Veterinary Specialists, Ringwood, Hampshire, United Kingdom

BJÖRN P. MEIJ, DVM, PhD
Diplomate, European College of Veterinary Surgeons; Department of Clinical Sciences of Companion Animals, Faculty of Veterinary Medicine, Utrecht University, Utrecht, The Netherlands

SARAH A. MOORE, DVM
Diplomate, American College of Veteninary Intetnal Medicine (Neurology); Assistant Professor, Neurology and Neurosurgery, Department of Veterinary Clinical Sciences, College of Veterinary Medicine, The Ohio State University, Columbus, Ohio

NATASHA OLBY, VetMB, PhD
Diplomate, American College of Veterinary Internal Medicine (Neurology); Associate Professor, Department of Clinical Sciences, College of Veterinary Medicine, North Carolina State University, Raleigh, North Carolina

JOANE PARENT, DMV, MVetSc
Diplomate, American College of Veterinary Internal Medicine (Neurology); Professor, Département de Sciences Cliniques, Faculté de Médecine Vétérinaire, Université de Montréal, Québec, Canada

SIMON R. PLATT, BVM&S, MRCVS
Diplomate, American College of Veterinary Internal Medicine (Neurology); Diplomate, European College of Veterinary Neurology; RCVS Specialist in Veterinary Neurology; Associate Professor, Department of Small Animal Medicine and Surgery, College of Veterinary Medicine, University of Georgia, Athens, Georgia

VALERIE F. SAMII, DVM
Diplomate, American College of Veterinary Radiology; Adjunct Professor, Department of Veterinary Clinical Sciences, College of Veterinary Medicine, The Ohio State University, Columbus, Ohio

VERONIKA M. STEIN, DVM, PhD
Diplomate, European College of Veterinary Neurology; Department of Small Animal Medicine and Surgery, University for Veterinary Medicine Hannover, Hannover, Germany

BEVERLY K. STURGES, DVM, MS
Department of Surgical and Radiological Sciences, School of Veterinary Medicine, University of California at Davis, Davis, California

ANDREA TIPOLD, DVM
Diplomate, European College of Veterinary Neurology; Professor for Neurology, Department of Small Animal Medicine and Surgery, University for Veterinary Medicine Hannover, Hannover, Germany

DICCON R. WESTWORTH, BVSc (Hons)
VCA Animal Care Center of Sonoma County, Rohnert Park; Assistant Clinical Professor, Department of Surgical and Radiological Sciences, School of Veterinary Medicine, University of California at Davis, Davis, California

FRED A. WININGER, VMD, MS
Diplomate, American College of Veterinary Internal Medicine (Neurology); Assistant Professor of Veterinary Neurology and Neurosurgery, Department of Veterinary Medicine and Surgery, College of Veterinary Medicine, University of Missouri, Columbia, Missouri

Contents

FORTHCOMING ISSUES

November 2010

Current Topics in Canine and Feline Infectious Diseases

Stephen C. Barr, BVSc, MVS, PhD,
Guest Editor

January 2011

Organ Failure in Critical Illness

Tim Hackett, DVM, MS,
Guest Editor

March 2011

Kidney Failure and Renal Replacement Therapies

Mark Acierno, MBA, DVM, and
Mary A. Labato, DVM,
Guest Editors

RECENT ISSUES

July 2010

Topics in Cardiology

Jonathan A. Abbott, DVM,
Guest Editor

May 2010

Immunology: Function, Pathology, Diagnostics, and Modulation

Melissa A. Kennedy, DVM, PhD,
Guest Editor

March 2010

Obesity, Diabetes, and Adrenal Disorders

Thomas K. Graves, DVM, PhD,
Guest Editor

RELATED INTEREST

Veterinary Clinics of North America: Exotic Animal Practice
September 2007 (Vol. 10, No. 3)
Neuroanatomy and Neurodiagnostics
Lisa A. Tell, DVM, Dipl. ABVP—Avian, and Marguerite F. Knipe, DVM, Dipl. ACVIM (Neurology), *Guest Editors*

Preface
Spinal Diseases

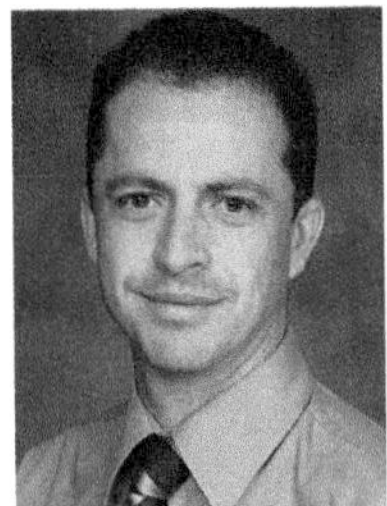

Ronaldo C. da Costa, DMV, MSc, PhD
Guest Editor

This *Veterinary Clinics of North America: Small Animal Practice* revisits Spinal Diseases after 18 years. Eighteen years is a long time. Enough time for one to be born, grow up, and head off to college. Not surprisingly, much has changed. For example, magnetic resonance imaging, now routinely used for spinal diseases, was in its infancy back in 1992.

Spinal problems are very common in practice. The articles were selected to provide clinicians with the knowledge and insights to be successful in their approach, diagnosis, and treatment of common spinal conditions of dogs and cats. For this purpose, experts from 6 countries representing 15 academic and private institutions have contributed the most current information to this issue.

We start by reviewing the fundamentals of clinical neurology with an article presenting the diagnostic approach and lesion localization of patients with spinal diseases. A fundamental principle in the approach to the neurologic patient is that lesion localization always comes first, and only thereafter can specific differential diagnoses and a diagnostic plan be considered. To facilitate this goal and enhance the reader's skills in lesion localization, the first article contains numerous online videos, and the reader is strongly advised to take advantage of this feature. The next article introduces the differential diagnoses in a straightforward approach based on lesion localization that identifies the main spinal diseases to be considered. The following article focuses on the advantages and disadvantages of computed tomography and magnetic resonance imaging in the diagnosis of spinal diseases, followed by 10 comprehensive articles covering the most common and important diseases of the spine, such as intervertebral disc disease. Cats are special, and the issue concludes with an article on feline spinal diseases.

It was an honor and a privilege to serve as the Guest Editor for this issue and to work with such a distinguished team of experts. I am indebted to all the contributors who sacrificed their personal time to share their knowledge and experience. Our profession is very grateful for their contributions. I thank John Vassallo for his patience and

Vet Clin Small Anim 40 (2010) xiii–xiv
doi:10.1016/j.cvsm.2010.07.002

assistance throughout this long process. I also thank my parents, my beautiful wife, Luciana, and my kids, Felipe and Rafaela, for once again "understanding" that Dad was busy. Finally, I thank God for one day long ago placing an epileptic dog in my path, which has since changed the way I see veterinary medicine.

The goal of all of us involved in this project was to bring you "simply the best." We hope you will enjoy it!

Ronaldo C. da Costa, DMV, MSc, PhD
Department of Veterinary Clinical Sciences
College of Veterinary Medicine
The Ohio State University
601 Vernon Tharp Street
Columbus, OH 43210, USA

E-mail address:
dacosta.6@osu.edu

Clinical Approach and Lesion Localization in Patients with Spinal Diseases

Joane Parent, DMV, MVetSc

KEYWORDS

- Spinal disease • Vertebral disease • Lesion localization
- Neck and back pain • Ataxia • Paresis/paralysis

In most cases, it is the owner's complaint that raises the suspicion of vertebral column disease. The history is taken to collect information about time of onset and progression of clinical signs as it relates to the reason of presentation. The physical and ophthalmologic examinations provide information about the general health of the animal and about the presence of systemic signs that could be related or compound the neurologic disease. The neurologic examination brings into light the neurologic deficits and leads to lesion localization. Once these steps have been completed, the differential diagnosis is established based on lesion localization, history, and the animal's signalment. The diagnostic workup is then planned, keeping in mind the most probable causes. Minimum database and ancillary laboratory diagnostic tests, imaging, cerebrospinal fluid (CSF) analysis, electrodiagnostics, and biopsies may all be necessary to reach the final diagnosis.[1] Each of these steps are covered in more detail in the following paragraphs.

OWNER'S COMPLAINT

A complaint of back or neck pain, difficulty or inability walking, and incoordination or presence of lameness that does not respond to medical treatment should all alert the clinician to a possible spinal/vertebral problem. Incoordination, wobbliness, and drunken gait all relate to neurologic gait. Dragging of the rear paws and assistance to get into the car or up the stairs may harbor rear-end weakness related to a vertebral/spinal disorder. A lameness in which no abnormality is found on radiographs or joint aspiration and that fails to respond to symptomatic treatment should be investigated for spinal nerve/nerve root disease and secondary spinal cord involvement.

Département de Sciences Cliniques, Faculté de Médecine Vétérinaire, Université de Montréal, 3200 rue Sicotte, St-Hyacinthe, Québec J2S-2M2, Canada
E-mail address: joane.parent@umontreal.ca

Vet Clin Small Anim 40 (2010) 733–753
doi:10.1016/j.cvsm.2010.07.001
vetsmall.theclinics.com
0195-5616/10/$ – see front matter

History

The time of apparition of the first clinical sign, the rapidity of onset, the progression of the disease (deterioration, status quo, or improvement), and if the animal is in pain give important clues toward possible causes. The length of the history is also an important factor for prognosis, which helps to decide how rapidly and aggressively the problem should be addressed. Generally, there is an expected time course with the different categories of neurologic diseases. Vascular events (as in fibrocartilaginous embolic myelopathy), as a rule, are acute in onset with stabilization of the clinical signs within hours of onset. The animal may cry out at the time of the event but the owner, following the event, does not report the dog as being in pain. The clinical signs in inflammatory diseases progress usually over a few days or more, with presence of pain if there is bone, disc, dorsal root, or meningeal involvement. In these instances, nonspecific systemic signs, such as inappetence and lethargy, may also be present. Tumors are usually more chronic in onset with signs that worsen over a few weeks to a few months, usually in the order of 6 to 12 weeks. With such gradual onset, it is not rare that sudden deterioration occurs just before presentation. Intervertebral disc disease can do it all, from acute to chronic. Pain is a salient feature of intervertebral disc disease. Cervical spondylomyelopathy may go unnoticed until exacerbation following a traumatic event occurs, and then there may be rapid progression or deterioration over a few days. In most cases, the disease is progressive over a few weeks to months, whereas degenerative myelopathy is insidious in onset progressing over many months. If 1 limb is primarily affected, the owner's complaint pertains to lameness. However, if there is more than 1 limb affected, the tendency is to speak of difficulty for the animal to walk, rear-end weakness, or incoordination.

The presence of neck or back pain deserves more attention because it plays a determining role in the establishment of the differential diagnosis. The most common complaint associated with vertebral column pain is reluctance for the animal to move (eg, climb stairs, or get onto the bed, couch, or car). Arching of the back, stiffness of the neck, inability to bend the head down to eat, yelping when picked up, and shaking are other frequently reported complaints. Clinicians should not accept at face value the complaint of pain without questioning the owner on the observations that lead to this conclusion. Dogs with generalized weakness may be interpreted as painful. An example is the dog with the generalized form of myasthenia gravis (Video 1). The dog advances, frequently sitting on its rear end, with stiff, short, and rapid steps usually more pronounced in the hind limbs giving an impression of a painful rear end, when in fact, the animal has never cried in pain when moved, carried, or picked up. Painful vertebral diseases appear to be less frequent in cats as compared with dogs.[2] In dogs and cats, when there are concomitant neurologic deficits, owners may focus on the gait abnormality and not volunteer that pain is present until asked.

Once the suspicion of spinal/vertebral disease is raised, it is important to evaluate if the disease is limited to the nervous system or if it is of a more systemic nature. Lethargy, weight loss, decreased appetite, vomiting, diarrhea, coughing, or sneezing, to name the most frequent, are signs that should alert the clinician to the possibility of a systemic illness. In dogs and cats, infectious and metastatic diseases are the most common illnesses to secondarily affect the vertebral column and its structures. In these instances, the neurologic disease is only a sign of a more serious problem even if the animal is presented with vertebral column disease as the chief presentation.

CONSIDERATION OF THE ANIMAL'S SIGNALMENT

The species, breed, and age of the animal are especially useful in the establishment of the differential diagnosis. As an example, intervertebral disc (IVD) disease is uncommon in cats, whereas it is the most common cause of spinal pain and neurologic deficits in the dog. Multiple genetic breed-associated neurologic diseases have now been recorded in dogs and cats. A recent chart listing all known syndromes[3] should be consulted whenever patients display an unusual neurologic presentation. Intervertebral disc disease is more common in chondrodystrophic breeds and should not be diagnosed in any dog younger than 2 years of age without a spinal diagnostic workup. Primary tumor or metastatic disease of the vertebral canal and its content remains a consideration in the older dog (>6 years) and cat (>8 years). Crucial in listing the possible causes of the animal's present problem, the age of the animal is kept in mind during examination because some age-related physical (eg, osteoarthritis) and ophthalmologic (eg, cataract, iris atrophy) abnormalities may interfere with the results of the neurologic examination.

PHYSICAL AND FUNDUSCOPIC EXAMINATIONS

The overall animal's condition (weight and hair coat) is assessed and the vital parameters taken, the mouth and mucous membranes examined, followed by palpation of the lymph nodes, thoracic auscultation with simultaneous femoral pulse examination, and abdominal palpation. Particular attention must be given to the musculoskeletal system because some orthopedic problems may have the appearance of a spinal disorder. The best example is the bilateral cruciate rupture in dogs, which may be misinterpreted as hind-limb paresis secondary to vertebral canal disease (Video 2). The ocular examination, especially as it relates to the retinas, can be done with the neurologic examination. The optic nerves and retinas are projections of the brain tissue and as such may be involved in any of the central nervous system (CNS) inflammatory diseases. Although dogs with primary disease of the vertebral column often do not have clinical signs or physical abnormalities indicative of other system involvement, there are several adult and geriatric patients that suffer from other ailments than the ones for which they are presented. The older German shepherd dog presenting with abnormal gait may suffer from concomitant hip dysplasia, degenerative joint disease, chronic cruciate rupture, lumbosacral pain, fibrotic myositis, IVD disease, and facets arthritis, yet the presenting complaint may relate to a nonpainful degenerative myelopathy. The presence of these other problems, unrelated to the spinal cord disease, likely has an effect on the overall animal's condition and adds to the complexity of the interpretation of the nervous system examination.

NEUROLOGIC EXAMINATION

Lesion localization is the most important element of neurologic disease. Although the evaluation of the gait, postural reactions, and spinal reflexes is more pertinent to vertebral/spinal disease, in all cases of suspected nervous system disease, a neurologic examination should always be carried out in its entirety. As an example, the Horner syndrome found on cranial nerve examination of the dog presented with traumatic avulsion of the brachial plexus adds invaluable information for prognostication. The Horner syndrome, in this instance, is indicative of root avulsion offering little chance for regeneration. For the purpose of this article, only abnormalities of the examination that directly relate to the evaluation of the spinal cord are discussed. Many patients with vertebral column pain have no other neurologic abnormality yet have significant spinal cord disease.[4,5]

Cranial Nerve Examination

The most common abnormality observed with an impact on lesion localization in spinal diseases is the presence of a Horner syndrome. Indeed, the pathway for the sympathetic innervation of the eye runs along the white matter of the cervical (C) cord to reach the gray matter of the thoracic (T) spinal cord segments, T1, T2, T3, to exit the vertebral canal by way of these respective ventral roots. On funduscopy, there may be retinitis or other abnormalities indicative of inflammatory noninfectious (granulomatous meningoencephalomyelitis) and infectious diseases. The presence of other cranial nerve deficits may be indicative of a diffuse or multifocal lesion or of a separate problem. The results must be interpreted in the light of the history and presenting complaint.

Gait and Posture

The evaluation of the gait and posture is pivotal to the localization of the lesion in spinal disease. It must be done with attention answering specific questions while observing the animal walking. With the use of a food treat, the dog is made to walk with its head elevated to accentuate the deficits by removing visual input.

Questions to answer while evaluating gait and posture[a]

1. Is the animal able to walk?
2. Is the gait normal?
3. Which limbs are affected (one limb, both hind limbs, the hind and front limbs, or the ipsilateral limbs)?
4. Is there presence of ataxia?
5. If there is ataxia, of which type (vestibular, cerebellar, or proprioceptive)?
6. Is there postural abnormality (neck curvature, low head carriage, arched back, and so forth)?

In cats with abnormal gait, it is sometimes necessary to have the owner video the animal in the home environment because, in the examination room, the cat may refuse to walk or walks crouched close to the ground falsifying the interpretation. If the dog is presented with a complaint of an inability to walk, it is important to encourage the animal to walk/move with an energetic voice before the animal tires out. The first few seconds that follow the command are crucial because in the weakened animal, the effort is so intense that movements, if any, are observable only for a few seconds. The presence of voluntary movements has great impact on prognosis and cost. In spinal cord disease, weakness (paresis) is present concomitantly with ataxia but weakness can be difficult to appreciate in the early stages of the disease. By far, the most sensitive test to evaluate for presence of proprioceptive ataxia remains the gait, not the proprioceptive positioning test (knuckling the paw over). In spinal cord disease, proprioceptive ataxia precedes deficits in proprioceptive positioning testing.

The observation of the posture adds useful information toward lesion localization. A stiff neck or an arched back in the dog is usually indicative of vertebral column pain. If

---

[a] *Adapted from* Parent J. The canine and feline neurological examination CD Rom. Scientific content: Joane Parent. System: I.C.Axon. 2001. ISBN 0-88955-511-7; with permission.

the arc of the arched back is centered to the thoracolumbar region, the disease is usually in the T10 to L2 region, whereas when the rear end of the animal is kept under, low lumbar (L) or lumbosacral (LS) disease is more likely. In the laterally recumbent animal, a Schiff-Sherrington posture (extension of neck and front limbs, with hind limb paralysis) indicates a T3 to L5 lesion.

Postural Reactions

Hopping and proprioceptive positioning are routinely and consistently done because they are easily performed in all sizes of dogs and cats. Although not specific for proprioceptive loss and of little localizing value, in the author's opinion the proprioceptive positioning reaction is, after the evaluation of the gait, one of the best tests to evaluate proprioception in the ambulatory dog. However, the test must be done appropriately (Video 3) and the results interpreted in light of the rest of the neurologic findings. Also named *paw replacement test*, its delay or absence is not specific of a particular function loss. Indeed, a paralyzed animal with motor polyneuropathy does not replace the paw because of motor neuron involvement, not because of proprioceptive loss. Generalized weakness from non-neurologic problems frequently causes this test to be delayed or absent. Musculoskeletal problems, such as degenerative joint disease, hip dysplasia, cruciate rupture, and arthritis, may all cause undue knuckling without true proprioceptive deficits. In the cat, paw placement is replaced by the lateral tactile placing reaction (see Video 3) if the cat does not let the examiner knuckle the paw over. When performed appropriately, the proprioceptive positioning test is a sensitive evaluator of proprioception in ambulatory patients, but will never replace a keen observation of the gait. Hopping (Video 4) is helpful to ascertain asymmetry between sides.

Spinal Reflexes

Presence of proprioceptive ataxia and weakness localizes the neurologic lesion to the spinal cord, whereas the nature of the spinal reflexes and muscle tone provides information about the location of the lesion along the neuraxis. The reflexes to be evaluated include the extensor and flexor (withdrawal) reflexes for the front and hind limbs, the cutaneous trunci reflex, the perineal reflex, and, although absent in the normal animal, the crossed extensor reflex. The extensor reflex of the front limb evaluates the radial nerve, which is responsible for weight bearing by allowing extension of the articulations for the entire front limb. The extensor reflex is assessed in the ambulatory dog by evaluating the ability of the dog to stand on its front limbs. In the laterally recumbent dog, the extensor reflex is elicited by stimulating, with a hand, the palmar face of the paw to cause extension of the limb (Video 5). The hind limb extensor tone is elicited as in the front limbs when the animal is standing or made to stand on the hind limbs, and by the evaluation of the patellar reflex. The patellar reflex assesses the femoral nerve, responsible for weight bearing in the hind limbs, and sensation of the medial face of the limb. The patellar reflex (Video 6) is frequently technically difficult to obtain. If the reflex is absent, it does not necessarily equate lower motor neuron (LMN) disease. Indeed, experimentally, in dogs, severing the L5 *dorsal* root causes loss of the patellar tendon reflex yet motor function and tone remain normal, whereas severing the L5 *ventral* root results in hyporeflexia, hypotonia, and LMN weakness.[6] The flexor or withdrawal reflex is easy to elicit but difficult to interpret. Pinching a toe causes withdrawal of the limb in the normal animal. All articulations should flex. The strength with which the animal withdraws the limb varies in relation to the severity of the lesion. In upper motor neuron (UMN) disease, the withdrawal is weak but complete (ie, each articulation flexes), whereas in LMN, the reflex is incomplete or absent (ie, there is decreased or absent flexion of the articulations). Although the term withdrawal reflex is used, it cannot be considered a true reflex whenever voluntary movements are present. Dogs often inhibit the withdrawal of their limb making it necessary to use a strong stimulus, one that hurts, to elicit the withdrawal or flexor reflex. Musculoskeletal diseases and other non-neurologic generalized weaknesses interfere with the strength with which an animal is able to pull its limb away from the examiner. The strength of the withdrawal reflex should always be interpreted in light of the patients' general health and other neurologic findings. The withdrawal reflex in the front limb evaluates the subscapular, axillary, musculocutaneous, median, and ulnar nerves. Sensation is provided to the dorsal aspect of the paw primarily by the radial nerve and to the ventral aspect by the median nerve. Pinching any toe should lead to a withdrawal of the limb. The withdrawal reflex in the hind limb evaluates primarily the sciatic nerve. Pinching the lateral toe causes flexion of the stifle, hock, and toes (Video 7). Distally, the sciatic nerve is divided into 2 branches, the peroneal nerve (primarily from L6, L7 spinal segments) and the tibial nerve (primarily from spinal segments L7, S1 [sacrum 1]). The peroneal nerve is responsible for the flexion of the hock and extension of the toes, and the tibial nerve for the extension of the hock and flexion of the toes. The sciatic nerve is responsible for the sensation of the lateral part of the limb. When assessing the hind-limb withdrawal reflexes, the lateral then the medial toes must be stimulated to evaluate nociception on all faces of the limb. The presence of the crossed extensor reflex is normal at the walk. As one limb flexes, the contralateral limb extends in preparation to support more of the animal's weight that is not supported by the flexed limb. Its presence is abnormal in the recumbent animal (normal in neonates) and is always indicative of a UMN lesion (Video 8). A crossed extensor reflex can be observed with cervical or thoracolumbar lesion, in the front or hind limbs, and is usually indicative of severe and mostly chronic lesions. The perineal reflex evaluates the pudendal nerve, which innervates the striated muscles of the external sphincter of the anus and urethra and the skin of the perineum. Touching the perineal region causes the tail to flex, evaluating the sensory part of the reflex. The motor part of the reflex (ie, the contraction of the anal sphincter), although observable concomitantly with the tail flexion, is best assessed with rectal examination. Although multiple attempts may be necessary to elicit the cutaneous trunci reflex, in most dogs a reflex can be obtained (Video 9). In cats, the reflex is frequently absent. The afferent (sensory) limb of the reflex (ie, the regional spinal nerve and spinal cord white matter upward to the level of the eighth cervical and first thoracic spinal segments) synapses on the cell bodies of the lateral thoracic nerve (the efferent limb of the reflex) causing contraction of the cutaneous trunci muscle. Touching the skin along the back stimulates a dermatome that results in an impulse that ascends to the spinal cord by way of the spinal nerve innervating this dermatome, then enters the spinal cord and ascends bilaterally to the C8, T1 segments, such as pinching the skin on one side causes contraction of both lateral thoracic nerves. Depending on the location of the lesion, the sensory (spinal cord) or the motor part (gray matter and lateral thoracic nerve) of the reflex may be affected. The reflex is useful in localizing lesion in spinal cord disease as long as the lesion is severe and above L1. The ascending fibers for this reflex are located deeper within the fasciculus proprius and as such are more resilient. Also, because the dermatome innervated by the T13 spinal nerve is located vis-à-vis the L4 lumbar vertebra, lower spinal nerves have their dermatomes over the pelvis, rendering this test less useful for lesions below L1. The reflex is also useful in the evaluation of gray matter damage at C8 and T1 spinal segments or for C8 and T1 ventral root avulsion (LMN signs).

The maintenance of muscle tone is a function of spinal reflexes (myotatic reflex or muscle stretch reflex). In LMN disease, reflexes and tone are decreased to absent.

The neurogenic atrophy that ensues is rapid to appear (within days). In UMN disease, reflexes and tone are normal to increased. The muscle atrophy is from lack of use (ie, not obvious in the early stage of the disease).

Nociception

With experience, one realizes that pain perception does not always need to be examined because many clues are gleaned during the examination to inform the clinician as to its presence. However, in many cases of severe spinal cord diseases, the evaluation of pain perception is crucial to prognosis. The expressions *deep* and *superficial* pain should probably not be used considering the nature of veterinary patients. The terms hypoesthesia, hyperesthesia, and anesthesia are preferable for decreased, increased, and absence of pain perception, respectively. In spinal cord diseases, the perception of pain is evaluated in the limbs first and, if there is anesthesia, the tail is stimulated. Much of the tail is autonomic in function and this system is more resilient. In dogs and cats with severe neurologic impairment, there may not be perception of pain per se. What the examiner may consider as a painful stimulus may only feel like a light touch or tingling sensation to the animal. For this reason, evaluation of pain perception should be done in a quiet environment, on patients that are calm and not distracted. Fear may also lead to a lack of response.

Vertebral Column Pain

Lastly, the vertebral column is evaluated for presence of pain. In the great majority of vertebral column diseases, the owner is aware that the animal is in pain. The examination confirms and localizes the painful region. Neck pain can be ascertained by observation of the neck posture as the animal walks around the room. The animal moves cautiously turning the entire body, not only the neck, when changing direction. When looking up, only the eyes lift not the head and neck. A food treat is used to entice the animal to turn the head and neck in each direction: up, down, right, and left. Undue manipulations of the neck are not necessary. Although rare and predominantly present in miniature breeds, the possibility of an atlantoaxial luxation/subluxation cannot be overlooked. Ventriflexion of the neck in such patients may have disastrous consequences. Pain may be present at all times or induced upon certain movement of the neck by the animal. Neck spasms can be transient and mistaken for paroxysmal events, such as seizure activity. Pressing on the lateral apophyses of the cervical vertebrae is not a reliable way to assess for presence of neck pain in dogs because many normal small to medium sized dogs react to this procedure with a contraction of the neck. Arching of the back and low head carriage are occasionally observed with neck pain. With back pain, the animal has a hunched back posture. Nerve root compression (as in lateral disc extrusion) causes focal pain, whereas diseases that affect bone, like tumors have a more regional, less localized pain. The common observations reported with lumbosacral pain are the animal's difficulty and caution in getting up or sitting down; pain when the lumbar region is touched during obedience; assistance to the animal to get into the car; reluctance for the dog to walk, jump, or run; and the inability to posture during defecation or urination. Characteristically, the dog walks away in a crouched posture while defecating or urinating. The animal may be worse after exercise, feature not present with thoracolumbar or cervical pain. It can be difficult to differentiate L7-S1 from L6-L7 intervertebral pain on clinical examination alone. The dog with pain at the L-S junction may resent the simultaneous extension or flexion of the hips or to be lifted by the base of the tail. Both manipulations accentuate the angle of the sacrum on the L7 vertebra. If there is concomitant osteoarthritis of the hips, it is preferable to uniquely perform tail lifting.

The findings of the neurologic examination are recorded on an appropriate neurologic examination form. Recording of the findings is important because it allows monitoring of the progression of the disease.

PROBLEM LIST AND DIFFERENTIAL DIAGNOSIS

Each of the problems isolated on history, physical, ophthalmologic, and neurologic examinations is listed by order of importance. If a single lesion can explain all neurologic abnormalities, it simplifies to list the spinal localization as one problem instead of including an exhaustive list of all neurologic abnormalities. The list of possible causes for the spinal disease is based on signalment, history, time of onset and progression of signs, lesion localization, presence or absence of vertebral pain, and systemic signs. With a purebred animal, it is recommended to look into a list of cat and dog breed-associated spinal diseases to rule out genetic or prevalent CNS disease.[3]

DATABASE AND ANCILLARY TESTS

The minimum clinicopathologic database includes a complete blood count, biochemical profile (including thyroxine and thyroid stimulating hormone), and urinalysis to evaluate the patients' general health, the presence of concomitant abnormalities suggestive of an infectious or neoplastic process, and to measure the risk anesthesia poses for patients. Titres and polymerase chain reaction (PCR) tests are requested for the suspected specific infectious diseases. In breeds at risk for bleeding disorders, coagulation testing is added if surgical treatment is a consideration.

Thoracic radiographs (3 views) are recommended in all patients older than 6 years of age, patients with cardiovascular or respiratory disease, and patients suspected of inflammatory or neoplastic CNS disease. If a cardiac murmur is present and discospondylitis is high on the list of possible causes, an echocardiography should be done to rule out endocarditis as a source of infection. Abdominal ultrasound should be performed in all older patients; patients with clinicopathologic abnormalities indicative of metabolic, endocrine, or neoplastic disease; and patients suspected of inflammatory or neoplastic CNS disease. If the orthopaedic examination reveals joint pain, radiographs of the region are taken, if not previously done. If the animal has been diagnosed with hip dysplasia or chronic cruciate rupture at a younger age, follow-up radiographs are repeated if there are no recent (<12 months) radiographs available. It is important that the general musculo-skeletal condition of patients be evaluated because of its impact on rehabilitation and ultimately on recovery.

NEUROIMAGING

Survey radiographs of the affected vertebral/spinal region are recommended to eliminate straightforward diseases, such as discospondylitis, bony tumors, and vertebral malformations. Advanced imaging is essential in most cases of spinal cord disease. Undoubtedly, MRI is superior to any other neuroimaging modality in the diagnosis of CNS disease, spinal cord included (see article on advanced imaging elsewhere in this issue). Elucidating the cause of neck pain when there is no other neurologic abnormality can be particularly challenging even with MRI. However, not all hospitals have a magnet powerful enough to obtain quality images, especially in large dogs. For intervertebral disc disease, CT may be preferable given its availability and short acquisition time. Myelography may be recommended if advanced imaging modality is not available and the situation is emergent.

CEREBROSPINAL FLUID ANALYSIS

The advent of MRI has decreased the need and frequency of CSF analysis. However, whenever an inflammatory disease is suspected, in the absence of abnormal findings on MRI and in the presence of a compressive lesion of unknown origin, CSF collection and analysis should be done. It should also be done before subarachnoid contrast injection with CT-myelography or myelography. Cerebrospinal fluid can be obtained from the cerebello-medullary or lumbar cistern (L5–L6). As a rule, the closer to the lesion, the more helpful is the analysis. The analysis should always include white and red cell counts, cytology, and protein concentration. If infectious disease is suspected, CSF protein electrophoresis, titres, and PCR can be added. Blood contamination may render the analysis unreliable.

ELECTRODIAGNOSTIC TESTING

Electrodiagnostic testing is of limited value in spinal cord disease. Electromyography (EMG) can be helpful in localizing involvement of a specific nerve root or spinal nerve when there is LMN disease. In such a case, denervation potentials can be recorded in the muscles innervated by the affected root or spinal nerve. Needle EMG study allows mapping of the muscles that have denervated potentials helping isolate the affected spinal nerve or root. This isolation can be particularly helpful in dogs with neck pain when no other neurologic abnormality is present. Magnetic motor-evoked potential is a sensitive, although nonspecific, tool in the diagnosis of cervical and thoracolumbar spinal cord abnormality.[7,8]

LESION LOCALIZATION IN PATIENTS WITH VERTEBRAL/SPINAL DISEASES

Anatomy and General Principles of Lesion Localization

The vertebral column is a bony canal that houses the spinal cord and the cauda equina. The cauda equina is this collection of nerve roots (sacral and caudal) resembling a horse's tail and located within the vertebral canal at the end of the spinal cord. In dogs and cats, there are 7 cervical, 13 thoracic, and 7 lumbar vertebrae followed by a sacrum, the fusion of the 3 sacral vertebrae, and a variable number of caudal vertebrae (6 to 23 in dogs). However, the number of spinal segments differs. The cervical vertebral canal contains 8 cervical spinal cord segments but 7 cervical vertebrae. As a consequence, cranial to vertebra C7, a spinal nerve exits *cranial* to the vertebra of the same number (**Fig. 1**), whereas caudal to vertebra C7, because of the addition of the C8 spinal segment, the spinal nerve exits *caudal* to the vertebra of the same number. The unequal relationship between vertebra and spinal segment takes dramatic proportion at the level of the lumbosacral enlargement (**Figs. 2** and **3**). The entire lumbosacral enlargement, spinal segments L4 to S3, is contained roughly within the vertebrae L4 and L5 in the dog (see **Fig. 2**), and L5 and L6 in the cat (see **Fig. 3**). The termination of the spinal cord, the filum terminale, is at the L6-L7 IVD space in medium-sized and large dogs, L7-S1 IVD space in small dogs (<7 kg), and over the body of S1 in most cats.[9,10]

The spinal cord consists of white and gray matter. The gray matter is located in the center of the spinal cord parenchyma and has the shape of a butterfly. The white matter situated peripherally to the gray matter is made primarily of myelinated axons, ascending axons (sensory fibers) going to and descending axons (motor fibers) coming from the brain. The gray matter is composed of nerve cell bodies. It is the center of the reflex arc. All sensory information from the peripheral nervous system enters the spinal cord by way of the dorsal horns, and all lower motor neurons exit the gray matter by way of the ventral horns. Roughly, the upper half of the spinal

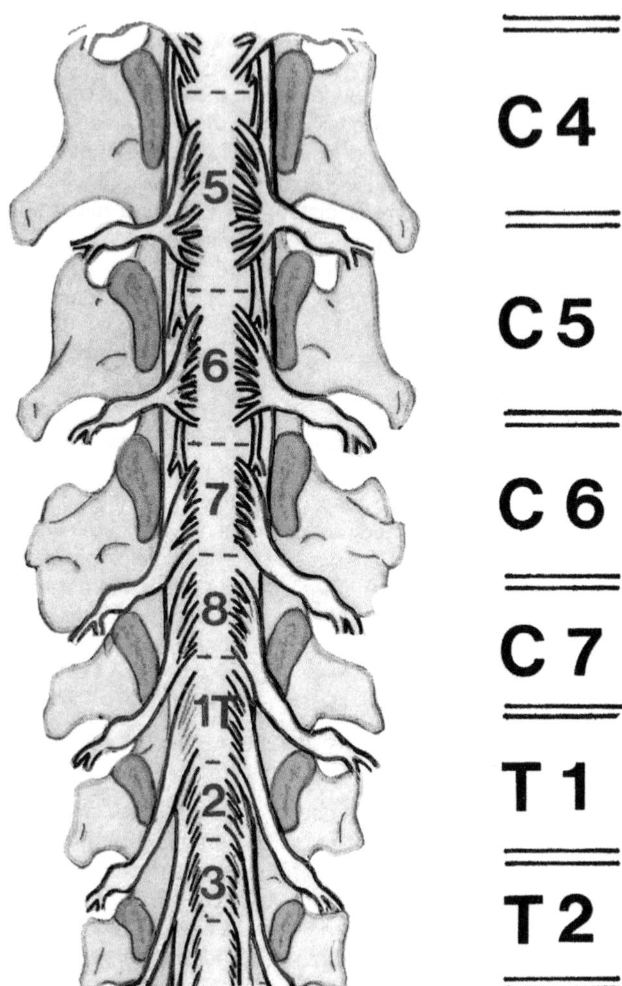

Fig. 1. Relation between vertebrae, spinal cord segments, and spinal nerve in the cervical region. C4 to T2 on the right represent vertebra number, whereas the numbers 5 to 3 on the left represent spinal cord segments. Cranial to C8, a given spinal nerve exits cranial to the vertebra of the same number. (*Courtesy of* Joane Parent, BSc, DMV, MVetSc, Montréal, Canada.)

cord, white and gray matter, is sensory in function, whereas the lower half is motor. With gray matter lesion, motor deficits are more obvious than sensory abnormalities. Total destruction of the ventral horn in one segment of the spinal cord causes loss of tone (hypotonia), some degree of flaccidity, and rapid wasting of the muscles innervated by that segment, with at least some degree of flaccid paresis.[11] The severity of the flaccid paresis is in relation to the number of spinal cord segments affected. Gray matter involvement, if the white matter is spared, causes neurologic deficits similar to those observed with peripheral nervous system lesion. A rare example of such a disorder is the spinal muscular atrophy in which the pathologic abnormalities are mainly restricted to the motor neurons of the ventral gray horns. Although it is

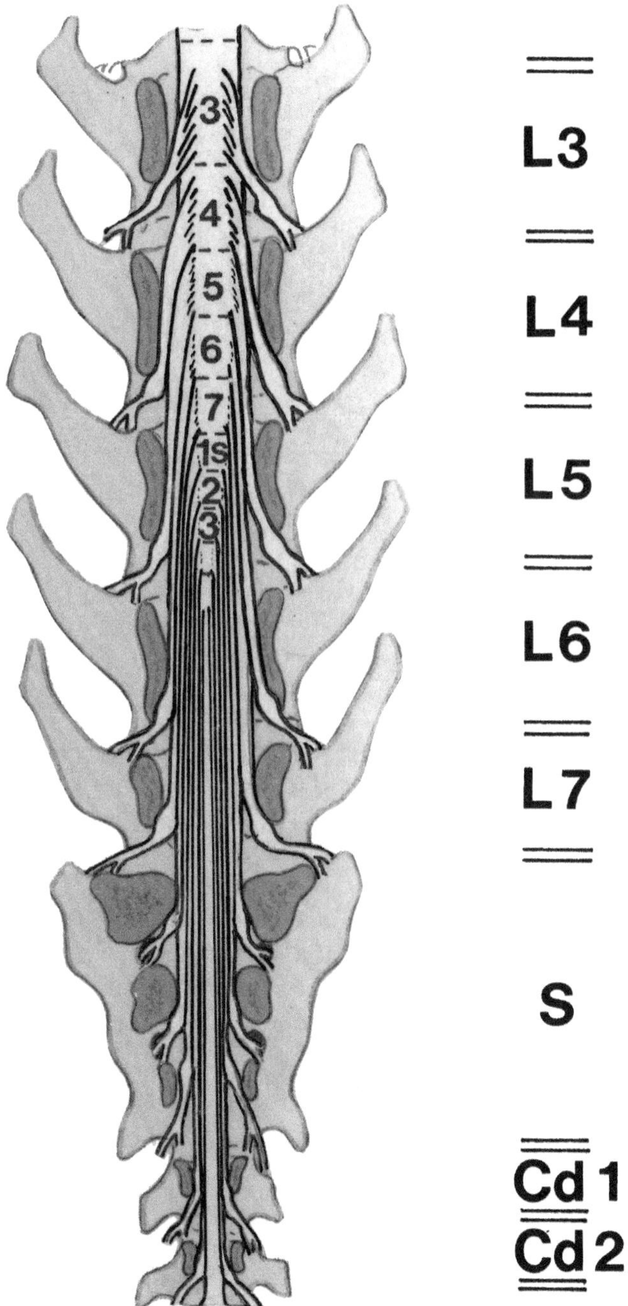

Fig. 2. Relation between vertebrae, spinal cord segments, and spinal nerves in the lumbosacral region in the dog. L3 to S on the right represent vertebra number. Numbers 3 to 3 on the left represent spinal cord segments. Caudal to C8, a spinal nerve of a given number exits caudal to the vertebra of the same number. The lumbosacral enlargement is contained within vertebra L4 and L5. Cd, caudal. (*Courtesy of* Joane Parent, BSc, DMV, MVetSc, Montréal, Canada.)

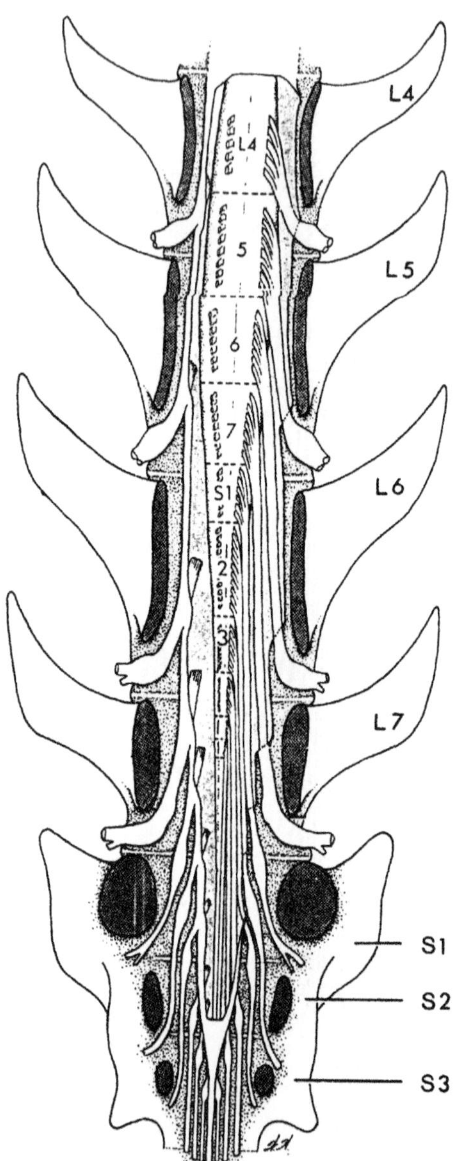

Fig. 3. Relation between vertebrae, spinal cord segments, and spinal nerves in the lumbosacral region in the cat. Numbers on the right represent vertebrae; numbers within spinal cord represent spinal cord segments. Caudal to C8, a spinal nerve of a given number exits caudal to the vertebra of the same number. The lumbosacral enlargement is contained primarily within vertebrae L5 and L6. (*Modified from* Kot W, Partlow GD, Parent JM. Anatomical survey of the cat lumbosacral spinal cord. Progress Vet Neurol 1993;4:76–80;with permission.)

a spinal cord disease, the clinical signs observed resemble those associated with motor polyneuropathies and consist of LMN paresis, tone and reflexes. Because of the intimate association between white and gray matter and the nature of spinal cord diseases in veterinary medicine, in the vast majority of cases white and gray matter are concomitantly affected. Spinal cord diseases between C1 and C5, and between T3 and L3, frequently affect white and gray matter, but because of the absence of limbs at that level, the gray matter signs cannot be appreciated.

Although multiple sensory modalities exist, only proprioceptive and nociceptive losses can be appreciated in veterinary patients. The salient feature of early spinal cord disease is the presence of proprioceptive ataxia. The proprioceptive fibers are the first white matter fibers to be impaired because of their larger size and rather superficial location. Their implication is closely associated, anatomically and timely, with involvement of the descending motor fibers, the UMNs. Involvement of the UMNs leads to variable degrees of paresis/paralysis and hypertonia and hyperreflexia secondary to the release of the tonic inhibitory effect of the UMNs on the LMNs, especially the ones that control the antigravity extensor muscles. There is some muscle wasting over time, which is caused by atrophy of disuse.

Clinically, regardless of the disorder affecting the spinal cord white matter, there is a sequence in which the neurologic signs usually appear based on the anatomy and organization of the spinal cord fibers. Proprioceptive ataxia is the primary feature to appear, which is closely associated to a decrease in purposeful movements that is displayed by weakness/paresis. As the disease progresses, UMN paralysis follows. Then there is involvement of the autonomic nervous system with the apparition of urinary and fecal incontinence. The last function to be lost is the nociception or perception of pain. Recovery occurs in a reverse manner with nociception being recovered first. It is helpful to remember this flow of events when a prognosis must be given or when the clinician wonders if there is urinary incontinence. If there are purposeful movements preserved, even if minimal, as a rule, urinary function remains.

Neck or back pain results from bone, disc, spinal nerve/root, or meningeal involvement. Neck and back pain alone, without neurologic deficits, may be associated in both instances with significant spinal cord compression.[4,5] Neck pain and back pain are never benign complaints.

The gray matter has greater energetic demand than the white matter because of the presence of nerve cell bodies. Acute spinal cord injury leads to central gray matter necrosis that gradually progresses to white matter necrosis, whereas progressive compressive injury tends to spare the gray matter. Generally speaking, the more acute the evolution of the neurologic white matter signs the greater the possibility of their reversibility as long as nociception is preserved. In the majority of compressive diseases of the spinal cord, the clinical signs are symmetric or mildly to moderately asymmetric if the compressive abnormality is lateralized. Only in inflammatory and vascular diseases (eg, fibrocartilaginous embolic myelopathy) can there be profound asymmetric neurologic signs.

C1 to C5 spinal cord: C1 to mid-C5 vertebrae

This region of the spinal cord is located within the vertebrae C1, C2, C3, and C4 to mid-C5 (see **Fig. 1**), with the C5 spinal nerve exiting at the C4-C5 IVD space. Except for the C1 segment, which is located within the first cervical vertebra, the cervical spinal segments are located cranial to their corresponding vertebra (see **Fig. 1**). The neurologic abnormalities associated with a spinal cord lesion between C1 and C5 involve all 4 limbs or mainly the ipsilateral limbs if the lesion is lateralized. The neurologic abnormalities vary from neck pain without neurologic deficits, ataxia and UMN weakness, tetraplegia, to death from respiratory failure. In the ambulatory animal, there are variable degrees of proprioceptive ataxia and UMN weakness involving front and hind limbs, but as a rule, the nature of the neurologic abnormalities is similar in the front and hind limbs. In the early stages of the disease, the ipsilateral limbs may move together as in pacing and the elbows may be slightly rotated outward. With extramedullary lesions, as is often the case, the nature of the gait is similar in all limbs but the ataxia and weakness are usually more pronounced in the pelvic limbs (Video 10). This weakness is in part because the pathways for the hind limbs are situated more superficially and damaged earlier and because as the animal weakens, the gravity center moves toward the rear end. With intramedullary lesions, the proprioceptive deficits are more pronounced in the front limbs than the hind limbs because of the more central location of the front limb's proprioceptive pathways (Video 11). These animals often scuff or frankly knuckle the front toes as they walk. In these instances, the list of possible causes should include preferentially parenchymal disorders, such as inflammatory (infectious or noninfectious) diseases; parenchymal space-occupying lesions (ependymoma); or other intramedullary lesions. Dogs with cervical subarachnoid diverticula (also called subarachnoid cyst) frequently have this clinical presentation because of the syringomyelia often present caudal to the diverticula.

As the cervical lesion progresses, the animal becomes unable to get up and, with continued progression, cannot assume sternal position unassisted or has difficulty keeping this position because of marked proprioceptive loss and UMN weakness. The reflexes and tone are normal to exaggerated, varying proportionally with the severity of the lesion and length of the history; the more severe and chronic the lesion is, the more tone and hyperreflexia is observed. If the animal is laterally recumbent at presentation yet is able to lift the head, the lesion is closer to vertebra C4 than C1. If the head cannot be lifted from the ground, the lesion is likely a high cervical lesion. In the recumbent animal, the front limbs may be held stiffly with marked extensor tone. In these dogs, it may be difficult to overcome the extensor tone when attempting to elicit the withdrawal reflex. A crossed extensor reflex can be observed in the front and hind limbs and is usually indicative of severe and mostly chronic lesions.

Marked lateralization of neurologic deficits, including neck curvature and Horner syndrome, provides strong diagnostic clues suggesting the presence of vascular or inflammatory disease. Neck curvature results from damage to the ipsilateral vestibulospinal tract. The neck curves toward the side of the lesion because of loss of facilitation of the extensor muscles on that side and concomitant loss of inhibition of opposite extensor muscles and inhibition of ipsilateral flexor muscles. Most commonly, this posture is acute and associated with inflammatory diseases but it can also be observed with fibrocartilaginous embolic myelopathy (FCEM). Only vascular and inflammatory diseases can affect these pathways unilaterally sparing the closely associated contralateral vestibulospinal tract. Neck curvature can be chronic and progressive, but in these instances the cause is usually different. In some central spinal cord syndromes, such as in syringomyelia and intramedullary tumors, there can be unilateral destruction of motor nuclei (gray matter) that innervate the paraspinal muscles leading to cervical scoliosis. The presence of a unilateral Horner syndrome is another lateralizing sign that can be observed with involvement of the sympathetic fibers in the lateral tecto-tegmental spinal tract of the upper cervical level. The sympathetic pathway for dilatation of the pupil runs along the entire cervical spinal cord white matter. The sympathetic system evolutionarily is more resilient to lesion. Horner syndrome is rarely encountered with compressive lesion of the spinal cord. It is with vascular disease (fibrocartilaginous embolic myelopathy) that it is the most prevalent.

The phrenic nerve, the only motor nerve supplying the diaphragm, arises from the C5, C6, and C7 spinal segments and nerves, with some dogs also having minor input from the C4 segment. A severe C1 to C5 cervical lesion may cause diaphragmatic and intercostal UMN paralysis leading to respiratory dysfunction and possibly death. In nonambulatory dogs, abdominal breathing is more frequently encountered with UMN intercostal than diaphragmatic involvement. When respiratory function is preserved in diseases affecting the C1 to C5 spinal cord, one can assume that purposeful movements are present, even if only minimally, and that urinary function is also preserved. If the disease is acute and can be treated such as in an extruded disc, the animal should regain the ability to walk rapidly. It is often the animal's size that limits survival in these cases.

Occasionally, the examiner cannot differentiate neck from back pain or cannot rule out the concomitant presence of back pain because the hunched posture is accompanied by a low head carriage. This factor should be taken into consideration when the differential diagnosis is established and workup planned.

The presence of lameness with neck diseases (root signature) is usually associated with cervical enlargement lesions, but because some dogs' brachial plexus receives contributions from spinal segment C5, lameness may on occasion be observed with C5-C6 intervertebral disease.

C6 toT2 spinal cord: mid-C5 to caudal T1 vertebrae

This area of the spinal cord gives origin to the brachial plexus. It encompasses the spinal cord segments C6, C7, C8, T1, and T2 with 24% of dogs also receiving input from spinal segment C5. The enlargement is contained within the caudal half of C5 vertebra, C6, C7, and T1 (see **Fig. 1**). The radial nerve, the largest nerve of the brachial plexus, originates from the spinal segments C7, C8, T1, and (T2) with 45% of the efferent fibers arising from C8, 29% from T1, and 21% from C7.[12] These spinal segments are located primarily within the vertebrae C6 and C7 (see **Fig. 1**). The suprascapular nerve originates primarily from the spinal segment C6 (IVD space C5-6) and innervates the infraspinatus and supraspinatus muscles involved in the extension and stabilization of the shoulder joint. The radial nerve with the suprascapular nerve is responsible for the ability of the animal to stand on its forelimb.[9] The other nerves of the brachial plexus (subscapular, axillary, musculocutaneous, median, and ulnar) are involved in the flexion of the limb and receive input from spinal segments C6, C7, C8, T1, and T2. The subscapularis and axillary nerves arise from C6 and C7 with 59% and 41% of their efferent fibers coming from C6 and C7, respectively.[12] They are responsible for the flexion of the shoulder joint. The musculocutaneous nerve originates from C6, C7, and C8 with 57% of the efferent fibers arising from C7, 26% from C6, and 16% from C8.[13] This nerve is responsible for the flexion of the elbow. The median and ulnar nerves originate primarily from C8 and T1 and are responsible for the flexion of the carpus and digits. For the median nerve, 38% of the efferent fibers arise from C8 and 46% from T1.[13] For the ulnar nerve, 24% come from C8 and 65% from T1.[13] In summary, the efferent fibers for the extension of the front limb originate in most part from the spinal cord segments C8 and T1 (ie, vertebrae C7), whereas the efferent fibers for flexion of the proximal articulations arise from C6 and C7 (ie, vertebrae C5 and C6) and for flexion of the distal articulations from C8 and T1 (ie, vertebrae C7). Clinically, the spinal segments of origin for the extension and flexion of the articulations of the front limbs are important in lesion localization at this level of the spinal cord.

Three other clinically relevant anatomic features not related to the thoracic limb, but that have an impact on lesion localization in this region of the cervical spinal cord, are the phrenic nerve innervating the diaphragm; the sympathetic fibers for pupil dilation; and the lateral thoracic nerve, the sole motor supply of the cutaneous trunci muscles. The phrenic nerve originates from the spinal cord segments C4, C5, C6, and C7, and diseases between C6-T2 may lead to diaphragmatic compromise from a LMN (gray matter) or UMN (white matter) lesion. Intercostal impairment can also be observed with severe UMN lesion causing abdominal breathing. Both combined can cause the animal's death by respiratory failure. Although the sympathetic pathway to the eye originates in the hypothalamus and runs along the entire brainstem and cervical cord, with CNS diseases, it is in the C6-T2 region that a lesion is most likely to cause a Horner syndrome by involvement of (1) the sympathetic preganglionic neuronal cell bodies located within the gray matter of T1, T2, and T3, or (2) the sympathetic fibers in the lateral tecto-tegmental spinal tract between C6 and T2. In vertebral canal disease, the Horner syndrome is usually partial, presented predominantly with a miosis, often subtle. The cutaneous trunci reflex is the third important structure extrinsic to the thoracic limb. The sensory pathway of the cutaneous trunci reflex runs within the thoracolumbar spinal cord white matter but the cell bodies of the motor part of the reflex are located within the gray matter of the spinal segments C8 and T1. An absence of the cutaneous trunci reflex may be observed with C8 and T1 gray matter lesions. The deficit can be bilateral but in most cases is unilateral.

Spinal cord lesions involving the cervical enlargement may involve mainly the white matter, white and gray matter, or rarely, the gray matter alone. The lesion may be at any level between the C5 and T1 vertebrae. With lesions in this area of the neck, the gait abnormalities vary greatly depending on the location, extent (white or gray matter), and progression of the disease. There may just be neck pain; neck pain with the presence of front-limb lameness; lameness only; ataxia with ipsilateral hemiparesis, tetraparesis, tetraplegia; and death from respiratory failure. Neck pain is frequently associated with spinal cord compression even in the absence of neurologic deficits.[5] The lameness may be the result of the compression/entrapment of nerve roots or spinal nerves and may be present with or without neck pain. A lameness that persists more than 6 to 8 weeks and that remains unresolved diagnostically should be investigated for presence of nerve sheath tumor and secondary spinal cord compression. When neurologic deficits other than lameness or neck pain are present, all limbs are affected, although at times quite asymmetrically.

In slowly progressive compressive diseases, such as in cervical spondylomyelopathy myelopathy or wobbler syndrome, the gray matter is often spared leading to proprioceptive ataxia and UMN weakness in all limbs without LMN signs in the front limbs even if the lesion is at the level of the cervical enlargement. The most frequent locations for lesion in this area of the vertebral canal are at the C5-C6 and C6-C7 IVD spaces. Frequently only the white matter is affected leading to characteristic gait abnormalities. If the lesion is at the C5-C6 IVD space (Video 12), all limbs are affected but the nature of the deficits differs between the front and hind limbs. In these instances, the front-limb gait is obviously neurologic because the lesion involves the release of most of the spinal segments giving rise to the brachial plexus resulting in UMN signs in the front and hind limbs. Concomitantly, reflexes and tone are normal to increased in all limbs. However, the spinal segment C6 is spared, which means that the UMNs controlling the radial nerve are more affected than the ones controlling the flexion of the front limb. As a result, the front limb is thrown forward in extension in the protracted phase of the gait. This extension results from the release over the inhibitory effect on the antigravity extensor muscles innervated by the radial nerve, which arises primarily from spinal segments C8 and T1 (vertebra C7).

If the lesion is at the C6-C7 IVD space (Video 13), the spinal segments C6 and C7, and possibly part of C8, are spared. In these instances, the front-limb gait has a characteristic short and stiff stepping motion. Ataxia and weakness in the hind limbs are evident but the neurologic deficits in the front limbs are subtle, seeming to be more the result of musculoskeletal abnormalities. As the disease progresses, there may be dragging or knuckling of the forepaws as the animal walks but the proprioceptive ataxia remains minimal. In the early stage of the disease, as in large dogs with caudal spondylomyelopathy, the involvement of the front limbs may be missed if not looked with scrutiny.

The deficits are easier to recognize if there is gray matter involvement superposed to the white matter lesion because there are LMN signs in the front limbs with hypotonic and hyporeflexic extensor or flexor reflexes.

T3 to L3 spinal segments: T2 to L3 vertebrae

This is the region of the spinal cord that is the most commonly affected in dogs because of the frequency of thoracolumbar disc extrusion in this species. This region of the spinal cord is located within the vertebrae T2 to L3 in dogs and T3 to L4 in cats. With lesions in this area, the neurologic abnormalities are limited to the hind limbs. The neurologic deficits vary greatly in relation to the location, severity, and duration of the disease. Significant spinal cord compression may exist with no other abnormality than back pain.[4] Arching of the back is usually indicative of back pain. Although there are no limbs to indicate involvement of the gray matter, as would be in millipedes, observation of the trunk position in relation to the rear end offers clues as to lesion localization between T3 and L3. The higher the lesion is along the thoracic region (T3–T10) the more obvious is the involvement of the trunk. Usually with lesions above T8 to 9, there is a wide excursion of the rear end (truncal ataxia) because more than half of the vertebral column proprioception is lost (Video 14). As severe paresis appears, the animal is unable to drag itself with its front limbs because the thoracic back muscles are necessary for this to occur (Video 15). With progression to paralysis, the animal is unable to sit on its front limbs even though the animal walks normally on its front limbs when assisted. With upper thoracic lesions, if the animal is ambulatory, there is lordosis from weakness of the back muscles (Video 16). The neurologic deficits progress from ataxia and spastic paresis, to spastic paralysis, then to urinary and fecal incontinence, and in severe cases, to anesthesia caudal to the lesion. Tone and reflexes progress from normal to exaggerated, and the limb reflexes may become clonic. A crossed extensor reflex can be observed in the hind limbs, and is usually indicative of severe and mostly chronic lesions.

Eight to 12 weeks following complete transverse myelopathy, spinal walking gradually develops. In true spinal walking, there is complete transverse myelopathy with paralysis and anesthesia caudal to the lesion. The spinal walking phenomenon is secondary to coordinated reflex patterns that develop within the spinal cord, without any input to or information from UMNs.[3] It is the result of loss of inhibition over the central pattern generator, which is the network of interconnected interneurons in the spinal cord gray matter that modulates motor neuron activity for the generation of gait.[14] This abnormal walking reflex is observed with stimulation of the hind limbs, pinching of the tail or anus, or when the dog defecates. A certain degree of spinal walking can also be observed in some ambulatory dogs and cats with slowly progressive T3 to L3 lesions. An automatism appears superposed to the hind limb motions even though the animal still has purposeful movements. The hind limb and front limb movements are not coordinated; the hind limbs advance at an automatic, steady, unchanged pace (similar to cross-country skiing) while the front limbs move normally (Video 17). With a T3 to L3 lesion, the spinal reflexes and muscle tone are normal to exaggerated with the occasional presence of crossed extensor reflexes. Crossed extensor reflexes are usually observed in chronic progressive spinal cord diseases or in severe acute intramedullary lesions.

The cutaneous trunci reflex plays an important role in lesion localization of this region of the spinal cord as long as the lesion is above L1. The dermatome innervated by the T13 spinal nerve is located approximately vis-à-vis the L4 lumbar vertebra, whereas the dermatomes corresponding to lower spinal nerves may end up over the pelvis, rendering the test less useful for lesions below L1. In FCEM, it is not uncommon that the reflex is absent unilaterally to a site above the main lesion.

Schiff-Sherrington posture can be observed with acute and severe thoracolumbar lesions. There is usually hind-limb paralysis. The posture is observed when the animal is in lateral recumbency. The front limbs and neck are held in extension (opisthotonus), while there is hypotonia but normal reflexes in the hind limbs. The posture may remain for 1 to 2 weeks. The posture can be mistaken for a cervical lesion but, except for the rigid extension of the front limbs, the front limbs are neurologically normal. The posture is the result of impairment of fibers originating from neurons in the lumbar gray matter primarily the L1 to L5 spinal segments. These fibers ascend along the thoracolumbar spine toward the cervical enlargement where they play an inhibitory role on the front-limb extensor motor neurons.[15] Schiff-Sherrington phenomenon can be observed with any acute and severe lesion below T3, but is most frequently observed with lesions in the T11 to L2 region because of the frequency of IVD diseases at this level.

Following acute traumatic events, spinal shock with atonia and areflexia caudal to the lesion, despite an UMN lesion, may be observed in primates and may last for many days. It is infrequently observed in dogs and cats. The hypotonia may be present but the reflexes can usually be elicited with a strong stimulus. Spinal shock, if observed, is usually present posttraumatically for a short time; by the time the animal is presented, it has disappeared.[15]

Severe spinal cord disease, where there is paralysis, may lead to urinary and fecal incontinence. With a lesion between T3 and L3, the deficits are UMN in nature. The animal cannot urinate. There is increased urinary sphincter tone (pudendal nerve release), making the emptying of the bladder difficult. Rarely, fecal incontinence, without urinary incontinence, is encountered with thoracolumbar lesion yet the animal is ambulatory, which is particularly true with subarachnoid diverticula.

With complete transverse myelopathy, there is anesthesia caudal to the lesion.

Lumbosacral enlargement: L4 and L5 vertebrae (dogs) and L5 and L6 vertebrae (cats)

In this region of the spinal cord, the spinal segments are short in relation to the corresponding vertebrae. Indeed, most of the lumbosacral enlargement, spinal segments L4, L5, L6, L7, S1, S2, and S3, are contained within vertebrae L4 and L5 in dogs, and L5 and L6 in cats (see **Figs. 2** and **3**). The spinal nerves exit caudal to their corresponding vertebrae. The neurologic deficits reflect damage to white and gray matter. The gray matter is particularly at risk because it occupies a large portion of the spinal parenchyma in this region. The ataxia, the result of white matter disease and which usually prevails with spinal cord disease, is subtle and may be masked by LMN deficits. Lower motor neuron deficits stand out in this region of the vertebral canal and, if patients are ambulatory, are best evaluated while patients are walking. Indeed, the evaluation of the reflexes complements the evaluation of the gait. The femoral, sciatic, and pudendal nerves are discussed at greater length because their involvement is of great localizing value in this region of the vertebral canal.

The femoral nerve originates from spinal segments L4, L5, and L6 and is responsible for sensory innervation of the medial face of the hind limb, stifle extension (weight bearing), and hip flexion. The patellar reflex is particularly important in the evaluation of the femoral nerve. The patellar reflex is a monosynaptic reflex and both neurons, sensory and motor, are necessary for transmission of the impulse and generation of the reflex (Video 18). The observer should ascertain which of the 2 neurons is involved. With a LMN femoral nerve injury, there is hyporeflexia or areflexia, hypotonia or atonia, *and* the inability to extend the stifle and flex the hip. However, if there is weight bearing or presence of extensor tone in the limb and hip flexion with limb withdrawal, yet the patellar reflex cannot be elicited, the areflexia is sensory in origin (likely L5 dorsal root lesion), which is not a sign of LMN dysfunction.

The sciatic nerve is the largest nerve of the animals' body. It originates from spinal segments L6, L7, S1, and S2. The sciatic nerve is divided into 2 branches, the peroneal nerve (primarily from spinal segments L6, L7), which is responsible for flexion of the hock and extension of the toes, and the tibial nerve (primarily from spinal segments L7, S1), which is responsible for extension of the hock and flexion of the toes. The sciatic nerve is responsible for sensation of the lateral part of the limb. With LMN sciatic nerve deficits, there is hypotonia or atonia and hyporeflexia or areflexia with inability to flex the stifle, hock, and digits. If the sciatic nerve is affected proximally but the femoral nerve is intact, there is pseudohyperreflexia of the patellar reflex from loss of sciatic nerve innervation to the antagonistic muscles of this reflex.[16] If the animal is ambulatory, the flexion of the hip brings the femur up, seeming to cause flexion of the stifle but this latter motion is passive; the stifle is dragged into flexion by the hip motion. All articulations should flex to conclude at the presence of a normal withdrawal reflex.

The pudendal nerve originates from the spinal segments S1, S2, and S3 and innervates the striated muscles of the external sphincter of the anus and urethra and the skin of the perineum. With a LMN lesion, there is urinary and fecal incontinence with atonic and areflexic sphincters. There may be anesthesia of the perineal region, unilaterally or bilaterally.

The neurologic abnormalities observed at the L4-L5 IVD space (dog) include low lumbar pain alone, subtle ataxia with LMN femoral and sciatic nerve involvement, LMN femoral and sciatic paralysis with or without LMN urinary incontinence (pudendal nerve involvement), and transverse myelopathy with LMN paralysis and anesthesia of the hind limbs, anus, and tail. If the lesion is focal, mainly at the IVD space, it may spare the sacral segments with a resulting UMN urinary incontinence with inability to void and a spastic urinary sphincter. Acute intervertebral disc extrusions or fractures at L4-L5 in dogs, or L5-L6 in cats can have devastating results. This area is frequently affected with FCEM. In this particular disease, although the deficits are at times frankly asymmetrical giving the impression that the disease is unilateral, in the author's experience it is rarely, if ever, unilateral at onset.

The prognosis is directly related to the severity and extension of the gray matter lesion. The greater the gray matter damage the more permanent the deficits because cell bodies do not regenerate.

Acute bilateral cruciate rupture may be mistaken for a neurologic disorder because the animal is unable to get up and has an absence of patellar reflexes from the inability to raise tension in the patellar tendons.

L5, L6, and L7 vertebrae and sacrum in dogs

At this level, the part of the spinal cord that controls limb function has ended. For this reason, diseases from the L5-L6 IVD space to the lumbosacral junction in dogs, and the L6-L7 and L-S in cats, lead to clinical signs similar to peripheral nervous system disorders. There is no ataxia but abnormal foot placement may be present from involvement of dorsal roots. Low lumbar pain often accompanies the disorders affecting this area of the vertebral canal. The arching of the back is centered on the low lumbar region. The deficits are usually less severe because roots are more resilient and because the size of the lumbar canal is large in relation to its neurologic content. It is unusual to have LMN fecal or urinary incontinence. There may be chronic licking of referred zone from related root irritation. Tail involvement, when present, is always indicative of vertebral canal disease.

The deficits may be limited to one side, as observed with neuritis or a nerve sheath tumor. There may be a discrepancy between sensory and motor deficits because the union of the dorsal and ventral roots to form the mixed spinal nerve occurs only at the intervertebral foramen. The prognosis is improved over a lesion at the L4 and L5 vertebrae because of the resilience of the roots as compared with cell bodies, but once axonal degeneration has occurred the prognosis becomes guarded because of the cell-body closeness.

L5 and L6 vertebrae (dogs) The neurologic structures contained within vertebrae L5 and L6 include the conus medullaris (sacral and caudal spinal segments) and the dorsal and ventral nerve roots L5, L6, L7, S1, S2, and S3. The neurologic deficits reflect involvement of femoral and sciatic nerve roots and sacral spinal segments and roots. The deficits include low lumbar pain alone, femoral and sciatic nerve paresis/paralysis, LMN urinary and fecal incontinence, and anesthesia of all faces of the hind limbs, perineum, and tail. With a lateralized lesion, the L5 spinal nerve can be entrapped causing an absent patellar reflex and collapsing of the limb under the animal's weight (Video 19).

L6 and L7 vertebrae (dogs) The neurologic structures in this region of the vertebral canal include the conus medullaris (sacral and caudal spinal segments) and the cauda equina (the collection of the sacral and caudal nerve roots). Moreover, along these structures the L6 and L7 dorsal and ventral nerve roots run toward their exit caudal to their corresponding vertebrae. In this particular location, the femoral nerve is entirely spared but sciatic, pudendal, and caudal nerves are at risk. The clinical signs include low lumbar pain, sciatic nerve dysfunction, LMN urinary and fecal incontinence, and anesthesia of the lateral face of the hind limbs, perineum, and tail. The most frequent presentation is low lumbar pain with a unilateral neurologic lameness from entrapment of 1 spinal nerve at the IVD space.

Lumbosacral junction (dogs) The lumbosacral junction is the most commonly affected area in this region of the vertebral canal. The neurologic structures found at the lumbosacral junction include the dorsal and ventral nerve roots of L7, S1, S2, and S3 and those that innervate the tail (the caudal nerve roots). The neurologic deficits reflect the involvement of the sciatic, pudendal, pelvic, and caudal nerves. The most common presentation is LS pain with no other neurologic deficits. The animal may have difficulty positioning to defecate and may walk while doing so. There may be formation of a lick granuloma from licking of a region of the lateral face of the hind limb from chronic irritation of the L7 root. The paw may knuckle over. Lateralized lesion causes lameness and, with progression, the lameness is frankly neurologic, having an exaggerated hip flexion while the hock remains straight because of loss of antagonistic muscle mass.

SUMMARY

In spinal cord diseases, the evaluation of the gait is pivotal to the localization of the lesion. The more precise the lesion localization, the less frustration there is in interpreting the results of the diagnostic tests. The list of possible causes is intimately linked to the animal's signalment, history, lesion localization, presence or absence of vertebral pain, and presence or absence of systemic signs. The findings must be evaluated in light of the presenting complaint.

SUPPLEMENTARY DATA

Supplementary data associated with this article can be found in the online version at DOI:10.1016/j.cvsm.2010.07.001.

REFERENCES

1. LeCouteur RA, Grandy JL. Diseases of the spinal cord. In: Ettinger SJ, Feldman EC, editors. Textbook of veterinary internal medicine. Diseases of the dog and cat. 6th edition. Philadelphia: W.B.Saunders Co; 2005. p. 842–87.
2. Marioni-Henry K, Vite CH, Newton AL, et al. Prevalence of diseases of the spinal cord of cats. J Vet Intern Med 2004;18:851–8.
3. Dewey CW, Bailey KS. Signalment, history, and the differential diagnosis: the first consideration. In: Dewey CW, editor. A practical guide to canine and feline neurology. Ames (IA): Wiley-Blackwell; 2008. p. 4–14, 44.
4. Sukhiani HR, Parent JM, Atilola MA, et al. Intervertebral disk disease in dogs with signs of back pain alone: 25 cases (1986-1993). J Am Vet Med Assoc 1996;209:1275–9.
5. Morgan PW, Parent JM, Holmberg DL. Cervical pain secondary to intervertebral disc disease in dogs: radiographic findings and surgical implications. Prog Vet Neurol 1993;4:76–80.
6. Wilson JW. Relationship of the patellar tendon reflex to the ventral branch of the fifth lumbar spinal nerve in the dog. Am J Vet Res 1978;39(11):1774–7.
7. da Costa RC, Poma R, Parent J, et al. Correlation of motor evoked potentials with magnetic resonance imaging and neurological findings in Doberman pinscher dogs with and without clinical signs of cervical spondylomyelopathy. Am J Vet Res 2006;67:1613–20.
8. Sylvestre AM, Cockshutt JR, Parent JM, et al. Magnetic motor evoked potentials for assessing spinal cord integrity in dogs with intervertebral disc disease. Vet Surg 1993;22:5–10.
9. Evans HE. The spinal nerves. In: Miller's anatomy of the dog. 3rd edition. Philadelphia: Saunders; 1993. p. 829–93.
10. Evans HE. Spinal cord and meninges. In: Miller's anatomy of the dog. 3rd edition. Philadelphia: Saunders; 1993. p. 806–7.
11. King AS. Somatic motor systems: general principles. In: Physiological and clinical anatomy of the domestic mammals. Oxford (UK): Oxford University Press; 1987. p. 138–9.
12. Sharp JW, Bailey CS, Johnson RD, et al. Spinal root origin of the radial nerve and of nerves innervating the shoulder muscles of the dog. Anat Histol Embryol 1991; 20:205–14.
13. Sharp JW, Bailey CS, Johnson RD, et al. Spinal nerve root origin of the median, ulnar, and musculocutaneous nerves and their muscle nerve branches to the canine forelimb. Anat Histol Embryol 1990;19:359–68.
14. De Lahunta A, Glass E. Upper motor neuron. In: Veterinary neuroanatomy and clinical neurology. 3rd edition. St Louis (MO): Elsevier; 2009. p. 200–20.
15. De Lahunta A, Glass E. Small animal spinal cord disease. In: Veterinary neuroanatomy and clinical neurology. 3rd edition. St Louis (MO): Elsevier; 2009. p. 248–9.
16. Bagley R. Clinical examination of the animal with suspected neurologic disease. In: Fundamentals of veterinary clinical neurology. Ames (IA): Blackwell Publishing; 2005. p. 81.

Differential Diagnosis of Spinal Diseases

Ronaldo C. da Costa, DMV, MSc, PhD*, Sarah A. Moore, DVM

KEYWORDS

• Spine • Spinal • Spinal cord • Nerve roots • Meninges
• Pain • Myelopathy • Radiculopathy

Neurologic diseases leading to gait problems are a common occurrence in small animal practice. Evaluating an ataxic, weak, or paralyzed patient can be an intimidating task, but a logical approach facilitates this process. A complete physical and neurologic examination enables the clinician to confirm that the patient has a neurologic problem and to localize the problem along the spine. The next step in the diagnostic approach is to develop a list of differential diagnoses. The patient's signalment and history often provide important clues to develop a logical list of differential diagnoses. This, in turn, provides the basis for developing a diagnostic plan. This article aims to facilitate the development of differential diagnoses lists for patients with spinal disorders. The authors' goal is to link the process of localizing a lesion with selecting the most likely diseases to develop a diagnostic plan. Detailed information about most of the differential diagnoses included herein can be found elsewhere in this issue.

DIAGNOSTIC APPROACH

The approach to patients with spinal disorders includes a thorough physical and neurologic examination aimed at localizing the lesion. Proper lesion localization is paramount for the diagnostic approach, because differential diagnoses and ancillary diagnostic tests are dependent on it (**Fig. 1**).

Classically, the spinal cord is divided into 4 major segments. The spinal cord segments do not match up with the vertebrae in the cervical and lumbar regions, and there are 7 cervical vertebrae but 8 cervical spinal cord segments. The main spinal cord divisions in terms of lesion localization are C1 to C5, C6 to T2, T3 to L3 and L4 to S3. Also, there are 2 subdivisions that are clinically relevant and may assist the clinician in considering the appropriate differential diagnoses and in selecting the most indicated ancillary tests. These subdivisions are the T2-T10 and L6-L7-S1vertebral regions.

Department of Veterinary Clinical Sciences, College of Veterinary Medicine, The Ohio State University, 601 Vernon Tharp Street, Columbus, OH 43210-1089, USA
* Corresponding author.
E-mail address: dacosta.6@osu.edu

Vet Clin Small Anim 40 (2010) 755–763
doi:10.1016/j.cvsm.2010.06.002

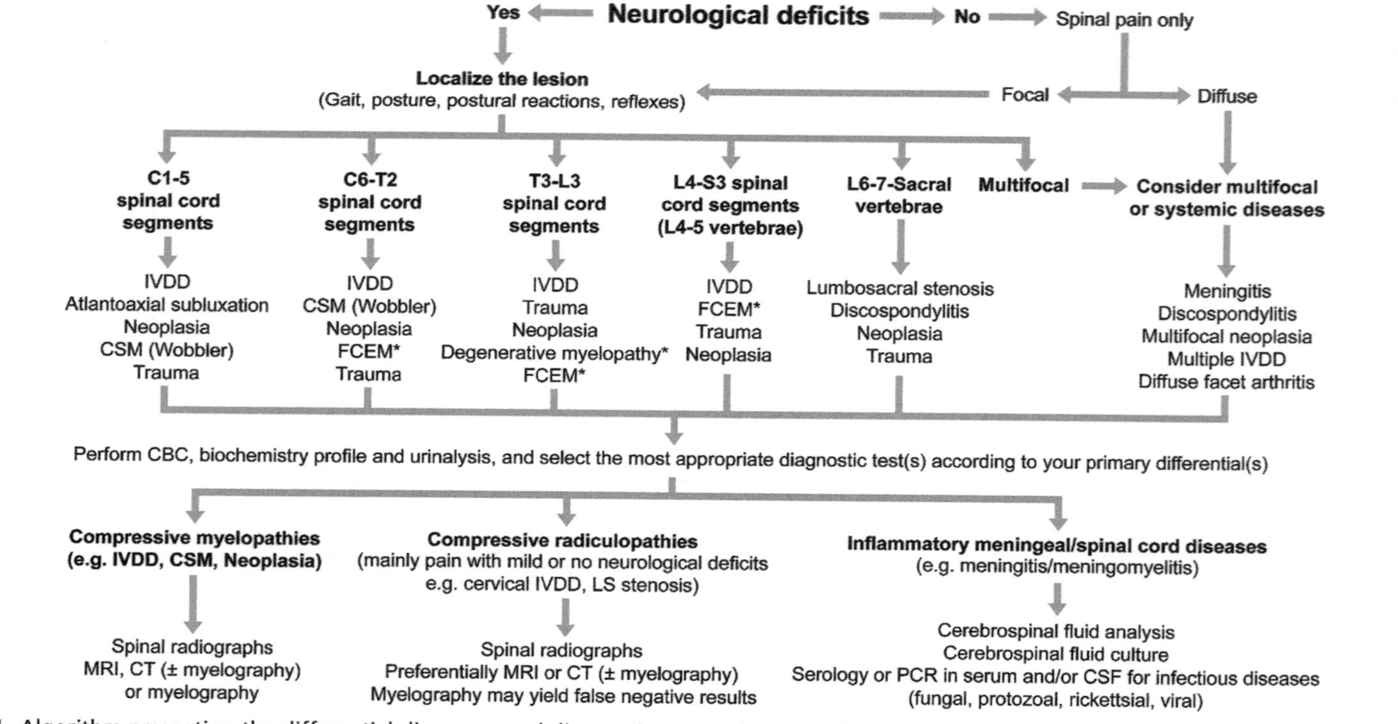

Fig. 1. Algorithm presenting the differential diagnoses and diagnostic approach to spinal problems according to lesion localization. (*), Nonpainful spinal cord diseases; CSF, cerebrospinal fluid analysis; CSM, cervical spondylomyelopathy; CT, computed tomography; IVDD, intervertebral disk disease; FCEM, fibrocartilaginous embolic myelopathy; MRI, magnetic resonance imaging; PCR, polymerase chain reaction.

The diseases presented in this article refer only to processes affecting the spinal cord or the vertebral column. Neuropathies, myopathies, and musculoskeletal conditions are not discussed. For specific information on the clinical features seen with lesions in each spinal cord segment or region, the reader is referred to the article on diagnostic approach and lesion localization of spinal disorders in this issue.

DIFFERENTIAL DIAGNOSIS

When approaching a case with spinal problems, the simplest approach once the lesion is localized is to consider differential diagnoses using the acronym lists based on pathophysiologic mechanisms. These acronyms are called VITAMIN-D or DAMNIT-V and are useful and practical ways to approach neurologic diseases. A list of common diseases according to the VITAMIN-D acronym is presented in **Table 1**.

Table 1
Common spinal diseases based on the VITAMIN-D acronym for dogs and cats

Disease Mechanism	Specific Diseases (Common Conditions in Bold)
Vascular	**Fibrocartilaginous embolic myelopathy** Epidural hemorrhage Spinal cord hemorrhage
Inflammatory/ Infectious	**Discospondylitis** (bacterial or fungal) **Meningitis (steroid-responsive meningitis-arteritis** or bacterial meningitis) **Meningomyelitis—infectious** (bacterial, fungal, rickettsial, viral), or **noninfectious** (unknown cause, granulomatous meningoencephalomyelitis) Spinal empyema Vertebral osteomyelitis
Trauma	**Spinal trauma** (fracture/luxations) Traumatic disk extrusion Traumatic atlantoaxial subluxation
Toxic	None
Anomalous	**Atlantoaxial instability** **Chiari-like malformation and syringomyelia** **Hemivertebra** Arachnoid cysts Multiple cartilaginous exostoses Spinal bifida Spinal dysraphism
Metabolic	None
Idiopathic[a]	Disseminated idiopathic skeletal hyperostosis
Neoplastic	**Primary or secondary spinal tumors**
Nutritional	Pathologic fractures because of metabolic bone disease Hypervitaminosis A (cats)
Degenerative	**Intervertebral disk degeneration** **Degenerative myelopathy** **Degenerative lumbosacral stenosis** Degenerative osteoarthritis of articular facets Extradural synovial cysts
Developmental	**Cervical spondylomyelopathy**

[a] Typically an incidental radiographic finding.

When using this acronym, it is useful to consider the signalment and history to develop appropriate differential diagnoses for the patient. For example, even though intervertebral disk disease is the most common spinal disease in dogs, it is not a reasonable differential diagnosis for a 6-month-old dog with chronic paraparesis. Some generalities should be considered when using the VITAMIN-D acronym. Young dogs are more likely to have congenital or inflammatory conditions. Acute presentations are usually caused by vascular or traumatic conditions. Chronic presentations are usually seen with degenerative or neoplastic processes. Another way to approach patients with spinal diseases is to develop a list of diseases that are known to affect specific spinal regions. This is useful because although many diseases affect several spinal regions (eg, intervertebral disk disease [IVDD], discospondylitis, fibrocartilaginous embolic myelopathy), many are region-specific (eg, atlantoaxial instability, cervical spondylomyelopathy, degenerative myelopathy). The primary differential diagnoses for the most common spinal diseases affecting each spinal region are presented in **Tables 2–5**. Some of the diseases listed are presented in only one table but can affect any spinal segment. For example, discospondylitis is more commonly seen in the lumbosacral area but can affect any vertebral region.

Once the list of differential diagnoses is prepared for the patient, the most probably causes should be ruled in or out based on appropriate diagnostic tests. The diagnostic approach exemplifying the diagnostic tests used to confirm common spinal diseases is presented in **Fig. 1**.

SPECIFIC SPINAL REGIONS

C1-C5 Spinal Cord Segments/Vertebrae C1 Through Mid-C5

Common diseases affecting the C1-C5 spinal cord segments in small breeds are atlantoaxial subluxation and cervical IVDD. Spinal pain is often present with these diseases. Primary differentials for large-breed dogs with C1-C5 lesions are IVDD, cervical spondylomyelopathy, and spinal neoplasia, mainly meningiomas. Trauma is also common and affects small and large breeds. Cervical pain without neurologic deficits affecting the C1-C5 regions is usually caused by steroid-responsive meningitis-arteritis, cervical IVDD, or discospondylitis. More information on the main clinical characteristics of each disease is presented in **Table 2**.

C6-T2 Spinal Cord Segments (Cervical Enlargement)/Vertebrae C5 Through T1

Frequent conditions seen at this region are cervical IVDD in large- and small-breed dogs and cervical spondylomyelopathy in large- and giant-breed dogs. Neoplasia, discospondylitis, osteomyelitis, trauma, and fibrocartilaginous embolic myelopathy can also occur in this region (see **Table 3**).

T3-L3 Spinal Cord Segments/Vertebrae T2 Through L3

Most spinal diseases in dogs and cats affect the T3-L3 spinal segments. IVDD (either extrusion or protrusion) is very common in this location. Other common diseases are degenerative myelopathy, spinal trauma, neoplasia, and fibrocartilaginous embolic myelopathy. If the lesion is localized to the mid-cranial thoracic region between the T2 and T10 vertebrae (based on the cutoff of the cutaneous trunci reflex and/or spinal pain), then a few diseases can be considered more likely. IVDD is rare at this region. The diseases that are more commonly seen between the T2 and T10 vertebrae are spinal neoplasia, discospondylitis, and hemivertebra. The differential diagnoses for the diseases affecting the T3-L3 spinal cord region are presented in **Table 3**.

Table 2
Differential diagnoses for common diseases affecting the cervical spine (C1-C5 spinal cord segments and cervical enlargement). These diseases cause proprioceptive ataxia, tetraparesis, and/or neck pain

	Breeds	Age	Onset	Neurologic Deficits	Spinal Pain
Atlantoaxial Instability (Subluxation)	Mainly toy or small; Yorkshire terriers, Poodles	Typically younger than 2 y	Acute or chronic	Common; obvious ataxia and tetraparesis	Present in most cases
Cervical IVDD (Extrusions)	Any; mainly small	Usually older than 2 y	Acute	Typically mild or not present	Severe
Cervical IVDD (Protrusion)	Any; mainly large	Middle-aged to old	Chronic	Mild-to-moderate	Present, but mild-to-moderate
Cervical Spondylomyelopathy (Osseous-Associated)	Giant breeds; Great Danes, Mastiffs	Usually younger than 3–4 y	Usually chronic but can be acute	Common; obvious ataxia and tetraparesis	Usually mild; seen in 50% of cases
Cervical Spondylomyelopathy (Disk-Associated)	Large; Dobermans, Weimaraners	Middle-aged to old dogs	Usually chronic but can be acute	Common; obvious ataxia and tetraparesis	Usually mild; seen in 50%–70% of cases
Fibrocartilaginous Embolic Myelopathy	Any; usually large	Any; commonly middle-aged	Acute	Common; usually strongly asymmetric	Absent (after 12–24 h)
Spinal Trauma	Any	Any	Acute	Common	Common
Steroid Responsive Meningitis-Arteritis	Boxers, beagles, Berneses, English pointers, Golden retrievers	Young; usually younger than 2 y	Acute or subacute	Uncommon	Severe

Table 3
Differential diagnoses for common diseases affecting the thoracolumbar spine (T3-L3 spinal cord segments). These diseases cause proprioceptive ataxia, paraparesis, or paraplegia, with normal-to-increased pelvic limb reflexes

	Breeds	Age	Onset	Neurologic Deficits	Spinal Pain
Degenerative Myelopathy	Mainly large; German shepherds, Boxers, Pembroke Welsh corgis	Older than 5 y	Chronic (months)	Common; obvious ataxia and paraparesis	Absent
Fibrocartilaginous Embolic Myelopathy	Any; usually large	Any; commonly middle-aged	Acute	Common; usually strongly asymmetric	Absent (after 12–24 h)
Hemivertebra	Screw-tailed breeds, French bulldogs, others	Young; usually younger than 1 y	Chronic	Common; paraparesis and ataxia	Rare
IVDD (Extrusions)	Any; mainly small	Usually older than 2 y	Acute	Typically moderate-to-severe	Moderate-to-severe
IVDD (Protrusion)	Any; mainly large	Middle-aged to old	Chronic	Mild-to-moderate	Usually present but mild
Meningomyelitis	Any	Any	Usually subacute (few days)	Variable, but signs are often asymmetric	Variable; can wax and wane
Spinal Neoplasia	Any; usually large	Any; commonly middle-aged to older	Chronic or subacute (2–3 d)	Common	Variable, but usually present
Spinal Trauma	Any	Any	Acute	Common	Common

Abbreviation: IVDD, intervertebral disk disease.

Table 4
Differential diagnoses for common diseases affecting the lumbosacral (L4-S3) spinal cord segments or vertebrae L4 through L5. These diseases cause mild proprioceptive ataxia, paraparesis, or paraplegia, with decreased-to-absent pelvic limb reflexes

	Breeds	Age	Onset	Neurologic Deficits	Spinal Pain
Degenerative Myelopathy	Mainly large; German shepherds, Boxers, Pembroke Welsh corgis	Older than 5 y	Chronic (months)	Ataxia and paraparesis. The decreased patellar reflex is usually a manifestation of a dorsal (sensory) radiculopathy, and not a lower motor neuron sign	Absent
Fibrocartilaginous Embolic Myelopathy	Any; usually large	Any; commonly middle-aged	Acute	Common; usually strongly asymmetric	Absent (after 12–24 h)
IVDD (Extrusions)	Any; mainly small	Usually older than 2 y	Acute	Typically moderate-to-severe	Moderate-to-severe
IVDD (Protrusion)	Any; mainly large	Middle-aged to old	Chronic	Mild-to-moderate	Usually present but mild
Meningomyelitis	Any	Any	Usually subacute (few days)	Variable; but signs are often asymmetric	Variable; can wax and wane
Spinal Neoplasia	Any; usually large	Any; commonly middle-aged to older	Chronic or subacute (2–3 d)	Common	Variable, but usually present
Spinal Trauma	Any	Any	Acute	Common	Common

Table 5
Differential diagnoses for common diseases affecting the vertebrae L6 through L7 and sacrum. These diseases may cause paraparesis with or without proprioceptive deficits but without proprioceptive ataxia because the spinal cord is not affected. Lameness is also frequently observed with asymmetric lesions in this area

	Breeds	Age	Onset	Neurologic Deficits	Spinal Pain
Lumbosacral Stenosis (Cauda Equina Syndrome)	Usually large breeds; German shepherds are overrepresented	Middle-aged to old	Chronic	Typically mild-to-moderate; can be severe in late stages; lameness may be the only sign	Often present, but may only be elicited with deep spinal palpation
Spinal Neoplasia	Any; usually large breeds	Any; commonly middle-aged to older	Chronic or subacute (2–3 d)	Common	Variable, but usually present
Discospondylitis	Any; usually large and giant breeds	Any; commonly young to middle-aged	Usually acute	Usually not present initially	Severe pain, sometimes not localizable
Spinal Trauma	Any	Any	Acute	Common	Common

L4-S3 Spinal Cord Segments (Lumbosacral Enlargement)/Vertebrae L4 Through L5 (Dogs)

This is a small spinal cord region, and most diseases affecting the T3-L3 spinal cord region can also affect this one (eg, IVDD, trauma, neoplasia). A disease that frequently affects this specific region is fibrocartilaginous embolic myelopathy. The main features of diseases affecting this region are shown in **Table 4**.

Vertebrae L6 Through L7 and Sacrum in Dogs

Problems affecting the caudal-lumbar region are very common in large-breed dogs. Spinal diseases affecting this region can appear similar to musculoskeletal disorders, because lameness may be the only clinical sign. The primary differential diagnoses for diseases affecting this region are degenerative lumbosacral stenosis, discospondylitis, neoplasia, and extradural synovial cysts. Spinal pain is often a consistent feature of diseases affecting the caudal-lumbar/lumbosacral spine. The main clinical features of the diseases affecting this region are presented in **Table 5**.

SUMMARY

A stepwise process facilitates the diagnostic approach to patients with spinal disorders. The VITAMIN-D system can be used to select the primary pathophysiologic mechanisms causing the patient's clinical signs. Using the acronym VITAMIN-D or the specific tables by lesion localization, the clinician may be able to go from a large list of diagnostic possibilities to a shorter list of diagnostic probabilities.

FURTHER READINGS

da Costa RC. Ataxia, paresis and paralysis. In: Ettinger SJ, Feldman EC, editors. Textbook of veterinary internal medicine. 7th edition. St Louis: Elsevier; 2010. p. 222–5.

de Lahunta A, Glass E. Veterinary neuroanatomy and clinical neurology. 3rd edition. St Louis (MO): Saunders-Elsevier; 2009.

Dewey CW. A practical guide to canine and feline neurology. 2nd edition. Ames (IA): Wiley-Blackwell; 2008.

Evans HE. Miller's anatomy of the dog. 3rd edition. Philadelphia: Saunders; 1993.

Lorenz MD, Kornegay JN. Handbook of veterinary neurology. 4th edition. St Louis (MO): Saunders; 2004.

Platt S, Olby N. BSAVA manual of canine and feline neurology. 3rd edition. Ames (IA): Blackwell; 2004.

Sharp NJH, Wheeler SJ, editors. Small animal spinal disorders diagnosis and surgery. 2nd edition. Philadelphia: Elsevier Mosby; 2005.

Advanced Imaging of the Spine in Small Animals

Ronaldo C. da Costa, DMV, MSc, PhD*, Valerie F. Samii, DVM

KEYWORDS

- Magnetic resonance imaging • Computed tomography
- Spinal • Spine • Myelopathy • Myelography • Dogs • Cats

Computed tomography (CT) and magnetic resonance imaging (MRI) are now routinely used in the diagnostic investigation of spinal diseases. This review discusses the fundamentals of CT and MRI, the technical aspects of both modalities, and the CT and MR imaging features of the most common spinal diseases.

Both CT and MRI offer significant advantages over survey radiographs and myelography. Whereas very few veterinary studies have been published demonstrating the benefits of CT or MRI over regular myelography, a wealth of data exists from studies on humans.[1] The few comparative veterinary studies confirm the findings seen in humans. The overall diagnostic sensitivity of MRI is superior to CT, and as such MRI can be used to image the vast majority of spinal disorders, with few exceptions (eg, spinal trauma caused by gun shot). Routine survey radiographs are always recommended before proceeding with advanced imaging because the area of interest may be more specifically localized, thus reducing scanning time, and severe spinal/osseous lesions, such as hemivertebrae or discospondylitis, may be identified without the need of advanced imaging studies. However, depending on the clinical status and treatment plan, advanced imaging may still be needed.

FUNDAMENTALS OF COMPUTED TOMOGRAPHY

Whereas conventional radiography produces summed images of an object, CT scanners rotate to divide an object and organize it into spatially consecutive, parallel image sections. Detectors that are aligned behind the patient opposite to the x-ray source measure the amount of x-ray attenuation. The CT computer not only collects but also stores this x-ray attenuation data and generates a matrix of values, depicted in various shades of gray. The major advantage of CT over radiographs is the improved spatial resolution.

Department of Veterinary Clinical Sciences, College of Veterinary Medicine, The Ohio State University, 601 Vernon L. Tharp Street, Columbus, OH 43210-1089, USA
* Corresponding author.
E-mail address: dacosta.6@osu.edu

Vet Clin Small Anim 40 (2010) 765–790
doi:10.1016/j.cvsm.2010.05.002
vetsmall.theclinics.com
0195-5616/10/$ – see front matter

In conventional CT, also known as single-slice CT, a series of equally spaced images are acquired sequentially through a specific region. The x-ray attenuation data is obtained on a slice-by-slice basis with the CT table advancing by predetermined set distances after each slice data acquisition. These units are no longer being manufactured but they are still used in many veterinary clinical settings.

With helical CT scanners, electrical slip ring contacts allow the gantry assembly to rotate continuously. By moving the table, and hence the position of the patient, during the scan, the data are acquired in a helical geometry around the patient. The advantage of this technology is that it significantly reduces scanning time. Multidetector technology permits CT scanners to acquire multiple slices or sections simultaneously and greatly increases the speed of CT image acquisition. The ability to obtain submillimeter slice thicknesses is also a characteristic feature of multidetector helical systems.

FUNDAMENTALS OF MAGNETIC RESONANCE IMAGING

Each nucleus with an odd number of protons and/or odd number of neutrons has a spin. Because protons carry an electric charge, the spin creates a magnetic field that has direction and finite strength. In the body, the "magnetic moments" of the protons point in all directions and cancel each other out. When the body is placed in a strong magnetic field, the magnetic moments of the protons will align parallel to the field direction (Z-axis).

This alignment, or magnetization, is then disrupted by radiofrequency pulses. As the nuclei recover their alignment by relaxation processes, they produce radio signals that are proportional to the magnitude of the initial alignment. Tissue contrast (ie, differences in signal) develops as a result of the different rates at which nuclei realign with the magnetic field.

The positions of the nuclei are localized during this process by the application of spatially-dependent magnetic fields called gradients. The signal is then read after a predetermined period of time has elapsed from the initial radiofrequency excitation. The signal is transformed by the computer into an image using a mathematical process known as Fourier transform.

Field strengths vary in the clinical MR units and range from 0.2 to 7.0 Tesla. Higher field strengths are available in research settings. In general, the higher the field strength, the higher the signal to noise ratio (SNR) and the faster the imaging times, to a limit. The field strength systems over 0.7 Tesla require more extensive shielding against external radiofrequency interference. Maintenance costs for these units are considerable.

CT VERSUS MRI

In general, CT provides superior spatial resolution and is better suited for imaging bone. Slice thicknesses as thin as 1 to 1.5 mm are possible in almost all available CT units. Thinner slice acquisitions (submillimeter) are possible with newer, multidetector systems. For CT this is a distinct advantage over MRI, for which such thin slice acquisitions are not currently possible because of decreases in SNR as slice thicknesses decrease. To some extent, high SNR is a factor of magnet field strength and the number of excitations (NEX) repeatedly collected over a sample volume of tissue. Although increasing NEX increases SNR, it also increases scan time. Other advantages of CT over MRI are decreased cost, fewer maintenance requirements and associated expense, and rapidity of imaging. Imaging patients under sedation is now possible with some of the newer scanners because of their rapid scan times. Because equipment costs and scanning times are less, client costs for CT are typically less than

MRI. CT can be used to successfully guide needle aspirations or biopsies once a lesion is localized, but this is not generally done with MRI guidance because of prolonged imaging times and the inability to use metal implements for tissue sampling.

MR provides superior contrast resolution and is better suited for imaging soft tissues, such as the spinal cord, nerve roots, and intervertebral discs. Images can be acquired in multiple planes whereas CT images can only be acquired in one plane (typically transverse). Although CT images can be reformatted into any plane desirable, including 3-dimensional, the image detail is slightly reduced on reformatted as compared with acquired images. The quality and conspicuity of the reformatted images is a factor of acquisition slice thickness; the thinner the slices acquired, the better the detail on reformatted images. Whereas myelography is still often used in conjunction with CT of the spine, this is not necessary with MRI because of the ability to alter tissue contrast by applying different acquisition sequences. Thus, the associated morbidity often accompanying myelography is avoided.

CT IMAGING TECHNIQUES

Positioning

- Dorsal recumbency (standard positioning for all spinal segments)
- Ventral recumbency for the cervical spine
  To avoid overextension of the neck in cases of atlantoaxial instability
  Useful for subtle intervertebral disc protrusions.

Plane of Acquisition

- Transverse
  Reformatted into sagittal and dorsal planar images.

Algorithm

Selection of the appropriate image algorithm before initiation of scanning is paramount and dependent on the tissue of interest. In most cases both bone and the soft tissues of spine, to include the spinal cord, intervertebral discs, and paralumbar musculature, will need to be assessed.

Technique

The choice of mA and kVp is determined by considering patient size and area imaged, patient exposure dose, SNR, and time, dictated by the necessity for tube cooling when using a higher mA. Most CT units are equipped with standard image protocols based on patient size that require little modification before scanning.

Field of View

Field of view (FOV) is specific to the spinal column and dependent on patient size.

Pitch (Specific to Helical Scanners)

Pitch is defined as the ratio of table speed per gantry (detector) rotation around the patient and slice thickness.

Slice Thickness

Slice thickness is specific to the region of the spinal column imaged and patient size. In general, the following parameters are recommended:

- 1 to 2 mm through intervertebral disc or localized lesion other than disc
- 3 to 5 mm through spinal column.

Initial images typically are acquired through a segment of spinal column based on neurolocalization of a lesion. This area may be scanned using larger slice thicknesses. Once an isolated lesion is identified, thinner slice acquisitions through the lesion may be acquired for greater lesion conspicuity. If looking specifically for intervertebral disc disease, the plane of imaging should be parallel to the intervertebral disc. Otherwise, transverse imaging perpendicular to the spinal column is advised. The desired imaging plane may be obtained by tilting the CT gantry.

MRI TECHNIQUES

Positioning

The same general principles of positioning apply as described for CT; however, straight spinal alignment is more important for MRI to allow direct comparison of multiple sites on sagittal images. The spinal segment(s) to be imaged must be in close contact with the radiofrequency coil for satisfactory SNR. As table surface coils designed for spinal imaging are used in most instances, patients are typically positioned in dorsal recumbency.

Plane of Acquisition

- Sagittal: Often used as the survey series to localize a specific site of pathology as a long segment of the spine can be imaged. The T2-weighted sequence is preferred for initial assessment for intervertebral disc disease, infection, or neoplasia.
- Dorsal
- Transverse: Typically limited to a specific site of pathology as imaging of extended lengths of spine in this plane is time intensive.

Image Sequences and Slice

- T2-weighted: Fluid, such as cerebrospinal fluid (CSF) or edema, will be hyperintense.
- T1-weighted: Fluid, such as CSF or edema, will be hypointense.
- FLAIR (fluid-attenuated inversion recovery): Pure fluid, such as normal CSF, will be hypointense whereas edema or abnormal fluids will be increased in intensity.
- STIR (short tau inversion recovery) or fat saturation: The typically hyperintense fat (on both T1- and T2-weighted sequences) will be of low signal intensity. If a sequence is T2-weighted, CSF can be more readily differentiated from epidural fat. If a sequence is T1-weighted, a contrast-enhancing lesion can be more readily differentiated from fat.
- Gradient echo (GRE): A fast sequence that is very sensitive to inhomogeneities in the magnetic field though less sensitive to motion artifact because of its speed of acquisition. It is often used to detect areas of hemorrhage, as excessive iron concentrations in hemorrhagic areas of the spinal cord will cause field inhomogeneity.

Recommended Standard Planes, Slice Thicknesses, and Sequences

- 2-mm thick T2-weighted sagittal images followed by 2-mm thick T1-weighted sagittal images. A 0.5-mm gap between slices, to avoid image cross-talk and resultant decreased signal to noise, or interleaved (no gap) acquisition is typical.
- 2- to 3-mm transverse images through the lesion identified on the sagittal images.
- 2-mm dorsal images for lateralized lesions identified on the prior sequences.

- T1-weighted images after intravenous gadolinium injection may be obtained in all 3 image planes according to the lesion characteristics.
- STIR, FLAIR, fat saturation, and GRE sequences may be necessary depending on lesion characteristics.

Field of View

FOV is defined as the vertical or horizontal distance across an image. It should be set specific to the spinal column, which is dependent on patient size. By decreasing FOV to a specific area, the SNR decreases and thus increases in sampling (NEX) or increases in slice width are necessary to maintain adequate spatial and contrast resolution. By increasing NEX, scan time is also increased.

Saturation Bands

As MRI is extremely sensitive to motion artifact secondary to respiration and blood flow, saturation bands may be placed over the abdomen and thorax to suppress the effects of motion from these areas during scanning.

Number of Excitements

NEX refers to the number of repeat signal samplings acquired in any given sequence. In general, the more times an area is sampled, the greater the SNR (improved tissue contrast). The downside is that the greater the NEX, the longer the overall imaging time. NEX values between 2 and 4 are typically required for field strengths over 1 Tesla.

CONTRAST IMAGING

Subarachnoid Nonionic Iodinated Contrast (CT only)

Indications include identification of nonmineralized extradural and intradural-extramedullary lesions. These indications may include intervertebral disc herniation, neoplasia, hematoma, granuloma/abscess, cyst (arachnoid or synovial), scar tissue, and empyema.

Intravenous Iodinated (CT) or Gadolinium Diethylenetriaminepentaacetic Acid (MRI) Contrast

Indications include identification of vascular lesions like those secondary to neoplasia, infectious/noninfectious inflammatory lesions other than related to intervertebral disc herniation, and vascular malformations.

CT AND MRI ARTIFACTS

A variety of artifacts are associated with both modalities, and it is beyond the scope of this article to discuss them. Both modalities are extremely sensitive to motion artifacts, MRI more so than CT. Many of the potential motion artifacts in CT can be overcome by the rapidity of imaging. Artifacts associated with metal implants or foreign bodies are also common to both modalities. In MRI, potentially deleterious effects to patients with pacemakers or small metallic shavings in or adjacent to critical sites are possible. Small shavings may move within the tissues, with the potential to penetrate, for instance, the spinal cord. For this reason, MRI of patients with gunshot injuries should be avoided.

NORMAL ANATOMY

The anatomic features of the spinal region being studied must be taken into consideration when interpreting advanced imaging studies. Each region of the vertebral column (cervical, thoracic, lumbar, and sacral) has specific anatomic features. A larger degree of anatomic variation is seen in the cervical vertebrae compared with other vertebral regions. Not only are the cervical vertebrae different, but also the shape and relationship of the spinal cord to the vertebral canal varies according to the location within the cervical column (**Fig. 1**).[2] The anatomic features of the cervical spine and lumbosacral spine have been reported in detail using CT, MRI, or both.[2–6]

Due to the exquisite sensitivity of MRI it is important to assess the imaging findings in the light of the patient's clinical signs and examination findings. The presence of asymptomatic spinal abnormalities is widely recognized in human medicine. The presence of multiple spinal abnormalities is commonly seen in aged dogs and cats. Clinically silent spinal cord compression, intervertebral disc degeneration, intervertebral disc protrusion, nerve root compression, intervertebral foraminal stenosis, and vertebral canal stenosis have all been reported without concurrent clinical signs in dogs.[2,4,7] Similarly, no correlation exists between the severity of spinal cord or nerve root compression and the severity of clinical signs.[8,9]

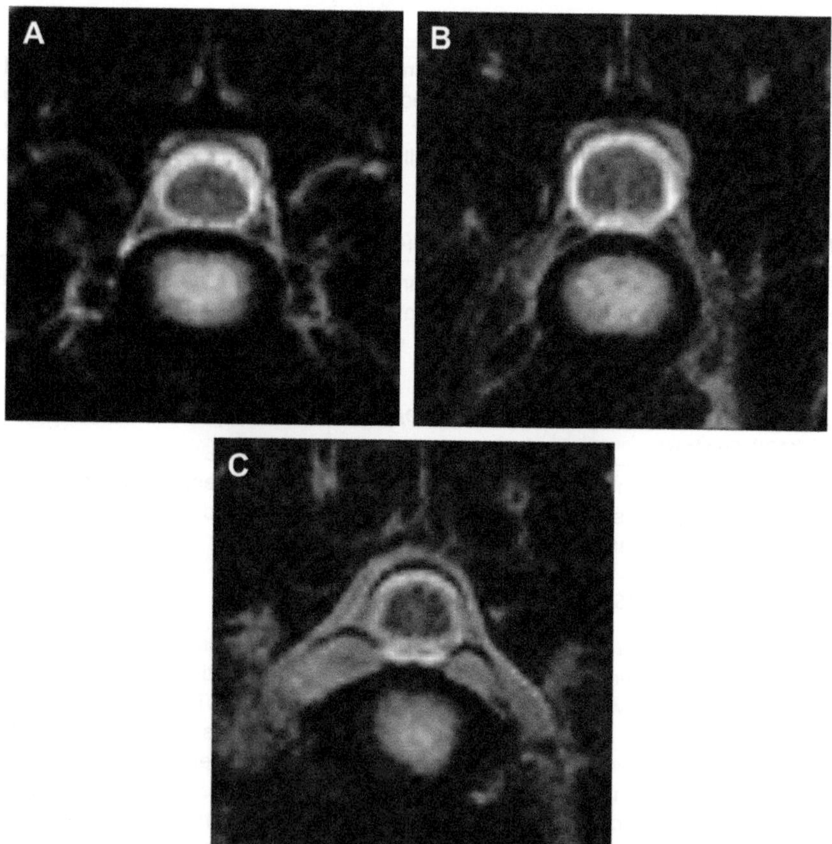

Fig. 1. Transverse T2-weighted MR images at the level of the C2-3 (*A*), C5-6 (*B*), and C7-T1 (*C*) intervertebral disks of a clinically normal Doberman Pinscher. Note the different shapes of the spinal cord at each cervical level. The normal spinal cord at C7-T1 has a trapezoid shape. (*From* da Costa RC, Parent JM, Partlow G, et al. Morphologic and morphometric magnetic resonance imaging features of Doberman Pinscher dogs with and without clinical signs of cervical spondylomyelopathy. Am J Vet Res 2006;67:1601–12; with permission.)

CONGENITAL SPINAL DISEASES

Atlantoaxial malformation and Chiari-like malformations are seen primarily in toy breed dogs and may be associated with severe clinical signs. Anatomic abnormalities associated with atlantoaxial malformation include odontoid process (dens) malformation, hypoplasia or aplasia, and/or weak or poorly developed supporting ligamentous structures of the odontoid process.[10] The result may be subluxation or luxation of the atlantoaxial articulation, usually resulting in ventroflexion and a widened angle or space between the dorsal lamina of the atlas and spinous process of the axis (**Fig. 2**). If the odontoid process is intact and normally or partially formed it may deviate dorsally within the spinal canal, resulting in severe compression of the spinal cord, exacerbated by increased ventroflexion of the cranial cervical spine (**Fig. 3**). Anatomic malformations associated with Chiari-like malformation include occipital hypoplasia and brainstem crowding. Atlanto-occipital overlapping with or without medullary kinking may be present (see **Fig. 2**B). Syringohydromyelia may or may not be seen.[11] CT is an excellent means of evaluating the size and shape of the odontoid process and in assessing for cranial over-riding of the atlas. MRI is sensitive for detecting secondary trauma to the spinal cord (hemorrhage, edema) secondary to instability at the articulations. MRI is also better suited for assessment of syrinx formation within the spinal cord (**Fig. 4**). Due to the naturally small size of the supporting ligamentous structures of the atlantoaxial articulation, these structures are typically not seen with either modality, even when normally formed.

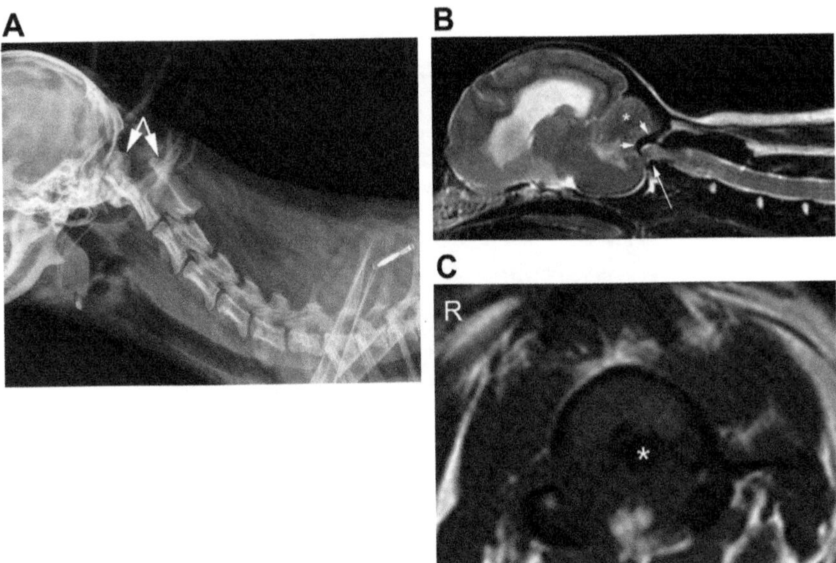

Fig. 2. Atlantoaxial subluxation. (*A*) Lateral radiograph showing increased distance between the dorsal lamina of the atlas and the spinous process of the axis (*arrows*). The odontoid process is normally formed but dorsally displaced. (*B*) Sagittal T2-weighted MR image in the same dog. The odontoid process is a hypointense structure ventral to the spinal cord (*long arrow*). A curvilinear hypointensity caudal to the cerebellum (*asterisk*) represents caudal occipital overlapping with medullary kinking (*short arrows*). (*C*) Transverse T1-weighted MR image through the odontoid process (*asterisk*) and the atlanto-occipital articulation in the same dog. The normally oval spinal cord has a "kidney-bean" shape secondary to ventral compression by the dorsally deviated odontoid process.

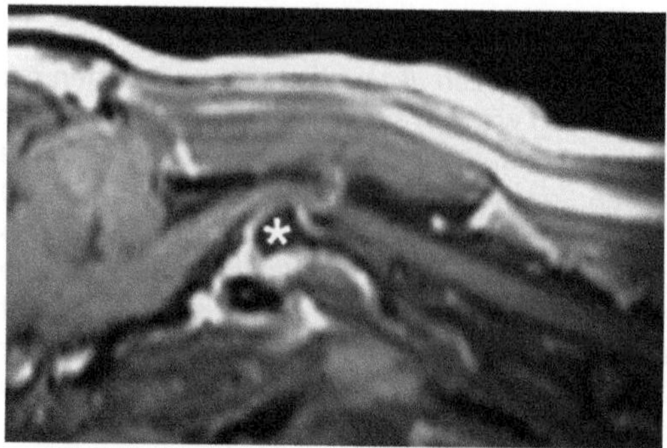

Fig. 3. Atlantoaxial subluxation. Sagittal T1-weighted MR image showing dorsal deviation of the odontoid process (*asterisk*) with resultant, severe spinal cord compression.

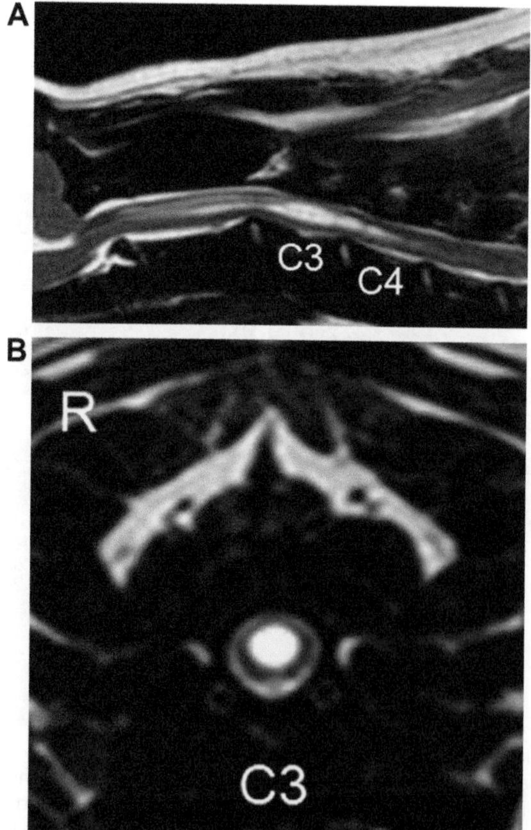

Fig. 4. Sagittal (*A*) and transverse (*B*) T2-weighted MR images through the cranial cervical spine of a dog with syringohydromyelia. A fusiform region of hyperintensity is present in the central spinal cord at the level of C3 and cranial C4 (*A*). There is a large, circular region of hyperintensity representing fluid in the central spinal cord secondary to syringohydromyelia (*B*).

Hemivertebrae are quite commonly recognized in brachycephaic, screwtail breeds. Besides the tail, the mid to caudal thoracic spine is often affected to varying degrees.[12,13] Hemivertebra results from abnormal, uneven growth between the two halves of one or more vertebrae during development, with often incomplete fusion between the halves. Because of the abnormal vertebral conformation, secondary spinal canal stenosis and spinal cord compression may occur. Also, inherent instability at the articulations at these sites is common, as articular process and vertebral end-plate conformation are compromised. One of the greatest challenges in imaging these patients is that most patients have associated, varying degrees of kyphosis, lordosis, and scoliosis. Achieving well-positioned planar images is difficult. CT is preferred for better definition of bone, particularly if a surgical stabilization process is being considered. If neurologic deficits are present, MRI is preferred for spinal cord imaging (**Fig. 5**). Other congenital vertebral anomalies include block vertebra, butterfly vertebra, transitional vertebra, and spina bifida (see the article by Westworth and Sturges elsewhere in this issue for further exploration of this topic). On rare occasions, herniation of the meninges (meningocele) or meninges and spinal cord (meningomyelocele) may be seen with spina bifida. Dermoid sinuses result from a congenital communication between the skin and spinal cord and may be seen in Rhodesian Ridgeback dogs, and occasionally in other breeds. MRI is the preferred imaging modality for assessment of meningoceles, myelomeningoceles, and dermoid cysts.

Spinal arachnoid cysts consist of outpouchings of the arachnoid matter or focal dilatations in the subarachnoid space that are filled with cerebrospinal fluid.[14] The use of the term "cyst" to describe these lesions is a misnomer, as these outpouchings are not lined by epithelium. These lesions are most commonly located in the dorsolateral area of the cervical spine, but may be seen ventrally and in other regions of the spine column; they may be bilaterally paired, having a bilobed appearance (**Fig. 6**).[15] There is still discussion as to whether these "pseudocysts" are congenitally acquired or

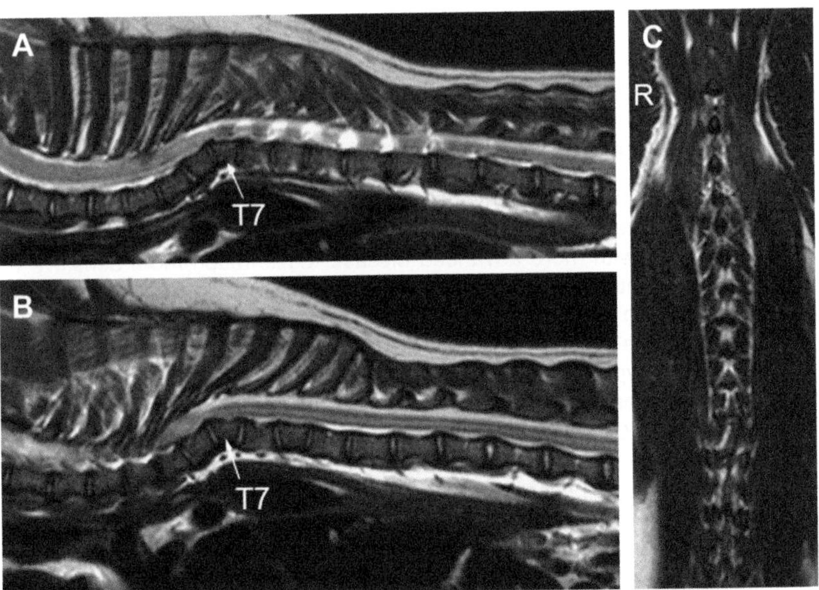

Fig. 5. Sagittal (*A, B*) T1-weighted and dorsal (*C*) T2-weighted MR images of the thoracolumbar spine of a French bulldog with severe lordosis and mild scoliosis secondary to T7, T8, and T9 hemivertebrae.

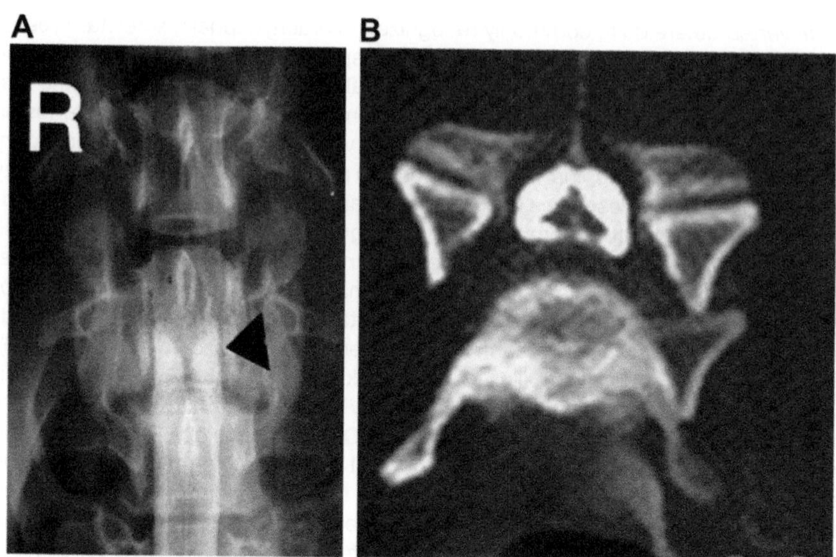

Fig. 6. Bilobed arachnoid cyst. Ventrodorsal myelogram of the caudal cervical spine (*A*) and a transverse postmyelogram CT image (*B*) made at the level of caudal C6. There is biaxially symmetric, focal dilatation of the contrast opacified subarachnoid space at the level of C6-7 (*arrowhead*).

possibly secondary to trauma or arachnoiditis-induced adhesions. Arachnoid adhesions resulting from chronic inflammation and microtrauma may be the instigating cause of pseudocyst development.[16] It has also been postulated that the arachnoid adhesions, rather than the subarachnoid outpouchings, are the cause of spinal cord compression and the resultant neurologic deficits.[16] As the Rottweiler breed is overrepresented, a genetic or hereditary component is likely in at least some patients.[14–16] An acquired arachnoid cyst has been reported in a cat.[17] CT myelography and MRI are equally adept at identifying cyst-like lesions of the subarachnoid space.

INFLAMMATORY SPINAL DISEASES

Discospondylitis has been, by convention, a radiographic diagnosis. Clinical signs often precede radiographic evidence of vertebral endplate lysis and medullary sclerosis, typically seen with more advanced disease. CT is much more sensitive than radiographs for identifying endplate osteolysis early in the course of disease (**Fig. 7**). MRI is much more sensitive for detecting soft-tissue inflammation of the disc that usually precedes bony changes. Also, early marrow changes in the affected vertebra (increased hyperintensity on T2-weighted images and contrast enhancement on T1-weighted images) may be seen with MRI prior to overt osteolysis. As such, MRI may be preferred to CT to screen for early cases of discospondylitis where bony changes are not observed radiographically.[18,19]

Myelitis and neuritis are best evaluated with pre- and post-intravenous contrast MRI (**Figs. 8** and **9**). Imaging features are very similar to, and are difficult to distinguish from, neoplasia. Cerebrospinal fluid analysis, surgical biopsy, and the patient's overall clinical picture may be necessary to confirm infectious or noninfectious inflammatory processes.

Epidural empyema is defined as the accumulation of purulent material within the spinal canal and may be the result of a penetrating wound, grass awn migration, or

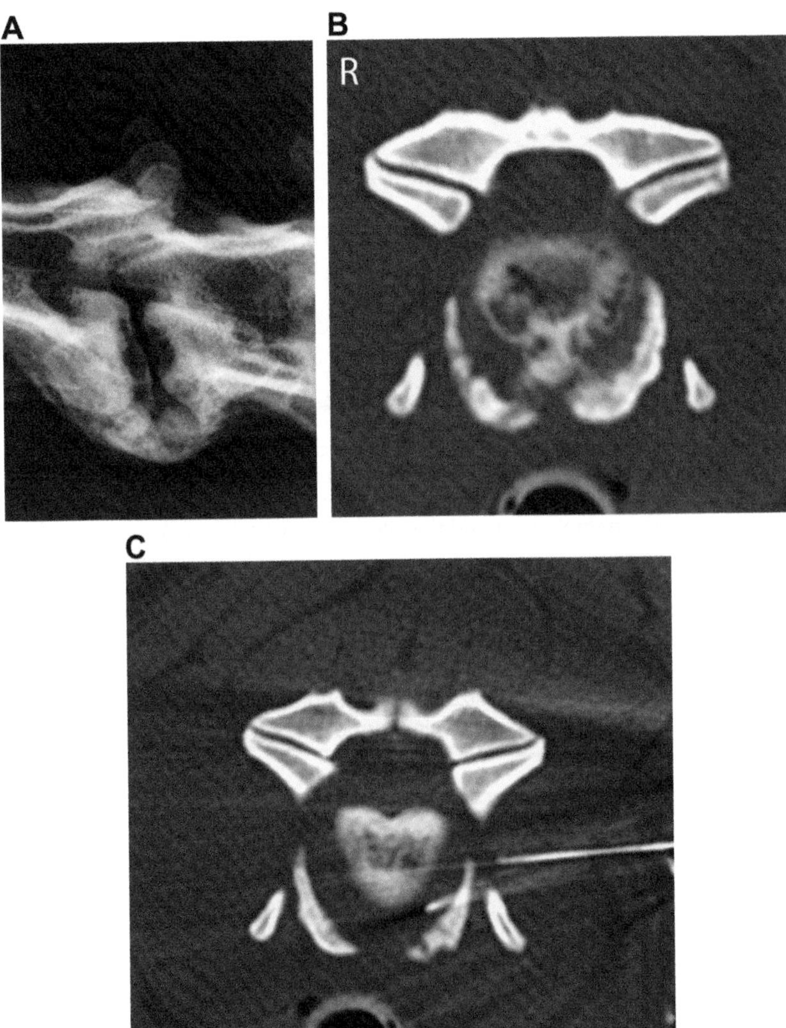

Fig. 7. C4-5 discospondylitis. A lateral radiograph (*A*) and a transverse CT image made through the C4-5 intervertebral disc space (*B*) show punctate to porous vertebral endplate lysis and extensive ventral spondylosis deformans. CT-guided placement of a spinal needle for aspirate sampling is shown (*C*).

systemic sepsis with discospondylitis that erodes into the spinal canal. Patients are typically pyrexic and have a rapid course of progressive myelopathy. Neurologic signs are secondary to the combined effects of regional tissue inflammation and spinal cord compression by an epidural mass effect. MRI is the preferred imaging test, again for its superior soft-tissue resolution.[20,21]

SPINAL NEOPLASIA

Spinal neoplasia is an important differential diagnosis for dogs presenting with either chronic or acute neurologic signs. Several classification systems are used to categorize spinal neoplasms. A common classification categorizes the tumors according to

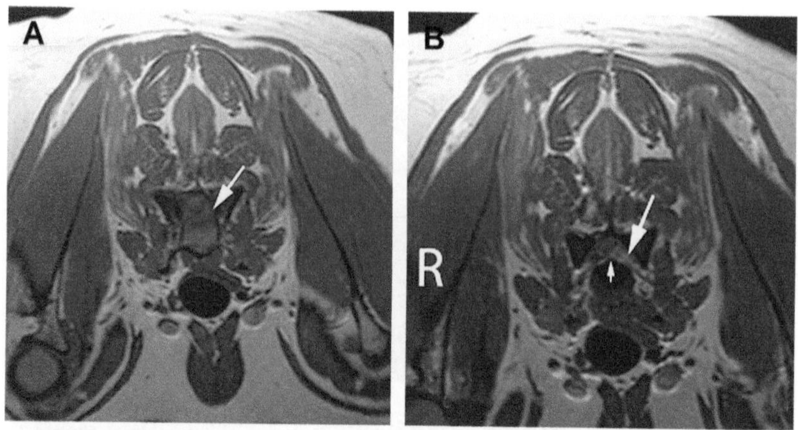

Fig. 8. C6-7 left-sided neuritis. Pre- (*A*) and post-intravenous contrast (*B*) transverse T1-weighted MR images made at the level of C6-7. There is thickening and diffuse contrast enhancement of the left C6-7 nerve root (*long arrow*). A slight dorsal protrusion of the hypointense C6-7 intervertebral disc is additionally present (*short arrow*).

the location into extradural, intradural-extramedullary, and intramedullary. Extradural tumors such as osteosarcoma and fibrosarcoma are the most common.[22]

Both CT and MRI are sensitive techniques for the diagnosis of spinal tumors. Due to the superior soft-tissue resolution, MRI is usually the preferred imaging method; however, CT is excellent for visualization of osseous lesions, which are commonly observed in spinal tumors. CT examination of spinal tumors will often require

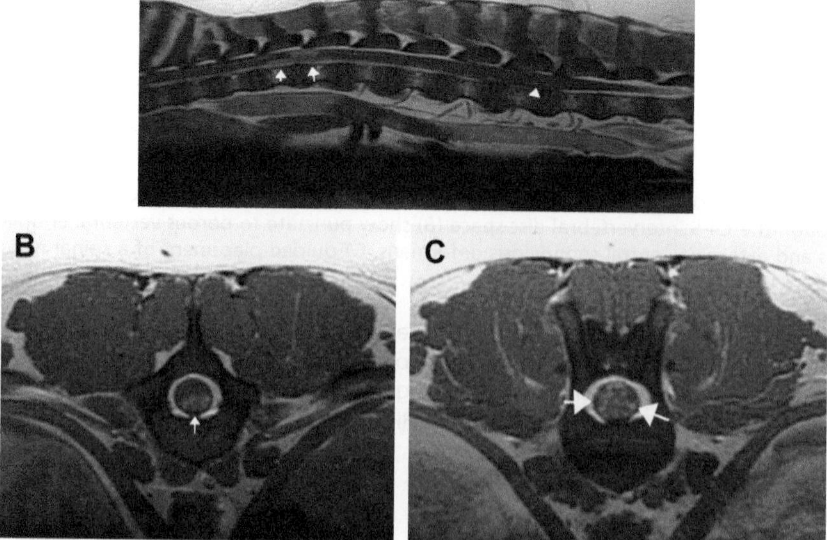

Fig. 9. Myelitis. Sagittal (*A*) and transverse (*B, C*) T1-weighted MR images after intravenous gadolinium injection showing the irregular areas of contrast enhancement in the spinal cord (*arrows*).

intravenous contrast injection to identify areas of contrast enhancement. Contrast injection into the subarachnoid space (myelography) may also be required.

A study comparing myelography and CT concluded that the lytic/proliferative osseous lesions were depicted more clearly on CT than on radiographs (**Fig. 10**).[23] Lytic and proliferative regions observed on imaging need to be differentiated from infections such as discospondylitis or vertebral osteomyelitis. As a general rule, lytic and proliferative lesions located in the vertebra itself are typical or neoplasia, whereas

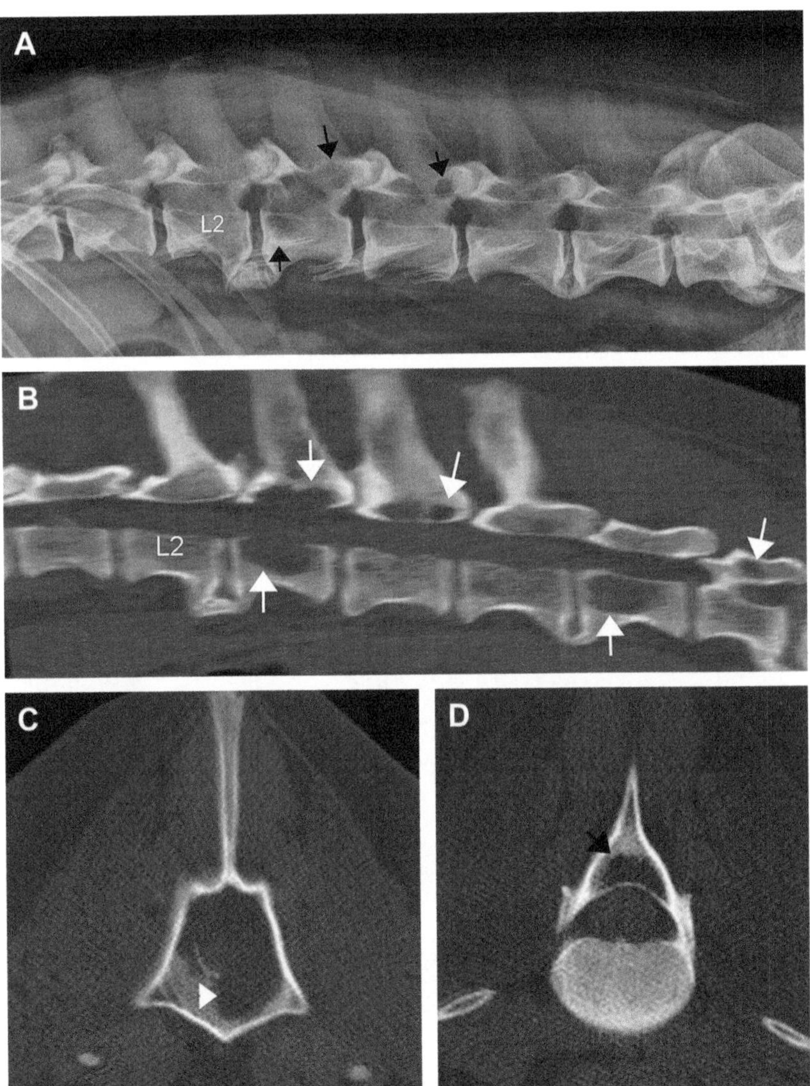

Fig. 10. Spinal neoplasia—multiple myeloma. (*A*) Lateral radiograph show multiple areas of osteolytic lesions (*arrows*). (*B*) Reformatted sagittal CT scan makes visualization of the lytic areas more evident and reveals other areas not previously identified (*arrows*). (*C*) Transverse CT image of L3 showing severe osteolysis (*arrowhead*). (*D*) Transverse CT image at the caudal aspect of L4 showing lysis of the dorsal lamina (*arrow*).

lytic/proliferative lesions centered at the disc space are caused by infections (discospondylitis). In one study, myelography was more useful in differentiating between intradural-extramedullary and intramedullary tumors than CT.[23] This same observation was made when comparing myelography and MRI in another study.[24] Careful evaluation of the images in all 3 planes (transverse, sagittal, and dorsal) may assist in defining the location of the tumor. Dorsal images are particularly useful. The MRI findings of spinal meningiomas, the most common intradural tumor, have been well described.[25,26] Most meningiomas are iso- to hyperintense on T1-weighted images and hyperintense on T2-weighted images.[24–26] Homogeneous, strong contrast enhancement and presence of dural tail are also consistently observed (**Fig. 11**).[24–26]

MRI findings for other spinal tumors have not been well described. Osseous tumors have very variable signal intensity, ranging from iso- to hyper- or hypointense on both T1- and T2-weighted images. Contrast enhancement is also variable. It is important to use fat suppression techniques (eg, STIR) when observing hyperintense lesions on T1- and T2-weighted images within osseous structures, as these changes may be caused by fat infiltration. Intramedullary tumors have more consistent imaging patterns. Due to the common presence of edema, hyperintensity on T2-weighted images and hypointensity on T1-weighted images, in relation to the surrounding spinal cord, is commonly observed. The pattern of enhancement is variable.

Primary or secondary nerve sheath tumors (NSTs) are the most common cause of neurogenic lameness. Approximately 45% of the tumors are located in the nerve roots proximal to the spinal cord while 55% are located in the plexus area or peripheral nerves.[27] This fact emphasizes the importance of using a larger FOV when imaging patients suspected of having NSTs. The imaging features of NSTs have been described using CT and MRI. The visualization of NSTs is facilitated using MRI. CT findings commonly observed in dogs with NSTs are rim enhancement and a hypodense center.[28] On MRI, nerve sheath tumors are consistently hyperintense on

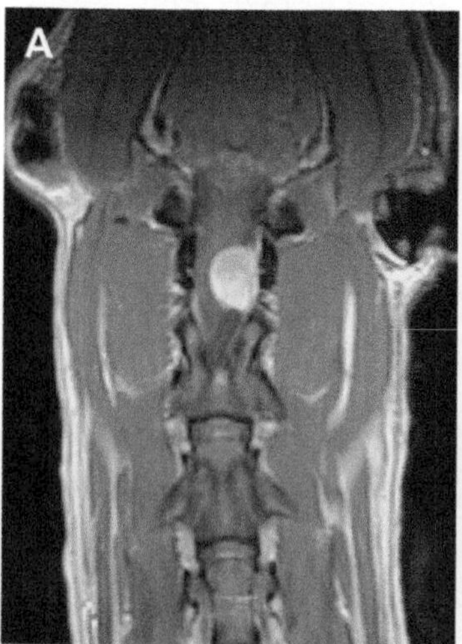

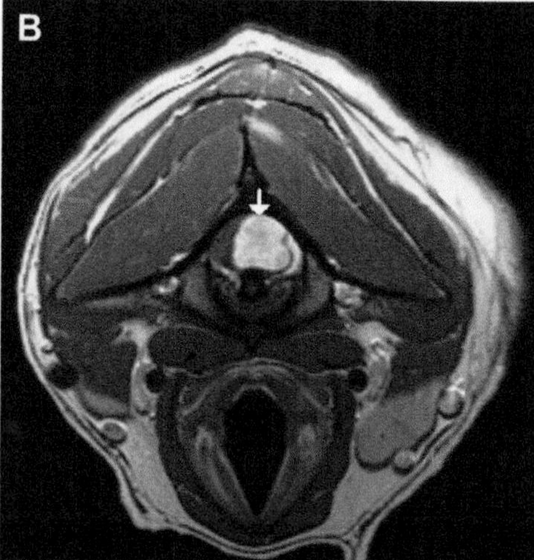

Fig. 11. Meningioma. T1-weighted MR images after intravenous gadolinium injection. (*A*) Dorsal and (*B*) transverse images show a large, mostly homogeneous, contrast-enhancing mass at the level of C1 and C2 (*arrow*). (*From* da Costa RC. In: Daleck, de Nardi, Rodaski, editors. Canine and feline oncology. São Paulo: Roca; 2009. p. 411–35 [in Portuguese]; with permission.)

T2-weighted images, hypointense on T1-weighted images, and show homogeneous or inhomogeneous contrast enhancement (**Fig. 12**). The tumor may appear as a diffuse brachial plexus nerve thickening or a circumscribed mass (**Fig. 13**).[29]

Biopsy is always needed to confirm the diagnosis of spinal tumors or NSTs, and to define the specific type of tumor. Depending on the location of the tumor, biopsy can be guided using CT or ultrasonography.[30]

INTERVERTEBRAL DISC DISEASE

Intervertebral disc disease (IVDD) is the most common spinal disease of dogs, and should be a differential diagnosis in any dog older than 1 year with spinal pain and myelopathic signs. A definitive diagnosis of IVDD requires myelography, CT myelography, or MRI. Noncontrast CT has been used in the diagnosis of acute IVDD for several years.[31] The normal spinal cord is surrounded by epidural fat, which can be seen on plain transverse CTs as an area of intermediate attenuation over the region of the intervertebral discs. Visualization of the spinal cord is more challenging over the vertebral bodies because of the lesser content of epidural fat. CT characteristics of acute intervertebral disc extrusion include hyperdense material within the vertebral canal, loss of epidural fat, and distortion of the spinal cord (**Figs. 14** and **15**). Chronic disc extrusions appear to be even more hyperattenuating, possibly because of progressive mineralization. Acute intervertebral disc herniations are often associated with epidural hemorrhage. Acute and subacute epidural hemorrhage can be seen as irregular linear hyperdense areas cranial and caudal to the herniated disc material. It is often difficult to distinguish between hemorrhage and extruded disc material because blood is often admixed with disc. If the extruded nucleus pulposus is not mineralized, identification of disc material is more difficult and has to be based on loss of epidural fat and displacement of the spinal cord. If surgery is planned, myelography should then be performed to precisely localize the site of extrusion.

It is important to reformat the transverse CT images for assessment of the cranial and caudal extent of disc herniation and to compare multiple sites of disc herniation.

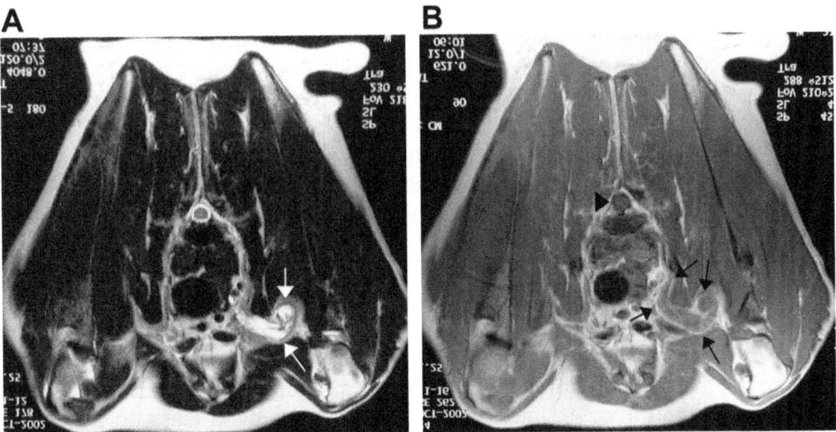

Fig. 12. Primary malignant nerve sheath tumor: distal location. (*A*) Transverse T2-weighted MR image reveals a large hyperintense mass at the level of the left axilla just lateral to the first rib (*arrows*). (*B*) Transverse T1-weighted MR image after intravenous gadolinium injection shows an inhomogeneously enhancing mass at the same level of *A* (*arrows*). Arrowhead indicates the spinal cord.

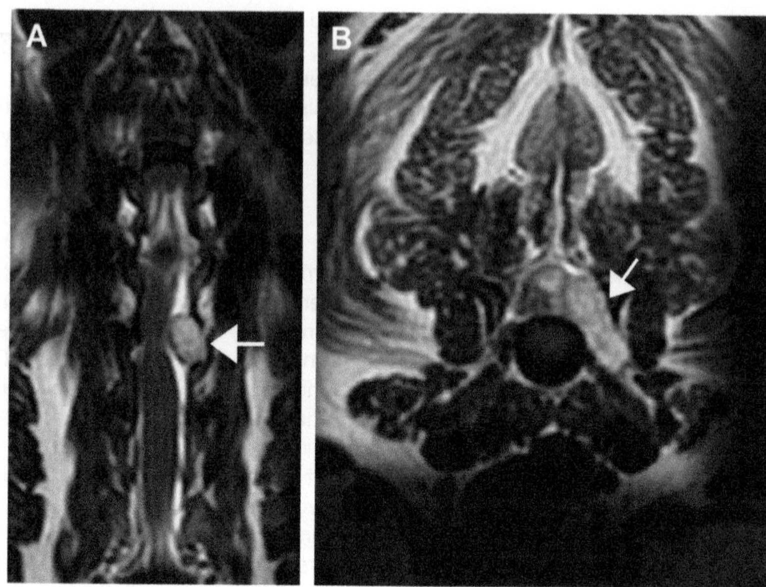

Fig. 13. Primary malignant nerve sheath tumor: proximal location. (*A*) Dorsal T1-weighted MR image after intravenous gadolinium injection shows an oval contrast-enhancing mass that appears to be displacing the spinal cord medially at the level of C5-6 (*arrow*). (*B*) Transverse T1-weighted MR image at the level of C5-6 shows a large contrast-enhancing mass involving the nerve roots and infiltrating into the spinal cord (*arrow*). (*From* da Costa RC. In: Daleck, de Nardi, Rodaski, editors. Canine and feline oncology. São Paulo: Roca; 2009. p. 411–35 [in Portuguese]; with permission.)

Recently, multiplanar reformatting was proposed as a useful technique to increase diagnostic certainty.[32]

Recent studies have compared myelography and CT in the diagnosis of IVDD in dogs. In one study with 182 dogs, noncontrast CT had a sensitivity of 81.8%, whereas myelography had a sensitivity of 83.6%.[33] Another study found a sensitivity of 90% for CT and 88% for myelography.[34] A study with 19 chondrodystrophic dogs found agreement with surgical findings in 94.7% of dogs using myelography, 100% using conventional CT, and 94.7% using helical CT.[35] It is possible that the differences in results among studies are related to the fact that the last study had only chondrodystrophic dogs that are predisposed to chondroid disc degeneration and disc mineralization. All of these studies focused on acute intervertebral disc herniations. The diagnostic sensitivity of plain CT in nonmineralized chronic, type II disc protrusions is currently unknown, but it is likely significantly less than the reported values for acute disc herniation. In chronic cases, CT myelography would likely be necessary. Of importance is that a normal CT does not rule out IVDD.

MRI allows clear visualization of intervertebral disc disease. The normal nucleus pulposus of the intervertebral disc appears a hyperintense ellipsoid area on sagittal T2-weighted images. Intervertebral disc degeneration leads to a decrease in signal intensity, and the degenerated disc becomes isointense to hypointense relative to the surrounding annulus fibrosus. The degree of brightness of the T2 signal of the nucleus pulposus correlates with the proteoglycan concentration but not with water or collagen concentration.[36] MRI allows detection of disc degeneration at earlier stages of the degenerative process, before mineralization

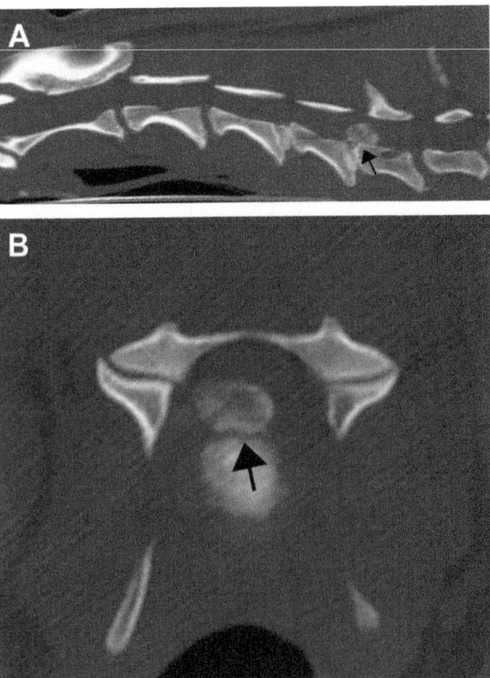

Fig. 14. Cervical intervertebral disc disease. (*A*) Reformatted sagittal CT image shows a large hyperdense area in the vertebral canal dorsal to the intervertebral disc space of C5-6 (*arrow*). Calcification is also seen at the C4-5 intervertebral disc space. (*B*) Transverse CT image reveals the large extradural hyperdense mass compressing and displacing the spinal cord dorsally (*arrow*).

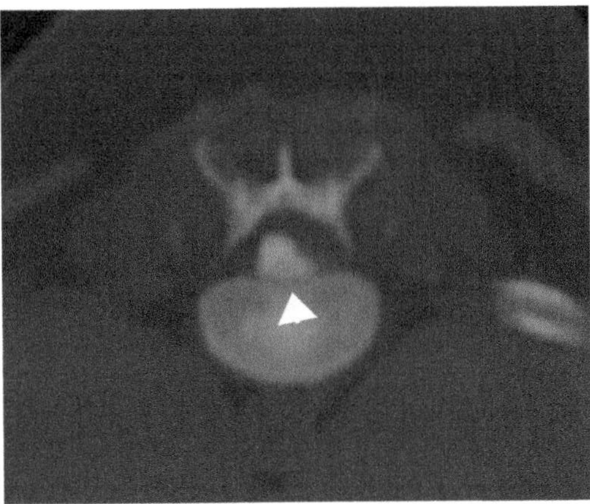

Fig. 15. Thoracolumbar intervertebral disc disease. Transverse CT image at the level of T12 shows a focal hyperdense mass compressing and displacing the spinal cord dorsolaterally (*arrowhead*).

occurs, which is when it can be visualized using CT and radiographs. It must be emphasized that disc degeneration per se does not lead to clinical signs, except in uncommon cases of discogenic spinal pain. MRI also allows visualization of the spinal cord, which facilitates comparison when multiple sites are affected (**Figs. 16** and **17**). The size of the spinal cord and vertebral canal varies according to different spinal locations, so the same degree of disc protrusion may lead to different degrees of spinal cord compression according to the spinal location. Sagittal and transverse images should be used concurrently to assess the severity and lateralization of spinal cord compression (see **Fig. 16**). It is common to observe lateralized disc extrusions causing nerve root compression, which may not be seen on mid-sagittal images. Parasagittal images allow visualization of lateralized disc herniations and nerve root compression. Hemorrhage associated with disc extrusion can cause a signal void on MR images.[37] GRE can confirm the presence of hemorrhage.

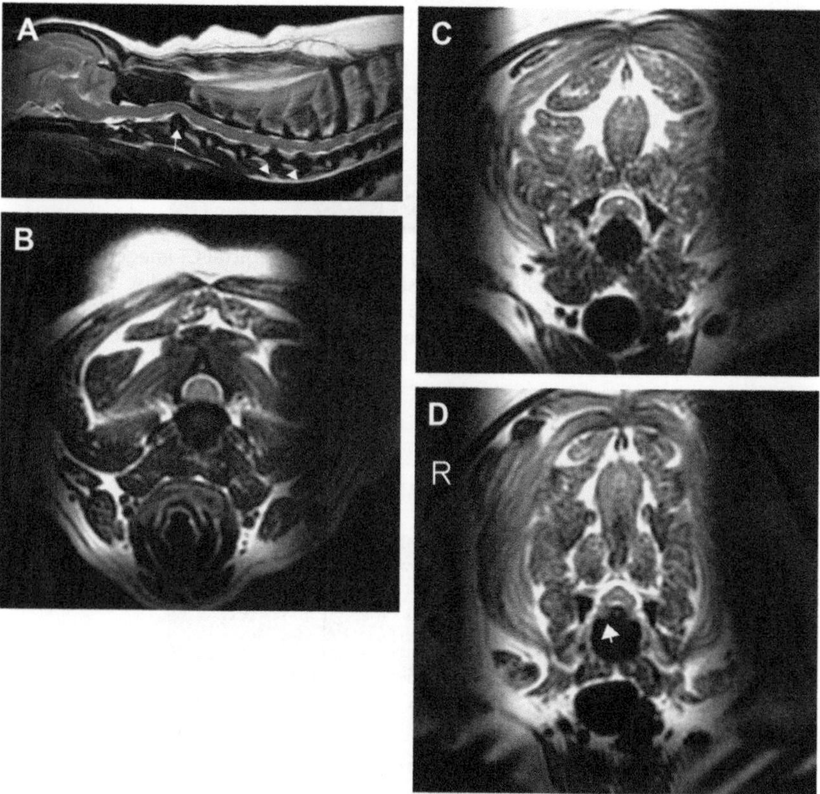

Fig. 16. Multiple sites of cervical intervertebral disc disease. (*A*) Sagittal T2-weighted MR image shows a large ventral extradural compressive lesion at the level of C2-3 (*arrow*), with less severe disc protrusions at C5-6 and C6-7. Intervertebral disc degeneration is seen at all these sites. (*B*) Transverse T2-weighted MR image at the level of C2-3 with a broad spinal cord compression. (*C*) Transverse T2-weighted MR image at the level of C5-6 shows a centrally located disc protrusion with dilation of the central canal of the spinal cord. (*D*) Transverse T2-weighted MR image at the level of C6-7 shows ventral compression of the spinal cord and nerve root on the right side (*arrow*). The nerve root compression was causing lameness of the right thoracic limb.

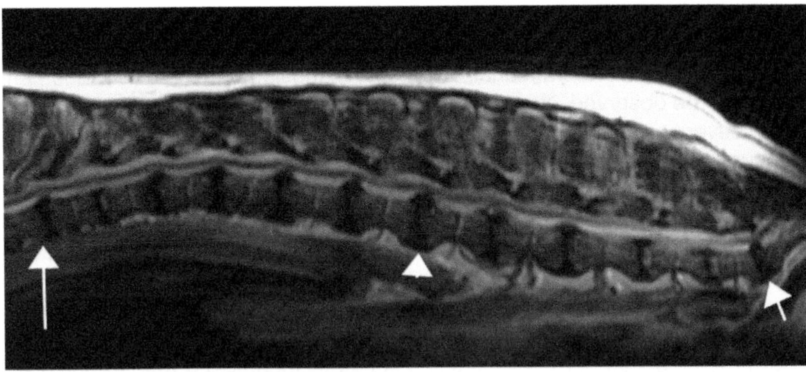

Fig. 17. Multiple sites of thoracolumbar intervertebral disc protrusion in a 9-year-old German Shepherd. Variable degrees of spinal cord compression are seen at almost every single disc space starting at T9-10 (*long arrow*). Compression is also seen at the lumbosacral space (*short arrow*). Intervertebral disc degeneration and spondylosis is also observed at multiple sites (*arrowhead*).

MRI also allows assessment of the spinal cord parenchyma and detection of spinal cord signal changes. In cases with multiple sites of spinal cord compression, identification of hyperintensity on T2-weighted images indicates the site with the worst compression. The spinal cord hyperintensity seen on T2-weighted images correlates with the severity of clinical signs.[38] The degree of severity of spinal cord compression, however, does not correlate with the severity of clinical signs.[38–40] Three studies in dogs have indicated that the presence and extension of spinal cord signal changes have prognostic implications.[39,41,42] A study suggested that areas of hyperintensity longer than 3 times the body of L2 were associated with poor prognosis, with only 20% of dogs with this signal change regaining ambulatory status.[41] The presence of hyperintensity was a more reliable prognostic indicator than absence of nociception.[41] Even in noncompressive intervertebral disc extrusions, the extent of spinal cord hyperintensity predicted the outcome.[42]

Chronic disc extrusions may be associated with inflammatory reaction surrounding the extruded disc, leading to a ring enhancement pattern surrounding the disc. The image may be mistaken as a granulomatous or neoplastic lesion. It is important to be aware of this imaging feature of IVDD to avoid misdiagnosing it as other conditions.[6] Intervertebral disc herniation can cause many different types of imaging patterns and should always be considered in the differential diagnosis for unusual MRI findings. In contrast to nonenhanced CT, normal MRI findings in all 3 imaging planes rule out the diagnosis of IVDD.

CERVICAL SPONDYLOMYELOPATHY

Cervical spondylomyelopathy (CSM) is characterized by static and dynamic spinal cord compressions. The disease is commonly caused by osseous compressions in young, giant breed dogs; and by disc protrusion in middle-aged to older large breed dogs. Both MRI and CT have been used in the diagnosis of CSM in dogs. When planning advanced imaging studies of the cases suspected of having CSM, it is important to plan the FOV to cover the entire cervical spine up to the third thoracic vertebrae. A recent study found compressions at T1-T2 and T2 associated with other cervical compressions in almost 10% of dogs.[43]

Noncontrast CT findings in dogs with CSM reveals the shape of the cervical vertebral canal, osteoarthritic changes in the articular processes, and mineralized disc herniation within the vertebral canal. Foraminal stenosis and lateralized disc herniations can also be observed. Noncontrast CT seems to be more valuable in evaluating dogs with severe osseous changes causing marked vertebral canal stenosis. CT after intravenous contrast injection allowed delineation of the venous sinuses dorsal to the vertebral bodies and appeared to be helpful in identifying asymmetric spinal cord compressions.[44] However, it is also less diagnostic than conventional myelography.[44] At present, noncontrast CT cannot be used as single diagnostic test for the diagnosis of CSM in dogs.

CT myelography allows cross-sectional images of the spinal cord area and provides superior visualization of areas of spinal cord compression as compared with myelography. Asymmetric spinal cord compression is readily identified (**Figs. 18** and **19**). CT myelography also allows detection of areas of spinal cord atrophy, seen as regular or irregular widening of the subarachnoid space with an altered spinal cord shape.[44] Spinal cord atrophy was seen in approximately 20% of dogs in a recent study.[43] It is unknown whether this finding has prognostic implications. CT myelography also allows easier visualization of synovial cysts that may be seen with osteoarthritic changes in giant breed dogs. CT myelography offers advantages over conventional myelography by establishing the exact location, degree, and lateralization of the compression.

MRI has been considered the best imaging technique for humans with cervical spondylotic myelopathy for more than 20 years.[45,46] CT myelography is still used in humans for equivocal cases where cervical radiculopathy secondary to foraminal stenosis is the main clinical problem.[47] The main advantage of MRI over CT myelography is the ability to directly visualize the spinal cord. This visualization allows detection of spinal cord signal changes that are helpful to determine the primary spinal cord lesion in cases with multiple compressions. Two recent studies indicate that multiple spinal compressions are seen in 63% of dogs with CSM.[43,48]

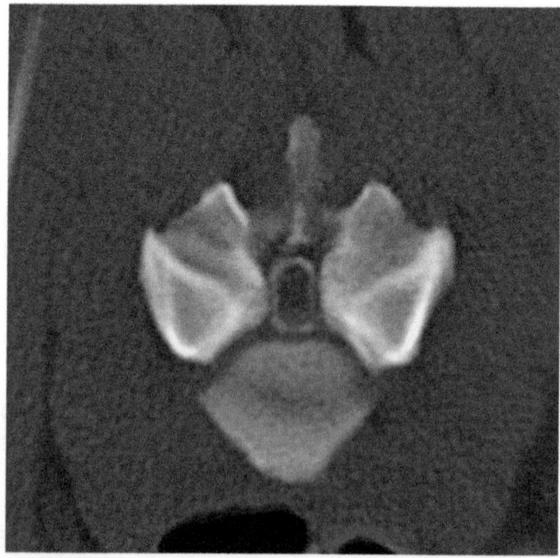

Fig. 18. Cervical spondylomyelopathy: osseous compression. Transverse CT-myelographic image at the level of C5-6 of a 1-year-old Great Dane showing bilateral spinal cord compression secondary to proliferative osteoarthritic lesions affecting both articular processes.

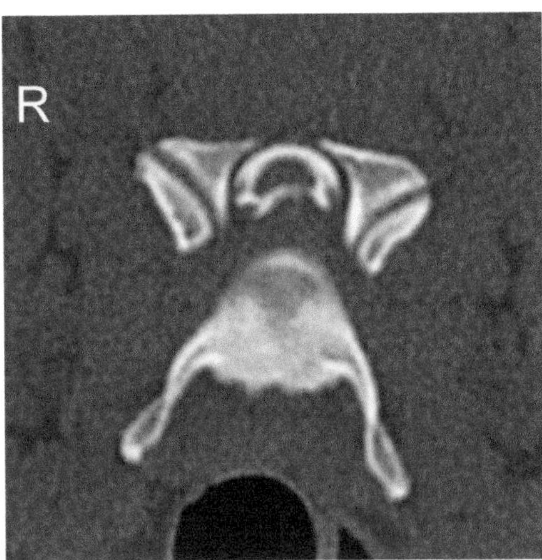

Fig. 19. Cervical spondylomyelopathy: disc-associated. Transverse CT-myelographic image at the level of the C5-6 of a 9-year-old Doberman with an asymmetric, disc-associated ventral spinal cord compression.

A recent study compared MRI and myelography for dogs with CSM. It was concluded that MRI allows identification of more sites of abnormalities than cervical myelography. Although myelography could identify the location of the lesion in most patients, MRI was more accurate in predicting the site, severity, and nature of the spinal cord compression. Spinal cord signal changes were seen in the majority of patients and provided assistance in precise lesion identification (**Fig. 20**).[49] The reader is referred to the discussion of CSM by Westworth and Sturges elsewhere in this issue for more information about imaging of CSM.

LUMBOSACRAL DISEASE

Lumbosacral (LS) disease, also known as degenerative lumbosacral stenosis (DLSS) or cauda equina syndrome, is a common disease of large breed dogs associated with nerve root compression at L6-L7 or L7-S1 vertebrae. Dogs with lumbosacral disease often present with lameness, paresis, and caudal lumbar or lumbosacral pain.

The CT findings in dogs with LS disease have been extensively studied by Jones and colleagues.[50,51] CT abnormalities observed are loss of epidural fat, increased soft-tissue opacity within the intervertebral foramen, bulging of the intervertebral disc, vertebral canal stenosis, and thickened articular processes. In noncontrast CT, the epidural fat surrounds the nerve roots and dural sac; however, with stenosis and compression, the epidural fat is lost and the compressive soft tissue becomes indistinguishable from adjacent nerves.[50] The use of intravenous contrast for CT evaluation of the LS area increased the sensitivity for detection of ventral and lateral compressions.[50] The use of subarachnoid contrast (myelography) associated with CT is not recommended for evaluation of the LS area because the contrast medium causes blooming and beam hardening artifacts, making interpretation difficult.[51]

The degree of lumbosacral compression detected using MRI has no correlation with the severity of clinical signs.[9] Fecal and urinary incontinence were observed in dogs

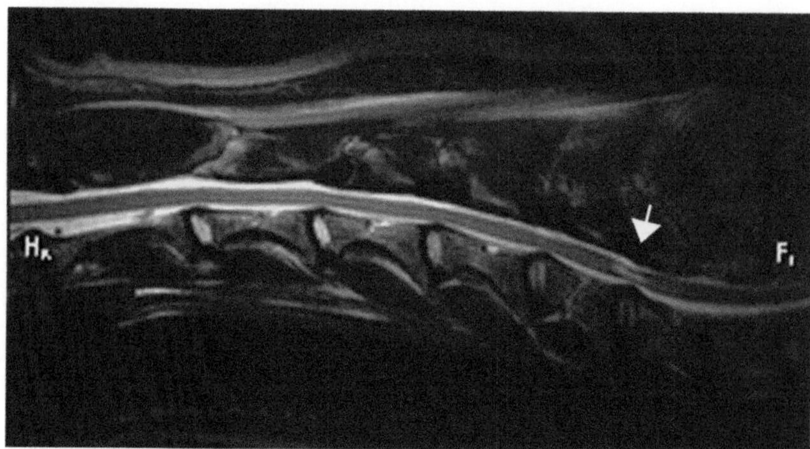

Fig. 20. Cervical spondylomyelopathy: disc-associated. Sagittal T2-weighted MR image showing ventral spinal cord compression at the level of C6-7 with spinal cord hyperintensity (*arrow*). The intervertebral discs C5-6, C6-7, and C7-T1 show the various stages of disc degeneration.

with minimal LS compression, whereas other dogs had severe compression of the LS region and showed pain only without neurologic deficits.[9] MRI usually reveals ventral compression caused by intervertebral disc degeneration and protrusion (**Fig. 21**). Intervertebral disc protrusion can be seen with loss of the normal bright hyperintense signal of the intervertebral disc.[9] Dorsal compression caused by joint capsule thickening, osteophyte formation, and hypertrophy of the ligamentum flavum can also be observed. Foraminal stenosis is an important component of the complex of the DLSS, and the parasagittal and transverse images should be carefully examined. Transverse images allow assessment of the dorsoventral diameter of the foramina while the parasagittal images allow evaluation of the craniocaudal diameter of the foramina. Dynamic studies of the LS spine can be performed[6]; however, criteria for testing and normal reference ranges have not been established and as such, interpretation of the results can be problematic.

CT and MRI findings for LS disease showed a high agreement between both modalities; however, the correlation between CT or MRI findings with surgical findings is low.[8,52] MRI and CT findings also had no correlation with outcome.[8] It is also important to bear in mind that clinically normal dogs can have imaging characteristics of LS diseases without clinical signs.[7]

SPINAL TRAUMA

No published data exist regarding the use of MRI in the evaluation of spinal trauma in small animals. The authors' experience indicates that MRI is a valuable tool in the evaluation of dogs with spinal trauma (**Fig. 22**). A study compared the diagnostic sensitivity of survey radiographs and CT in dogs with confirmed spinal fractures and luxations. Radiographs missed approximately 25% of the lesions detected on CT.[53] CT is the gold standard test for evaluation of spinal trauma in humans,[54] and should be used whenever possible in the evaluation of dogs and cats with spinal trauma.

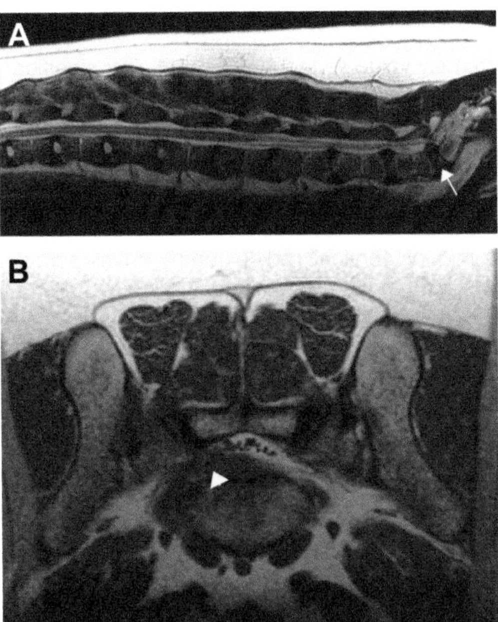

Fig. 21. Degenerative lumbosacral stenosis. (*A*) Sagittal T2-weighted MR image showing severe ventral compression at the level of L7-S1 (*arrow*). Milder compressions are also seen at L5-6 and L6-7, along with degeneration of the caudal lumbar intervertebral discs. (*B*) Transverse T2-weighted MR image at the level of the lumbosacral junction showing foraminal stenosis and nerve root compression secondary to asymmetric disc protrusion (*arrowhead*).

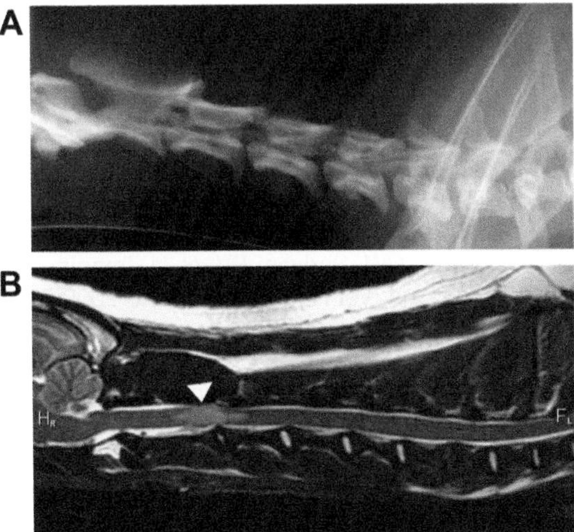

Fig. 22. Spinal trauma. (*A*) Lateral radiograph of the cervical spine of a dog hit by a car that was presented with nonambulatory tetraparesis. No abnormalities were detected on survey radiographs. (*B*) Sagittal T2-weighted MR image of the same dog showing an extensive area of hyperintensity within the spinal cord parenchyma between C2 and C3 (*arrow*) indicating spinal cord injury.

SUMMARY

CT and MRI are extremely valuable techniques that offer significant advantages over conventional radiographs and myelography. These techniques have allowed us to identify and characterize many spinal disorders. Our knowledge and ability to detect spinal disorders will continue to advance as these technologies evolve.

REFERENCES

1. Castillo M. Imaging of cervical radiculopathy, myelopathy, and postoperative changes. In: Castillo M, editor. Spinal imaging state of the art. 1st edition. Philadelphia: Hanley & Belfus, Inc; 2001. p. 207–19.
2. da Costa RC, Parent JM, Partlow G, et al. Morphologic and morphometric magnetic resonance imaging features of Doberman pinscher dogs with and without clinical signs of cervical spondylomyelopathy. Am J Vet Res 2006;67:1601–12.
3. Gomez MA, Jones JC, Broadstone RV, et al. Evaluation of the internal vertebral venous plexus, vertebral canal, dural sac, and vertebral body via nonselective computed tomographic venography in the cervical vertebral column in healthy dogs. Am J Vet Res 2005;66:2039–45.
4. Axlund TW, Hudson JA. Computed tomography of the normal lumbosacral intervertebral disc in 22 dogs. Vet Radiol Ultrasound 2003;44:630–4.
5. Jones JC, Wright JC, Bartels JE. Computed tomographic morphometry of the lumbosacral spine of dogs. Am J Vet Res 1995;56:1125–32.
6. Bagley RS, Gavin P, Holmes SP. Diagnosis of spinal disease. In: Gavin PR, Bagley RS, editors. Practical small animal MRI. Ames (IA): Wiley; 2009. p. 123–232.
7. Jones JC, Inzana KD. Subclinical CT abnormalities in the lumbosacral spine of older large-breed dogs. Vet Radiol Ultrasound 2000;41:19–26.
8. Jones JC, Banfield CM, Ward DL. Association between postoperative outcome and results of magnetic resonance imaging and computed tomography in working dogs with degenerative lumbosacral stenosis. J Am Vet Med Assoc 2000;216:1769–74.
9. Mayhew PD, Kapatkin AS, Wortman JA, et al. Association of cauda equina compression on magnetic resonance images and clinical signs in dogs with degenerative lumbosacral stenosis. J Am Anim Hosp Assoc 2002;38:555–62.
10. McCarthy RJ, Lewis DD, Hosgood G. Atlantoaxial subluxation in dogs. Compend Contin Educ Pract Vet 1995;17:215–26.
11. Cerda-Gonzalez S, Dewey CW, Scrivani PV, et al. Imaging features of atlanto-occipital overlapping in dogs. Vet Radiol Ultrasound 2009;50:264–8.
12. Bailey CS, Morgan JP. Congenital spinal malformations. Vet Clin North Am Small Anim Pract 1992;22:985–1015.
13. Jeffery ND, Smith PM, Talbot CE. Imaging findings and surgical treatment of hemivertebrae in three dogs. J Am Vet Med Assoc 2007;230:532–6.
14. Jurina K, Grevel V. Spinal arachnoid pseudocysts in 10 rottweilers. J Small Anim Pract 2004;45:9–15.
15. Rylander H, Lipsitz D, Berry WL, et al. Retrospective analysis of spinal arachnoid cysts in 14 dogs. J Vet Intern Med 2002;16:690–6.
16. Gnirs K, Ruel Y, Blot S, et al. Spinal subarachnoid cysts in 13 dogs. Vet Radiol Ultrasound 2003;44:402–8.
17. Sugiyama T, Simpson DJ. Acquired arachnoid cyst in a cat. Aust Vet J 2009;87:296–300.

18. Cherubini GB, Cappello R, Lu D, et al. MRI findings in a dog with discospondylitis caused by *Bordetella* species. J Small Anim Pract 2004;45:417–20.
19. Gonzalo-Orden JM, Altonaga JR, Orden MA, et al. Magnetic resonance, computed tomographic and radiologic findings in a dog with discospondylitis. Vet Radiol Ultrasound 2000;41:142–4.
20. De Stefani A, Garosi LS, McConnell FJ, et al. Magnetic resonance imaging features of spinal epidural empyema in five dogs. Vet Radiol Ultrasound 2008;49:135–40.
21. Nykamp SG, Steffey MA, Scrivani PV, et al. Computed tomographic appearance of epidural empyema in a dog. Can Vet J 2003;44:729–31.
22. Dernell WS, Van Vechten BJ, Straw RC, et al. Outcome following treatment of vertebral tumors in 20 dogs (1986-1995). J Am Anim Hosp Assoc 2000;36:245–51.
23. Drost WT, Love NE, Berry CR. Comparison of radiography, myelography and computed tomography in the evaluation of canine vertebral and spinal cord tumors in sixteen dogs. Vet Radiol Ultrasound 1996;37:28–33.
24. Kippenes H, Gavin PR, Bagley RS, et al. Magnetic resonance imaging features of tumors of the spine and spinal cord in dogs. Vet Radiol Ultrasound 1999;40:627–33.
25. McDonnell JJ, Tidwell AS, Faissler D, et al. Magnetic resonance imaging features of cervical spinal cord meningiomas. Vet Radiol Ultrasound 2005;46:368–74.
26. Petersen SA, Sturges BK, Dickinson PJ, et al. Canine intraspinal meningiomas: imaging features, histopathologic classification, and long-term outcome in 34 dogs. J Vet Intern Med 2008;22:946–53.
27. Brehm DM, Vite CH, Steinberg HS, et al. A retrospective evaluation of 51 cases of peripheral nerve sheath tumors in the dog. J Am Anim Hosp Assoc 1995;31: 349–59.
28. Rudich SR, Feeney DA, Anderson KL, et al. Computed tomography of masses of the brachial plexus and contributing nerve roots in dogs. Vet Radiol Ultrasound 2004;45:46–50.
29. Kraft S, Ehrhart EJ, Gall D, et al. Magnetic resonance imaging characteristics of peripheral nerve sheath tumors of the canine brachial plexus in 18 dogs. Vet Radiol Ultrasound 2007;48:1–7.
30. da Costa RC, Parent JM, Dobson H, et al. Ultrasound guided fine needle aspiration biopsy in the diagnosis of peripheral nerve sheath tumors in dogs. Can Vet J 2008;49:77–81.
31. Olby NJ, Munana KR, Sharp NJ, et al. The computed tomographic appearance of acute thoracolumbar intervertebral disc herniations in dogs. Vet Radiol Ultrasound 2000;41:396–402.
32. King JB, Jones JC, Rossmeisl JH Jr, et al. Effect of multi-planar CT image reformatting on surgeon diagnostic performance for localizing thoracolumbar disc extrusions in dogs. J Vet Sci 2009;10:225–32.
33. Israel SK, Levine JM, Kerwin SC, et al. The relative sensitivity of computed tomography and myelography for identification of thoracolumbar intervertebral disk herniations in dogs. Vet Radiol Ultrasound 2009;50:247–52.
34. Olby NJ, Munana K, Sharp NJ, et al. A comparison of computed tomography and myelography in the diagnosis of acute intervertebral disc disease in dogs. Proceedings of ACVIM Conference 1999;17:705.
35. Hecht S, Thomas WB, Marioni-Henry K, et al. Myelography vs. computed tomography in the evaluation of acute thoracolumbar intervertebral disk extrusion in chondrodystrophic dogs. Vet Radiol Ultrasound 2009;50:353–9.
36. Pearce RH, Thompson JP, Bebault GM, et al. Magnetic resonance imaging reflects the chemical changes of aging degeneration in the human intervertebral disk. J Rheumatol Suppl 1991;27:42–3.

37. Tidwell AS, Specht A, Blaeser L, et al. Magnetic resonance imaging features of extradural hematomas associated with intervertebral disc herniation in a dog. Vet Radiol Ultrasound 2002;43:319–24.
38. Besalti O, Pekcan Z, Sirin YS, et al. Magnetic resonance imaging findings in dogs with thoracolumbar intervertebral disk disease: 69 cases (1997–2005). J Am Vet Med Assoc 2006;228:902–8.
39. Levine JM, Fosgate GT, Chen AV, et al. Magnetic resonance imaging in dogs with neurologic impairment due to acute thoracic and lumbar intervertebral disk herniation. J Vet Intern Med 2009;23:1220–6.
40. Penning V, Platt SR, Dennis R, et al. Association of spinal cord compression seen on magnetic resonance imaging with clinical outcome in 67 dogs with thoracolumbar intervertebral disc extrusion. J Small Anim Pract 2006;47:644–50.
41. Ito D, Matsunaga S, Jeffery ND, et al. Prognostic value of magnetic resonance imaging in dogs with paraplegia caused by thoracolumbar intervertebral disk extrusion: 77 cases (2000–2003). J Am Vet Med Assoc 2005;227:1454–60.
42. De Risio L, Adams V, Dennis R, et al. Association of clinical and magnetic resonance imaging findings with outcome in dogs with presumptive acute noncompressive nucleus pulposus extrusion: 42 cases (2000–2007). J Am Vet Med Assoc 2009;234:495–504.
43. da Costa RC, Echandi RL, Beauchamp D. Computed tomographic findings in large and giant breed dogs with cervical spondylomyelopathy: 58 cases. J Vet Intern Med 2009;23:709.
44. Sharp NJ, Cofone M, Robertson ID, et al. Computed tomography in the evaluation of caudal cervical spondylomyelopathy of the Doberman pinscher. Vet Radiol Ultrasound 1995;36:100–8.
45. Modic MT, Ross JS, Masaryk TJ. Imaging of degenerative disease of the cervical spine. Clin Orthop Relat Res 1989;239:109–20.
46. Larsson EM, Holtas S, Cronqvist S, et al. Comparison of myelography, CT myelography and magnetic resonance imaging in cervical spondylosis and disk herniation. Pre- and postoperative findings. Acta Radiol 1989;30:233–9.
47. Song KJ, Choi BW, Kim GH, et al. Clinical usefulness of CT-myelogram comparing with the MRI in degenerative cervical spinal disorders: is CTM still useful for primary diagnostic tool? J Spinal Disord Tech 2009;22:353–7.
48. da Costa RC, Parent JM. Magnetic resonance imaging findings in 60 dogs with cervical spondylomyelopathy. J Vet Intern Med 2009;23:740.
49. da Costa RC, Parent JP, Dobson H, et al. Comparison of magnetic resonance imaging and myelography in 18 Doberman pinscher dogs with cervical spondylomyelopathy. Vet Radiol Ultrasound 2006;47:523–31.
50. Jones JC, Shires PK, Inzana KD, et al. Evaluation of canine lumbosacral stenosis using intravenous contrast-enhanced computed tomography. Vet Radiol Ultrasound 1999;40:108–14.
51. Jones JC, Sorjonen DC, Simpson ST, et al. Comparison between computed tomographic and surgical findings in nine large-breed dogs with lumbosacral stenosis. Vet Radiol Ultrasound 1996;37:247–56.
52. Suwankong N, Voorhout G, Hazewinkel HA, et al. Agreement between computed tomography, magnetic resonance imaging, and surgical findings in dogs with degenerative lumbosacral stenosis. J Am Vet Med Assoc 2006;229:1924–9.
53. Kinns J, Mai W, Seiler G, et al. Radiographic sensitivity and negative predictive value for acute canine spinal trauma. Vet Radiol Ultrasound 2006;47:563–70.
54. Holmes JF, Akkinepalli R. Computed tomography versus plain radiography to screen for cervical spine injury: a meta-analysis. J Trauma 2005;58:902–5.

The Pathogenesis and Treatment of Acute Spinal Cord Injuries in Dogs

Natasha Olby, VetMB, PhD

KEYWORDS

• Spinal cord trauma • Infarct • Methylprednisolone
• Polyethylene glycol • Primary damage • Secondary damage

Acute spinal cord injuries (SCIs) are an extremely common problem in veterinary medicine and can lead to permanent, severe neurologic deficits affecting motor, sensory, and autonomic function. The most common causes of acute SCI in dogs are acute intervertebral disk herniations, fibrocartilaginous embolism (FCE), and trauma. Cats suffer from similar diseases but at different frequencies, with trauma being more common than intervertebral disk herniations and thromboembolic events much more common than FCE. These specific topics are covered in other articles in this issue. There is a wealth of information on numerous experimental therapies targeting different pathophysiologic events, which are reviewed elsewhere,[1–3] and the number of human clinical trials completed or being performed is escalating.[4] By contrast, few placebo-controlled clinical trials have been performed in dogs (**Table 1**). This article discusses the pathophysiology of acute SCI in terms of the primary and secondary pathologic events that occur and describes the therapies that are currently clinically applicable.

The events that follow acute SCI are typically divided into primary and secondary damage, with the secondary damage developing over acute (0–48 hours), subacute (48 hours–2 weeks), and chronic phases.[1] Vascular injuries bypass the primary damage caused by physical trauma but induce the same secondary injury pathways.

PRIMARY DAMAGE

The initial acute traumatic injury inflicts mechanical damage to the spinal cord that causes contusion, shearing, acceleration or deceleration, and laceration.[1] The result is physical disruption of cell membranes causing hemorrhage and consequent ischemia and widespread neuronal and glial injury (**Fig. 1**). Herniated disk material,

Department of Clinical Sciences, College of Veterinary Medicine, North Carolina State University, 4700 Hillsborough Street, Raleigh, NC 27606, USA
E-mail address: Natasha_olby@ncsu.edu

Vet Clin Small Anim 40 (2010) 791–807
doi:10.1016/j.cvsm.2010.05.007 vetsmall.theclinics.com
0195-5616/10/$ – see front matter

Table 1
Canine clinical trials

Trial	Type of Trial	Findings
OFS Unit[66]	Blinded, placebo controlled in patients with grade 5[a] IVDD	Safe, improvement in sensory function
N-acetylcysteine[39]	Blinded, placebo controlled in nonambulatory patients with IVDD	No effect
4-AP[75]	Phase 1	Small therapeutic range; improved sensory, motor, and bladder functions
4-AP	Blinded, placebo controlled, underway in patients with chronic grade 5[a] SCI	Pending
t-Butyl derivative of 4-AP[10]	Phase 1	Safe; improved sensory, motor, and bladder functions
t-Butyl derivative of 4-AP	Blinded, placebo controlled, underway in patients with chronic grade 5[a] SCI	Ongoing
OEC Transplants[9]	Phase 1	Safe
OEC Transplants	Blinded, placebo controlled, underway	Ongoing
MPSS, PEG	Blinded, placebo controlled in patients with grade 5[a] IVDD	Ongoing

Abbreviations: 4-AP, 4-aminopyridine; IVDD, intervertebral disk disease; MPSS, methylprednisolone sodium succinate; OEC, olfactory ensheathing cells; OFS, oscillating field stimulator; PEG, polyethylene glycol.

[a] Paraplegic with no nociception.

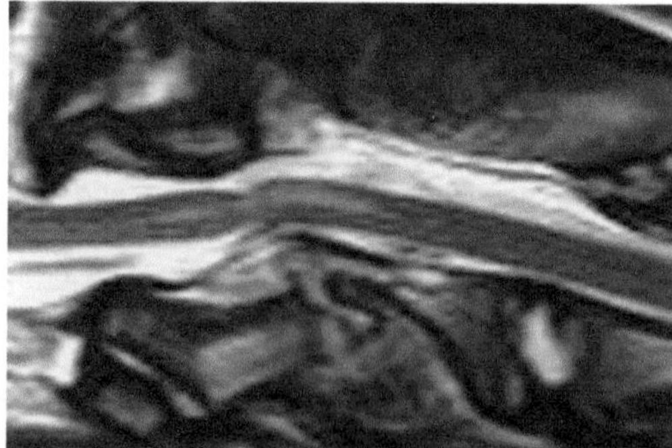

Fig. 1. T2-weighted sagittal magnetic resonance image of the cervical spine of a 1-year-old dog that fell from a balcony. The second cervical vertebra is fractured, causing a contusive injury to the overlying spinal cord. The region of hyperintensity represents accumulation of fluid (edema).

displaced vertebrae, or vertebral fragments and epidural hematomas cause ongoing compression (**Fig. 2**). Compression affects spinal cord perfusion by limiting arterial supply and occluding venous drainage and causes direct damage to myelin and axons.[5,6] In case of a displaced spinal fracture, the primary injury can cause complete physical transection of the spinal cord, with devastating results (**Fig. 3**). However, after acute disk herniations, the meninges usually remain intact, and even in clinically complete injuries, the subpial axons are spared, although they are often demyelinated and dysfunctional.[7,8] These physiologically dysfunctional but anatomically intact axons are the focus of much attention for the development of new therapies in patients with chronic paresis and are being targeted in dogs with SCI.[9,10]

Therapy for Primary Injury

Treatment of the primary injury focuses on prevention of further contusive injury by spinal stabilization, if indicated, and on decompression of the compressed spinal cord. The timing of decompression has been contentious, but a critical meta-analysis of preclinical studies and human clinical trials concluded that prompt decompression improves outcomes.[11] Clearly, this advice has to be tempered by evaluation of the systemic condition of the patient, particularly one that has just suffered a major trauma such as being hit by a car.

SECONDARY DAMAGE: THE ACUTE PHASE

Primary damage initiates a series of secondary events that cause an expanding zone of tissue destruction. These events include hemorrhage and destruction of the microvascular bed, rapid changes in intracellular ion concentration, excitotoxicity, free radical production, and inflammation. The end point of these destructive cascades is often apoptosis, which can continue for a long time after the injury.[1]

Vascular Changes

There is a close relationship between perfusion of the injured spinal cord and outcome, highlighting the central importance of maintaining blood flow to the region.[12] Primary damage to blood vessels causes hemorrhage and ischemia, but petechial hemorrhages continue to form during the first 24 hours after injury, frequently resulting in large zones of hemorrhage (**Fig. 4**).[12,13] Heme products are toxic to neurons, and the mass effect of hemorrhage further increases interstitial pressure and decreases perfusion of the region. Recent work has underlined the importance of upregulation of a gene called *Trpm4* in the genesis of secondary hemorrhage.[14] This gene encodes one of

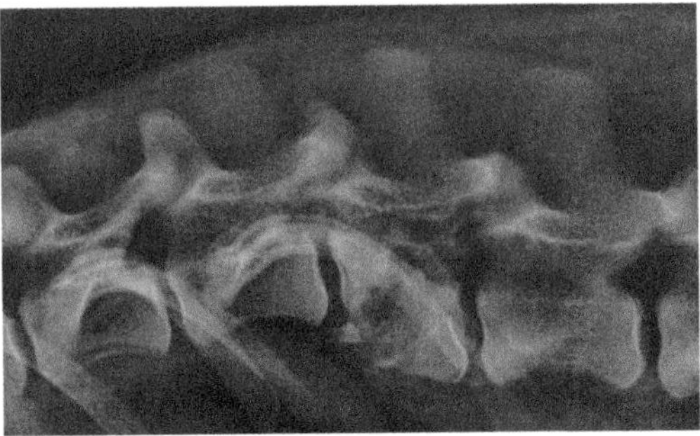

Fig. 2. Lateral radiograph of the thoracolumbar spine of a dog that was hit by a car. The first lumbar vertebra is fractured and displaced, causing distortion of the vertebral canal.

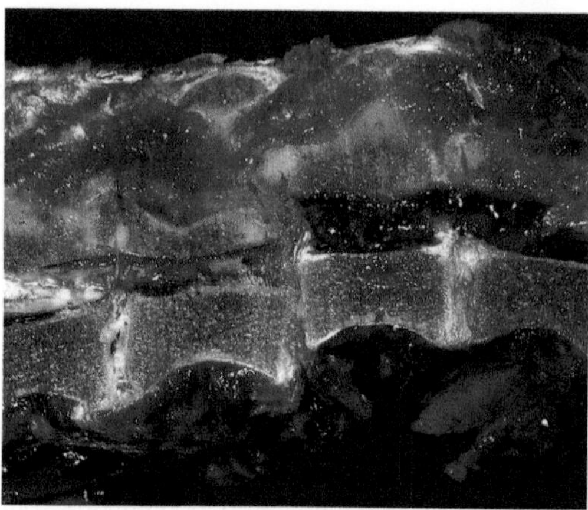

Fig. 3. Spine of a dog that was hit by a car. This sagittal section shows displacement of the vertebrae causing complete transection of the spinal cord.

a large family of transient receptor potential channels that is permeable to monovalent ions. *Trpm4* is normally expressed at low levels in the central nervous system (CNS), but expression is upregulated dramatically in capillary endothelial cells after SCI, causing ion entry, oncotic swelling, and cell death. Intravenous administration of antisense *Trpm4* resulted in a dramatic reduction of postinjury hemorrhage and lesion volume. This finding is the first to demonstrate a molecular mechanism for secondary vascular damage and can prove to be important in developing novel therapies. Many additional mechanisms play a role in the progressive decrease in perfusion of the injured spinal cord including free radical–induced damage to endothelial cell membranes, vasospasm by the release of neurotransmitters and inflammatory mediators, and increased interstitial pressure caused by cytotoxic and vasogenic edema.[12]

Severe SCI produces systemic effects on blood pressure causing hypertension followed after about 10 minutes by hypotension,[15] although this has not been recorded as a response to severe SCI caused by disk herniations in dogs (Olby N, VetMB, PhD, unpublished data, 2000). Perfusion of the normal spinal cord is maintained within narrow limits, but this autoregulatory ability is lost after injury and with compression.[16]

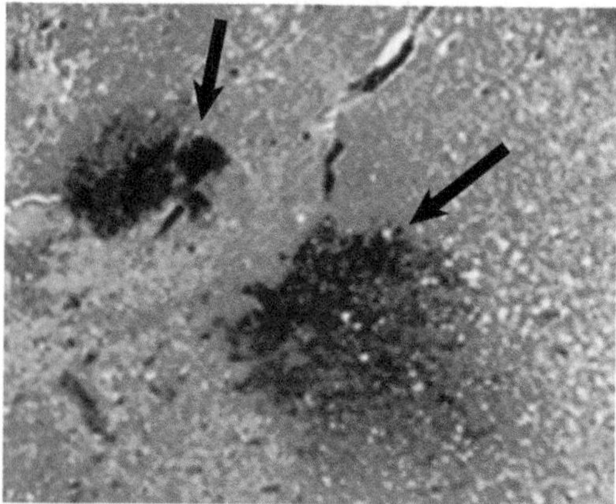

Fig. 4. Transverse section of the spinal cord of a dog that suffered a disk herniation. There is hemorrhage within the spinal cord parenchyma (*arrows*).

Loss of autoregulation coupled with systemic hypotension can worsen perfusion and therefore the outcome.

Therapy for spinal cord ischemia

It is extremely important to measure the systemic blood pressure of patients with SCI and to treat hypotension with fluids and pressors as appropriate. It is just as important to measure the partial pressure of oxygen in arterial blood and supplement with oxygen if the patient is hypoxemic. Prompt decompression of compressive lesions also aids in restoring perfusion. Although decompression may be associated with reperfusion injury, there is experimental evidence that decompression of the severely compressed spinal cord has an effect on the outcome.[17] After injury, focal swelling of the spinal cord can result in a compartment syndrome caused by the enclosing meninges, and it has been proposed that durotomy helps to relieve the resulting pressure, restoring perfusion. The effect of durotomy on the outcome of disk-induced canine SCI has been investigated prospectively[18] and more recently in a retrospective study.[19] Both studies failed to find a benefit of durotomy performed more than 2 hours after injury. Given the importance of maintaining spinal cord perfusion and the known effectiveness of cerebrospinal fluid (CSF) drainage in controlling intracranial pressure in patients with traumatic brain injury, it is logical that CSF drainage might improve outcome of SCI by controlling intra–spinal cord pressure. Recently, a pilot study in humans with SCI demonstrated the safety of lumbar CSF drainage,[20] and larger clinical trials are planned. This approach merits investigation in dogs.

Ionic Disturbances and Excitotoxicity

Damage to cell membranes alters permeability and results in an influx of chloride and cations.[1–3] In addition, extracellular concentrations of glutamate increase because of release from damaged neurons and a failure in normal, energy-dependent astrocytic reuptake. These excitatory amino acids interact with *N*-methyl-D-aspartate (NMDA), kainic, and α-amino-3-hydroxy-5-methyl-4-isoxazolepropionic acid receptors found on neurons and oligodendrocytes to produce rapid influx of sodium and a slower influx of calcium.[21] Failure of energy-dependent sodium-potassium ATPase exacerbates this effect. Increases in the levels of intracellular sodium result in cytotoxic edema, increasing swelling in the region, and thus worsening perfusion. Elevated levels of intracellular calcium activate enzymes such as calpain and caspase, causing necrosis and apoptosis, and phospholipase A_2, triggering eicosanoid production. Calcium also binds with phosphates, further depleting available energy. The resulting cell death is known as excitotoxicity.[21] Excitotoxicity plays an important role in neuronal and oligodendroglial cell death and continues to present a potential pharmacologic target for therapy for SCI. Elevated levels of glutamate in the CSF have been documented in dogs with naturally occurring SCI, and glutamate concentration has been correlated to injury severity,[22] suggesting that excitotoxicity is relevant in canine SCI.

Therapy for ion fluxes and excitotoxicity

Numerous experimental studies of calcium channel antagonists, such as nimodipine and nifedipine, suggested benefit, but a human clinical trial of nimodipine failed to demonstrate improved outcome.[23] Sodium channel antagonists have also shown benefit experimentally,[24] and the most effective of these drugs, riluzole, is being tested in a human phase 1 clinical trial. In spite of positive results with numerous different drugs that antagonize NMDA and non-NMDA receptors,[3,21] there are no clinically proven excitotoxicity-specific therapies available, in part because of the unacceptable side effects.[4] Gacyclidine (GK11) is an NMDA antagonist with tolerable side effects, but it failed to show a benefit at the 1-year follow-up in a human clinical trial.[25]

Free Radical–Induced Damage

Since the demonstration of the importance of oxygen-derived free radical–induced damage in mediating secondary injury,[26] free radical–induced damage has received intense scrutiny and has been reviewed in detail.[27] Reactive oxygen species (ROS) are produced by ischemic conditions, elevated intracellular calcium concentrations, copper and iron within heme, and the inflammatory reaction. ROS damage membranes by lipid peroxidation, causing glial, neuronal, and endothelial damage; nitrate and oxidize proteins and nucleic acids; and cause inhibition of mitochondrial respiration by interactions with specific mitochondrial enzymes.[28] ROS production peaks within the first 12 hours of injury, and levels remain elevated for at least a week; thus therapies that target ROS production must be administered early in the injury cascade to have significant effect. Intravenous administration of methylprednisolone sodium succinate (MPSS), 30 mg/kg, followed by continuous rate infusion (CRI), 5.4 mg/kg/h, for 24 hours is believed to exert neuroprotective effects through the inhibition of lipid peroxidation.[29] MPSS was evaluated in the landmark placebo-controlled, blinded National Acute Spinal Cord Injury (NASCIS) trials reported in the 1980s and 1990s.[30–33] The first trial failed to demonstrate a beneficial effect with MPSS.[33] Escalating the dose of MPSS in the second trial also failed to show benefit. However, secondary analysis of a subset of the data demonstrated a small benefit when treatment was initiated within 8 hours of injury, and the same benefit was demonstrated in the final NASCIS trial.[30–32] However, there is much controversy associated with the conclusions of these trials[34–36]; the benefits reported are minimal, analysis of the data is open to question, and the side effects associated with these high doses of MPSS in humans are significant. A derivate of MPSS, tirilazad mesylate, a 21-aminosteroid designed to have the free radical scavenging effects without the glucocorticoid effects, failed to show benefit over MPSS in human clinical trials.[30,31]

Recent interest has focused on the peroxynitrite radical, a reactive nitrogen species (RNS) that is formed from interaction between the nitrite and superoxide radicals. This RNS is believed to play a central role in oxidative damage after SCI, and its effects can be mitigated with specific inhibition of peroxynitrite using uric acid or tempol.[28,37] Clinical trials of these inhibitors are not yet underway.

Therapy for free radical–induced injury

Although many veterinarians treat acute SCI with MPSS using the NASCIS protocol, data on MPSS use in dogs with SCI are limited. Two trials in experimental models of canine SCI failed to demonstrate an effect with MPSS,[17,38] although both studies were likely underpowered. A blinded, placebo-controlled study of MPSS in dogs with acute disk herniations is currently underway (see **Table 1**) and may help to resolve whether MPSS is beneficial in the treatment of acute canine SCI. A blinded, controlled clinical trial using the antioxidant *N*-acetylcysteine in dogs with acute disk herniations has been completed and has failed to show any benefit,[39] and an experimental study evaluating dimethyl sulfoxide and ϵ-aminocaproic acid also failed to show benefit in dogs.[40]

Inflammatory Reaction

The SCI-induced inflammatory reaction is extremely complex and has both beneficial and deleterious effects.[41] Inflammatory mediators such as tumor necrosis factor α and interleukin-1β are produced by microglial cells within minutes of injury. These mediators increase the permeability of the blood–spinal cord barrier, result in the production of toxic chemicals such as nitric oxide, and recruit inflammatory cells. The matrix metalloproteinases (MMPs) are endogenous zinc endopeptidases that are important in the degradation of extracellular matrix and wound healing. Production of MMP-9 after SCI has been shown to damage the blood–spinal cord barrier, increase neutrophil infiltration, and limit recovery after SCI. Antagonism of MMP-9 improves outcome.[42] MMP-9 activity has been measured in the CSF of normal dogs and dogs with naturally occurring SCI,[43] and increased activity was detected in spinal cord injured dogs with signs lasting for more than 24 hours. This mechanism therefore seems to be relevant to canine SCI patients.

Neutrophils invade the SCI lesion within hours and tend to disperse within a week,[41] although there are species differences. Macrophage invasion is slower, peaking at around 4 days and lasting for weeks to months. The secondary peak in cellular infiltration coincides with a new wave of axonal loss and demyelination.[44] Both populations of invading cells remove cellular debris, potentially enhancing the environment for axonal regeneration and sprouting, but they also cause secondary, bystander damage. It has been proposed that infiltration of a subset of circulating monocytes (macrophages) is vital to recovery,[45,46] and a human clinical trial evaluating the injection of autologous macrophages (ProCord) is underway. B- and T-lymphocyte infiltration also occurs, and B cells have been shown to produce damaging autoantibodies.[47] More recently, it has been recognized that SCI causes a systemic depression of lymphocyte function, leading to the argument that SCI should be considered a multiorgan system problem.[48]

Therapy for inflammation

There are no proven therapies in clinical use that specifically target the inflammatory response following SCI, despite the numerous experimental studies showing that antagonism of inflammatory mediators or inhibition of infiltration of neutrophils or macrophages[41] can improve outcome of SCI. There has been a lot of interest in the immunophilin family of drugs (that includes cyclosporin A and FK 506 [tacrolimus]), and several experimental studies suggest that these drugs improve outcome of SCI. There is 1 report of a human SCI clinical trial using tacrolimus, but the results have not been published.[4] The use of corticosteroids, and more specifically, dexamethasone, to decrease edema is widespread in veterinary medicine, but there are little data to support this use. There are experimental studies that failed to show a benefit from dexamethasone in rodents and dogs.[49,50] Recent retrospective analyses of dogs with surgically treated intervertebral disk herniations also failed to show benefit from dexamethasone administration[51,52] and reported a high incidence of adverse effects associated with this drug.[51]

Apoptosis

After acute SCI, neurons, glial, and endothelial cells die by necrosis or apoptosis. While there are little data available for dogs, in humans, neurons typically die by necrosis and are difficult to rescue once this process has been initiated.[53] Oligodendrocyte death is a prominent feature of the early phase of acute SCI and continues for extended periods after injury, contributing to demyelination and loss of function.[54,55] Unlike that of neurons, oligodendrocyte death frequently occurs through apoptosis as the result of activation of the Fas receptor by microglial cells expressing the Fas ligand and by p75 neurotrophin receptor signaling. Activation of the Fas receptor triggers the caspase cascade, resulting in apoptosis.[56] This process can be blocked by intravenous administration of soluble Fas receptor, improving outcome and underlining the importance of this particular biochemical cascade in the evolution of secondary tissue damage.[57] The presence of demyelinated axons at the lesion epicenter in dogs with naturally occurring

SCI[7] suggests that anti-apoptotic therapies may be effective in dogs, although there are no clinically proven therapies available at present.

Multimodal Therapies for the Acute Phase of SCI

It is clear that many different pathologic processes play a collaborative role in the development of tissue damage in the acute phase after SCI. It is therefore logical to target multiple different aspects of these pathways to optimize outcome. An exhaustive review of the different experimental therapies described is beyond the remit of this article but is provided elsewhere.[2] In the 1990s, there was a lot of interest in opioid antagonists, thyrotropin-releasing hormone (TRH) analogues, and gangliosides.[3] Naloxone, TRH, and ganglioside GM1 have been evaluated in human clinical trials and have failed to produce more improvement than MPSS, and these drugs have not been pursued further. Recent interest has focused on several drugs with multiple effects (minocycline, erythropoietin, melatonin) and on hypothermia. Another intriguing field of investigation is the effect of calorie restriction.[58] Some of these approaches are being evaluated in ongoing human clinical trials,[4] but none have been evaluated clinically in dogs.

Polyethylene Glycol

Recently, substances that fuse membranes (fusogens) have been advocated for treatment of acute SCI.[59] Polyethylene glycol (PEG) is a hydrophilic polymer, or fusogen, that, on intravenous administration, targets damaged membranes.[60] The surfactant properties of PEG helps to seal damaged membranes, preventing intracellular leak of ions and subsequent axonal disruption and thus reducing many of the injury cascades. In an experimental model of SCI in guinea pigs, there is rapid recovery of somatosensory-evoked potentials and of the cutaneous trunci reflex after treatment with PEG.[61] A phase 1 clinical trial of PEG (3500 Da, 30% wt/wt in saline) has been completed in dogs with paralysis and loss of nociception caused by acute disk herniations.[62] The drug was administered at a dose of 2 mL/kg twice at an interval of 45 minutes. No adverse effects were reported, and 60% of the dogs recovered function. However, this preliminary study was not blinded and included a historical control group with an unusually low recovery rate. The reported recovery rate with PEG is similar to that of prior reports of dogs with the same severity of injury treated with surgery alone.[63–65] Efficacy still needs to be proved in a blinded, controlled trial, but this therapy shows promise as a safe and effective treatment. A placebo-controlled trial is ongoing in dogs with naturally occurring SCI (see **Table 1**).

Oscillating Electrical Field

Electrical fields promote axonal regeneration, and to harness this phenomenon, the Center for Paralysis Research at Purdue University developed an implant that could generate an oscillating electrical field across the SCI site. The investigators performed a blinded, placebo-controlled clinical trial in dogs with disk herniations and demonstrated an improvement in sensory function.[66] A phase 1 trial in 10 human patients also generated promising results,[67] but it is unclear whether a larger clinical trial will ensue and whether the implant will be developed commercially.

SECONDARY INJURY—SUBACUTE AND CHRONIC PHASES

After the initial wave of degeneration, the lesion starts to stabilize. There are largely abortive attempts at axonal regeneration; a glial scar composed of hypertrophied astrocytic processes forms at the borders of the lesion; and necrotic debris are removed by macrophages, leaving a cystic cavity (**Fig. 5**). If the meninges are damaged in the initial mechanical injury, fibroblasts tend to infiltrate the lesion, making an even denser scar. Over time, disturbances in CSF flow at the site of the lesion can result in the development of syringomyelia, which can cause further problems. Although this phenomenon has not been described in the veterinary literature, the author has seen it in many patients (**Fig. 6**). Another phenomenon that can occur is the development of a subarachnoid cyst at the site of injury.[68] Syringomyelia and subarachnoid cysts can cause further neurologic deterioration months to years after injury.

Failure of Axonal Regeneration

CNS axons fail to regenerate successfully because of a weak intrinsic response and because of a nonpermissive environment. Over the last decade, understanding of the intrinsic and environmental factors that inhibit regeneration has escalated, leading to the identification of new therapeutic targets. Intrinsically, mature CNS neurons express low levels of cyclic adenosine monophosphate (AMP); increasing cyclic AMP levels increases axonal regeneration.[69] Extrinsically, myelin and astrocytes express factors that inhibit axonal extension.[70] Myelin of CNS expresses several different inhibitory factors (eg, Nogo and myelin-associated glycoprotein) that act through the Nogo receptor, NgR.[1,71] Activation of NgR ultimately results in modifications of the actin cytoskeleton, causing collapse of the growth cone. An intermediary step in this cascade that is of clinical interest is the Rho-ROCK signaling pathway.[72] Targeting the inhibitory proteins with antibodies and inactivating Rho with the C3 enzyme of *Clostridium botulinum* eliminates the inhibitory effects of myelin and improves outcome.[1] Both strategies are now in human clinical trials, although there are significant concerns about possible unwanted side effects associated with increased axonal sprouting at the site of the lesion, such as neuropathic pain.[4] Astrocytes also express a group of inhibitory factors, the chondroitin sulfate proteoglycans.[70] These molecules can be digested directly with a bacterial enzyme called chondroitinase ABC, producing an improvement in outcome. Treatment with this enzyme has been coupled with cellular transplants and with rehabilitative exercises with interesting results.[69] This approach has not yet reached clinical trials.

Therapy for the Chronic Lesion: Restoring Function to Demyelinated Axons

The persistence of demyelinated axons across the site of a lesion offers a potential therapeutic opportunity. Function can potentially be restored to these axons by using

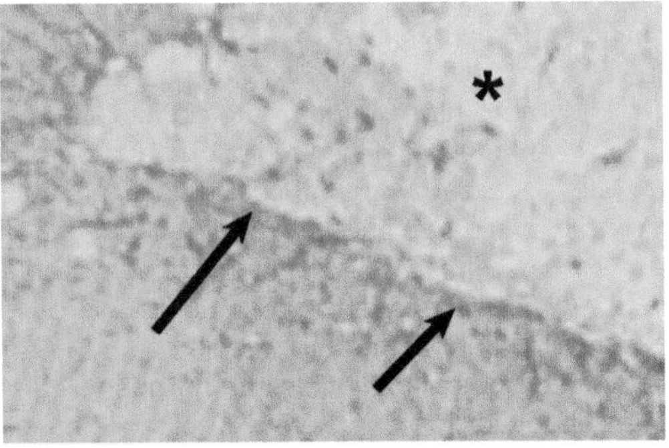

Fig. 5. Glial fibrillary acidic protein (GFAP) immunostaining of a transverse section of the spinal cord 1 month after injury. Note the intense GFAP staining at the border of the lesion (*arrows*). An asterisk is placed within the cavity of the lesion.

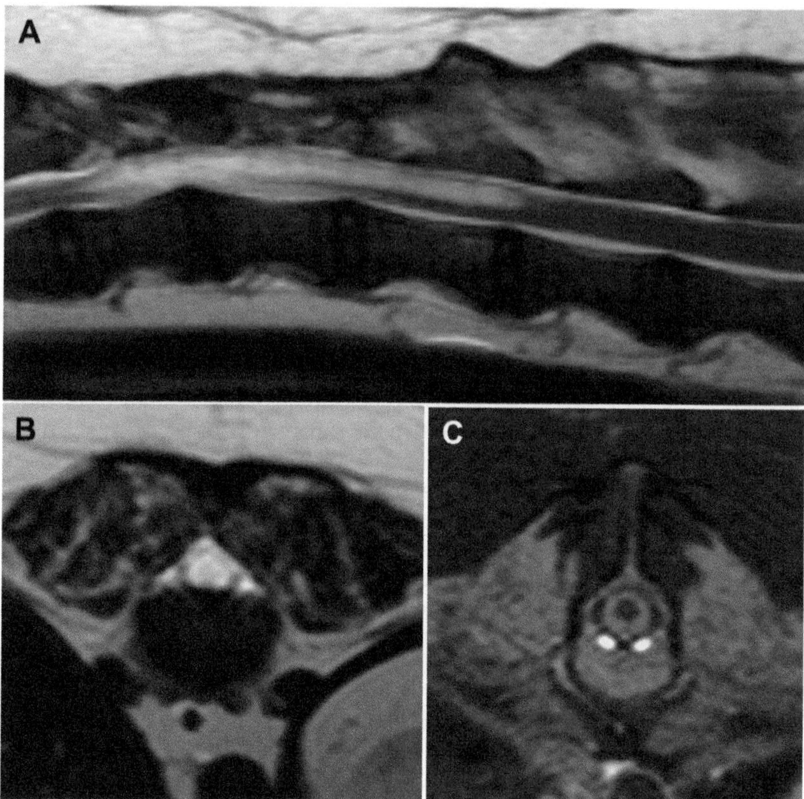

Fig. 6. (*A*) T2-weighted sagittal magnetic resonance image of the spinal cord of a dog showing a large syrinx extending from the original injury site. The dog suffered an acute disk herniation before 2 years previously and was treated surgically. After a slow recovery, the dog's neurologic status stabilized, but she then developed worsening weakness associated with severe spasticity. (*B*) Axial T2-weighted image of the site of the disk herniation; the entire cross-sectional area is hyperintense, consistent with fluid accumulation. (*C*) T1-weighted post–gadolinium fat suppression image from just caudal to the site of the disc herniation showing the syrinx cavity extending along the spinal cord.

potassium channel blockers[73,74] or by remyelination after transplantation of Schwann cells, olfactory ensheathing cells (OECs), or a variety of different stem cells programmed to produce oligodendrocytes or Schwann cells.[1] Demyelination of axons exposes underlying rapidly activating voltage-gated potassium channels, producing an outward potassium current that blocks action potential propagation.[73,74] 4-Aminopyridine (4-AP) has been used to block these potassium channels specifically, restoring conduction to demyelinated axons in addition to improving synaptic transmission and muscle strength.[74] These pharmacologic effects produce an electrophysiologic and functional improvement in experimental models of SCI, in human and canine patients with chronic SCI, and in multiple sclerosis.[75–77] However, the clinical use of 4-AP has been limited by significant side effects, such as tremors and seizures, when used at clinically effective doses. Derivatives of 4-AP have been evaluated in dogs with naturally occurring SCI and have been shown to be safe[78] and to improve gait in a pilot study of dogs with chronic paresis.[10] A blinded, placebo-controlled clinical trial comparing 4-AP with one of its derivatives is ongoing (see **Table 1**).

Cellular Transplantation Therapy

Cellular transplantation approaches are currently receiving a lot of interest and are being investigated in dogs with naturally occurring SCI. Full reviews of this area can be found elsewhere.[1,79] Transplanted cells may be used to replace damaged tissue, promote host axonal regeneration, or play a neuroprotective role. Schwann cells and OECs have been used to remyelinate and to support regeneration of host axons. Both cell types provide a peripheral myelin environment that is permissive to axonal regeneration. Schwann cells are attractive because they can be expanded in culture from host nerve biopsies, and they have been shown to promote host regeneration in numerous models of SCI. However, reintegration of the regenerating axon back into the spinal cord caudal to the lesion is limited.[80] This can be mitigated by combining Schwann cells with chondroitinase ABC or OEC[80] and this approach deserves evaluation in dogs. OECs have the advantage of promoting regeneration of axons back into the spinal cord, a feature that is thought to relate to the normal role of these cells in bridging the CNS and peripheral nervous system.[9,79] OECs can be harvested from canine nasal mucosa, allowing for generation of autologous cells,[81] and use of these cells is being evaluated in human clinical trials.[4] After initial excitement, the optimism surrounding these cells is somewhat abating, but these cells have been transplanted safely into the spinal cord of dogs with naturally occurring lesions,[9] and a canine clinical trial is ongoing (see **Table 1**).

A variety of different stem cells are being used to treat SCI, and many have reached human clinical trials across the world, in spite of extremely variable and confusing results in experimental studies.[4] Adult-derived stem cells present an attractive therapy because they can be harvested from the patient to produce autologous transplants.[82] These so called stem cells have been derived from skin, fat (adipose-derived stem cells), bone marrow (bone marrow stromal and hematopoietic stem cells), and umbilical cord blood and are collectively called mesenchymal stem cells or stromal cells. These cell populations can be cultured in conditions that induce neural differentiation, although there is debate about the true functionality of cell populations produced in this way. Reports of neural lineage cells from canine mesenchymal stem cells are starting to appear.[83–85] Although frequently called stem cells, these cells do not have the true pluripotent potential of an embryonic stem cell, and their ability to replicate is limited. There are numerous, often conflicting reports of the effect of transplanting these cells into spinal cord lesions in the first 2 weeks after injury. There are also reports of administering them intrathecally and intravenously. The observation that few transplanted cells survive within the lesion supports the theory that they may play a neuroprotective role and underlines the importance of evaluating the published literature carefully. Umbilical cord blood–derived mesenchymal stem cells have been transplanted into an experimental model of canine SCI and have improved outcome with no evidence of adverse effects.[83]

Neural stem cells can be derived from embryos or adults, and the procedure has been described in dogs.[84–86] These cells can be differentiated into neuronal or glial lineages, and there are numerous published reports of transplanting neural stem cells into different models of SCI.[1,79] The approach that has proved the most consistently successful to date is the induction of differentiation of neural stem cells to produce oligodendroglial precursors, which in turn produce oligodendrocytes capable of myelination after transplantation.[79] A human clinical trial testing this therapy is currently underway in the United States, the first Food and Drug Administration approved trial of its kind in the country. The most recent development is the ability to generate true pluripotential stem cells, analogous to embryonic stem cells, by reprogramming adult fibroblasts.[87] The resulting cells are called induced pluripotential stem cells, and they open up the potential of using cells with all the benefits of embryonic cells, with the added benefit of being derived from the patient rather than an embryo. Of course, they are also associated with some of the same problems as embryonic stem cells, such as the potential to produce tumors because of their unlimited ability to replicate.

Stem cell transplantation has really caught the attention and imagination of the public, and it is now possible to obtain a wide variety of stem cell transplants in different countries. The number of anecdotal reports of dramatic clinical recoveries is also increasing. However, with some notable exceptions, experimental studies to date have produced conflicting data, and carefully controlled human clinical trials are difficult to perform when patients are undergoing a surgical intervention. As stem cell transplantation therapies become popular in veterinary medicine, there exists the opportunity to perform ground-breaking clinical trials to establish their true worth.

SUMMARY

Although the understanding of the pathophysiology of SCI continues to grow, this has yet to translate to novel, clinically proven therapies in companion animals. Basic factors such as blood pressure, oxygenation, and spinal cord decompression remain central to effective therapy for acute SCIs. Placebo-controlled clinical trials of neuroprotective drugs and therapies aimed at the chronic lesion are underway in dogs, and it is likely, after a long period of stagnation, that our ability to successfully treat acute SCIs will improve in the near future.

REFERENCES

1. Rowland JW, Hawryluk GW, Kwon B, et al. Current status of acute spinal cord injury pathophysiology and emerging therapies: promise on the horizon. Neurosurg Focus 2008;25(5):E2.
2. Baptiste DC, Fehlings MG. Pharmacological approaches to repair the injured spinal cord. J Neurotrauma 2006;23(3–4):318–34.
3. Olby NJ. Current concepts in the management of acute spinal cord injury. J Vet Intern Med 1999;13:399–407.
4. Hawryluk GW, Rowland J, Kwon BK, et al. Protection and repair of the injured spinal cord: a review of completed, ongoing, and planned clinical trials for acute spinal cord injury. Neurosurg Focus 2008;25(5):E14.
5. Fish CJ, Blakemore WF. A model of chronic spinal cord compression in the cat. Neuropathol Appl Neurobiol 1983;9:109–19.
6. Shi R, Blight AR. Compression injury of mammalian spinal cord in vitro and the dynamics of action potential conduction failure. J Neurophysiol 1996;76:1572–80.
7. Smith PM, Jeffery ND. Histological and ultrastructural analysis of white matter damage after naturally-occurring spinal cord injury. Brain Pathol 2006;16:99–109.
8. Griffiths IR. Spinal cord injuries: a pathological study of naturally occurring lesions in the dog and cat. J Comp Pathol 1978;88(2):303–15.
9. Jeffery ND, Lakatos A, Franklin RJ. Autologous olfactory glial cell transplantation is reliable and safe in naturally occurring canine spinal cord injury. J Neurotrauma 2005;22(11):1282–93.
10. Olby NJ, Humphrey J, Spinapolice K, et al. Phase 1 clinical trial of 4-aminopyridine derivatives in dogs with chronic myelopathies [abstract]. J Vet Intern Med 2008;22:722.

11. Furlan JC, Noonan V, Cadotte DW, et al. Timing of decompressive surgery after traumatic spinal cord injury: an evidence-based examination of pre-clinical and clinical studies. J Neurotrauma 2010. [Epub ahead of print].
12. Tator CH, Fehlings MG. Review of the secondary injury theory of acute spinal cord trauma with emphasis on vascular mechanisms. J Neurosurg 1991; 75(1):15–26.
13. Balentine JD. Pathology of experimental spinal cord trauma. I. The necrotic lesion as a function of vascular injury. Lab Invest 1978;39(3):236–53.
14. Gerzanich V, Woo SK, Vennekens R, et al. De novo expression of Trpm4 initiates secondary hemorrhage in spinal cord injury. Nat Med 2009;15(2):185–91.
15. Guha A, Tator CH. Acute cardiovascular effects of experimental spinal cord injury. J Trauma 1988;28(4):481–90.
16. Griffiths IR, Trench JG, Crawford RA. Spinal cord blood flow and conduction during experimental cord compression in normotensive and hypotensive dogs. J Neurosurg 1979;50(3):353–60.
17. Rabinowitz RS, Eck JC, Harper CM Jr, et al. Urgent surgical decompression compared to methylprednisolone for the treatment of acute spinal cord injury: a randomized prospective study in beagle dogs. Spine (Phila Pa 1976) 2008; 33(21):2260–8.
18. Parker AJ, Smith CW. Functional recovery from spinal cord trauma following delayed incision of spinal meninges in dogs. Res Vet Sci 1975;18(1):110–2.
19. Loughin CA, Dewey CW, Ringwood PB, et al. Effect of durotomy on functional outcome of dogs with type I thoracolumbar disc extrusion and absent deep pain perception. Vet Comp Orthop Traumatol 2005;18(3):141–6.
20. Kwon BK, Curt A, Belanger LM, et al. Intrathecal pressure monitoring and cerebrospinal fluid drainage in acute spinal cord injury: a prospective randomized trial. J Neurosurg Spine 2009;10(3):181–93.
21. Park E, Velumian AA, Fehlings MG. The role of excitotoxicity in secondary mechanisms of spinal cord injury: a review with an emphasis on the implications for white matter degeneration. J Neurotrauma 2004;21(6):754–74.
22. Olby NJ, Sharp NJ, Muñana KR, et al. Chronic and acute compressive spinal cord lesions in dogs due to intervertebral disc herniation are associated with elevation in lumbar cerebrospinal fluid glutamate concentration. J Neurotrauma 1999;16(12):1215–24.
23. Petitjean ME, Pointillart V, Dixmerias F, et al. Medical treatment of spinal cord injury in the acute stage. Ann Fr Anesth Reanim 1998;17:114–22.
24. Ates O, Cayli SR, Gurses I, et al. Comparative neuroprotective effect of sodium channel blockers after experimental spinal cord injury. J Clin Neurosci 2007; 14(7):658–65.
25. Tadie M, D'Arbigny P, Mathe J, et al. Acute spinal cord injury. Early care and treatment in a multicenter study with gacyclidine. Soc Neurosci 1999;25:1090.
26. Demopoulos HB, Flamm ES, Pietronigro DD, et al. The free radical pathology and the microcirculation in the major central nervous system disorders. Acta Physiol Scand Suppl 1980;492:91–119.
27. Genovese T, Cuzzocrea S. Role of free radicals and poly (ADP-ribose)polymerase-1 in the development of spinal cord injury: new potential therapeutic targets. Curr Med Chem 2008;15(5):477–87.
28. Xiong Y, Hall ED. Pharmacological evidence for a role of peroxynitrite in the pathophysiology of spinal cord injury. Exp Neurol 2009;216(1):105–14.
29. Hall ED. The neuroprotective pharmacology of methylprednisolone. J Neurosurg 1992;76(1):13–22.

30. Bracken MB, Shepard MJ, Holford TR, et al. Administration of methylprednisolone for 24 or 48 hours or tirilazad mesylate for 48 hours in the treatment of acute spinal cord injury. Results of the Third National Acute Spinal Cord Injury Randomized Controlled Trial. National Acute Spinal Cord Injury Study. JAMA 1997; 277(20):1597–604.
31. Bracken MB, Shepard MJ, Holford TR, et al. Methylprednisolone or tirilazad mesylate administration after acute spinal cord injury: 1-year follow up. Results of the third National Acute Spinal Cord Injury randomized controlled trial. J Neurosurg 1998 Nov;89(5):699–706.
32. Bracken MB, Shepard MJ, Collins WF, et al. A randomized, controlled trial of methylprednisolone or naloxone in the treatment of acute spinal-cord injury. Results of the Second National Acute Spinal Cord Injury Study. N Engl J Med 1990;322(20):1405–11.
33. Bracken MB, Shepard MJ, Hellenbrand KG, et al. Methylprednisolone and neurological function 1 year after spinal cord injury. Results of the National Acute Spinal Cord Injury Study. J Neurosurg 1985;63(5):704–13.
34. Coleman WP, Benzel D, Cahill DW, et al. A critical appraisal of the reporting of the National Acute Spinal Cord Injury Studies (II and III) of methylprednisolone in acute spinal cord injury. J Spinal Disord 2000;13(3):185–99.
35. Hurlbert RJ. Methylprednisolone for acute spinal cord injury: an inappropriate standard of care. J Neurosurg 2000;93(Suppl 1):1–7.
36. Nesathurai S. Steroids and spinal cord injury: revisiting the NASCIS 2 and NASCIS 3 trials. J Trauma 1998;45(6):1088–93.
37. Scott GS, Cuzzocrea S, Genovese T, et al. Uric acid protects against secondary damage after spinal cord injury. Proc Natl Acad Sci U S A 2005;102(9):3483–8.
38. Coates JR, Sorjonen DC, Simpson ST, et al. Clinicopathologic effects of a 21-aminosteroid compound (U74389G) and high-dose methylprednisolone on spinal cord function after simulated spinal cord trauma. Vet Surg 1995;24:128–39.
39. Baltzer WI, McMichael MA, Hosgood GL, et al. Randomized, blinded, placebo-controlled clinical trial of N-acetylcysteine in dogs with spinal cord trauma from acute intervertebral disc disease. Spine (Phila Pa 1976) 2008; 33(13):1397–402.
40. Parker AJ, Smith CW. Lack of functional recovery from spinal cord trauma following dimethylsulphoxide and epsilon amino caproic acid therapy in dogs. Res Vet Sci 1979;27(2):253–5.
41. Donnelly DJ, Popovich PG. Inflammation and its role in neuroprotection, axonal regeneration and functional recovery after spinal cord injury. Exp Neurol 2008; 209(2):378–88.
42. Noble LJ, Donovan F, Igarashi T, et al. Matrix metalloproteinases limit functional recovery after spinal cord injury by modulation of early vascular events. J Neurosci 2002;22(17):7526–35.
43. Levine JM, Ruaux CG, Bergman RL, et al. Matrix metalloproteinase-9 activity in the cerebrospinal fluid and serum of dogs with acute spinal cord trauma from intervertebral disk disease. Am J Vet Res 2006;67(2):283–7.
44. Blight AR. Delayed demyelination and macrophage invasion: a candidate for secondary cell damage in spinal cord injury. Cent Nerv Syst Trauma 1985;2(4): 299–315.
45. Shechter R, London A, Varol C, et al. Infiltrating blood-derived macrophages are vital cells playing an anti-inflammatory role in recovery from spinal cord injury in mice. PLoS Med 2009;6(7):e1000113.

46. Kigerl KA, Gensel JC, Ankeny DP, et al. Identification of two distinct macrophage subsets with divergent effects causing either neurotoxicity or regeneration in the injured mouse spinal cord. J Neurosci 2009;29(43):13435–44.
47. Ankeny DP, Guan Z, Popovich PG. B cells produce pathogenic antibodies and impair recovery after spinal cord injury in mice. J Clin Invest 2009; 119(10):2990–9.
48. Popovich P, McTigue D. Damage control in the nervous system: beware the immune system in spinal cord injury. Nat Med 2009;15(7):736–7.
49. Parker AJ, Smith CW. Functional recovery from spinal cord trauma following dexamethazone and chlorpromazine therapy in dogs. Res Vet Sci 1976; 21(2):246–7.
50. Arias MJ. Treatment of experimental spinal cord injury with TRH, naloxone, and dexamethasone. Surg Neurol 1987;28(5):335–8.
51. Levine JM, Levine GJ, Boozer L, et al. Adverse effects and outcome associated with dexamethasone administration in dogs with acute thoracolumbar intervertebral disk herniation: 161 cases (2000–2006). J Am Vet Med Assoc 2008; 232(3):411–7.
52. Ruddle TL, Allen DA, Schertel ER, et al. Outcome and prognostic factors in non-ambulatory Hansen Type I intervertebral disc extrusions: 308 cases. Vet Comp Orthop Traumatol 2006;19(1):29–34.
53. Beattie MS. Inflammation and apoptosis: linked therapeutic targets in spinal cord injury. Trends Mol Med 2004;10(12):580–3.
54. Crowe MJ, Bresnahan JC, Shuman SL, et al. Apoptosis and delayed degeneration after spinal cord injury in rats and monkeys. Nat Med 1997;3(1):73–6.
55. Emery E, Aldana P, Bunge MB, et al. Apoptosis after traumatic human spinal cord injury. J Neurosurg 1998;89(6):911–20.
56. Casha S, Yu WR, Fehlings MG. Oligodendroglial apoptosis occurs along degenerating axons and is associated with FAS and p75 expression following spinal cord injury in the rat. Neurosci 2001;103(1):203–18.
57. Ackery A, Robins S, Fehlings MG. Inhibition of Fas-mediated apoptosis through administration of soluble Fas receptor improves functional outcome and reduces posttraumatic axonal degeneration after acute spinal cord injury. J Neurotrauma 2006;23(5):604–16.
58. Plunet WT, Streijger F, Lam CK, et al. Dietary restriction started after spinal cord injury improves functional recovery. Exp Neurol 2008;213(1):28–35.
59. Borgens RB, Bohnert D. Rapid recovery from spinal cord injury after subcutaneously administered polyethylene glycol. J Neurosci Res 2001;66: 1179–86.
60. Shi R, Borgens RB. Anatomical repair of nerve membranes in crushed mammalian spinal cord with polyethylene glycol. J Neurocytol 2000;29:633–43.
61. Shi R, Borgens RB. Acute repair of crushed guinea pig spinal cord by polyethylene glycol. J Neurophysiol 1999;81:2406–14.
62. Laverty PH, Leskovar A, Breur GJ, et al. A preliminary study of intravenous surfactants in paraplegic dogs: polymer therapy in canine clinical SCI. J Neurotrauma 2004;21(12):1767–77.
63. Olby NJ, Harris T, Muñana K, et al. Long term functional outcome of dogs with severe thoracolumbar spinal cord injuries. J Am Vet Med Assoc 2003;222: 762–9.
64. Scott HW, McKee WM. Laminectomy for 34 dogs with thoracolumbar intervertebral disc disease and loss of deep pain perception. J Small Anim Pract 1999; 40:417–22.

65. Duval J, Dewey C, Roberts R, et al. Spinal cord swelling as a myelographic indicator of prognosis: a retrospective study in dogs with intervertebral disc disease and loss of deep pain sensation. Vet Surg 1996;25:6–12.
66. Borgens RB, Toombs JP, Breur G, et al. An imposed oscillating electrical field improves the recovery of function in neurologically complete paraplegic dogs. J Neurotrauma 1999;16(7):639–57.
67. Shapiro S, Borgens R, Pascuzzi R, et al. Oscillating field stimulation for complete spinal cord injury in humans: a phase 1 trial. J Neurosurg Spine 2005;2(1):3–10 [erratum in: J Neurosurg Spine 2008;8(6):604].
68. Skeen TM, Olby NJ, Muñana KR, et al. Spinal arachnoid cysts in 17 dogs. J Am Anim Hosp Assoc 2003;39(3):271–82.
69. Hannila SS, Filbin MT. The role of cyclic AMP signaling in promoting axonal regeneration after spinal cord injury. Exp Neurol 2008;209(2):321–32.
70. Fawcett JW. Overcoming inhibition in the damaged spinal cord. J Neurotrauma 2006;23(3–4):371–83.
71. Giger RJ, Venkatesh K, Chivatakarn O, et al. Mechanisms of CNS myelin inhibition: evidence for distinct and neuronal cell type specific receptor systems. Restor Neurol Neurosci 2008;26(2–3):97–115.
72. Kubo T, Yamaguchi A, Iwata N, et al. The therapeutic effects of Rho-ROCK inhibitors on CNS disorders. Ther Clin Risk Manag 2008;4(3):605–15.
73. Blight AR. Effect of 4-aminopyridine on axonal conduction-block in chronic spinal cord injury. Brain Res Bull 1989;22:47–52.
74. Nashmi R, Fehlings MG. Mechanisms of axonal dysfunction after spinal cord injury: with an emphasis on the role of voltage-gated potassium channels. Brain Res Brain Res Rev 2001;38:165–91.
75. Blight AR, Toombs JP, Bauer MS, et al. The effects of 4-aminopyridine on neurological deficits in chronic cases of traumatic spinal cord injury in dogs: a phase I clinical trial. J Neurotrauma 1991;8:103–19.
76. Hayes KC, Potter PJ, Wolfe DL, et al. 4-Aminopyridine-sensitive neurologic deficits in patients with spinal cord injury. J Neurotrauma 1994;11:433–46.
77. Goodman AD, Cohen JA, Cross A, et al. Fampridine-SR in multiple sclerosis: a randomized, double-blind, placebo-controlled, dose-ranging study. Mult Scler 2007;13:357–68.
78. Olby NJ, Smith DT, Humphrey J, et al. Pharmacokinetics of 4-aminopyridine derivatives in dogs. J Vet Pharmacol Ther 2009;32(5):485–91.
79. Rossi SL, Keirstead HS. Stem cells and spinal cord regeneration. Curr Opin Biotechnol 2009;20(5):552–62.
80. Fortun J, Hill CE, Bunge MB. Combinatorial strategies with Schwann cell transplantation to improve repair of the injured spinal cord. Neurosci Lett 2009; 456(3):124–32.
81. Ito D, Ibanez C, Ogawa H, et al. Comparison of cell populations derived from canine olfactory bulb and olfactory mucosal cultures. Am J Vet Res 2006;67(6): 1050–6.
82. Schaffler A, Buchler C. Concise review: adipose tissue-derived stromal cells-basic and clinical implications for novel cell-based therapies. Stem Cells 2008; 25:818–27.
83. Lim JH, Byeon YE, Ryu HH, et al. Transplantation of canine umbilical cord blood-derived mesenchymal stem cells in experimentally induced spinal cord injured dogs. J Vet Sci 2007;8(3):275–82.
84. Lim JH, Olby NJ, Mariani CL. Neural stem cell sources in adult dogs [abstract]. ACVIM Forum. In: Proceedings of ACVIM. J Vet Intern Med 2009;23:742.

85. Kamishina H, Cheeseman J, Clemmons R. Nestin-positive spheres derived from canine bone marrow stromal cells generate cells with early neuronal and glial phenotypic characteristics. In Vitro Cell Dev Biol Anim 2008;44:140–4.
86. Milward EA, Lundberg CG, Ge B, et al. Isolation and transplantation of multipotential populations of epidermal growth factor-responsive, neural progenitor cells from the canine brain. J Neurosci Res 1997;50(5):862–71.
87. Takahashi K, Yamanaka S. Induction of pluripotent stem cells from mouse embryonic and adult fibroblast cultures by defined factors. Cell 2006;126(4):663–76.

Vertebral Fracture and Luxation in Small Animals

Nick D. Jeffery, BVSc, PhD, FRCVS

KEYWORDS

• Spinal • Fixation • Therapy • Spinal cord injury

Vertebral fractures and luxations (VFL) are a major cause of neurologic injury in small animal patients. These injuries are most commonly associated with severe external trauma, occurring in approximately 6% of cases presented with neurologic deficits indicative of spinal cord dysfunction,[1,2] but there is also a sizeable minority of affected animals that present following fracture of an abnormal bone (ie, pathologic fractures).

VFL almost invariably cause pain and neurologic deficits. Neurologic deficits result from compression or contusion of neural tissue, while pain may arise because of neural compression or through direct mechanical injury and instability of mesenchymal tissues. Impact injury to the spinal cord inevitably results in tissue destruction, the severity of which is highly variable and is discussed in more detail in the article by Natasha Olby elsewhere in this issue. In addition, persistent compression of the spinal cord or the nerve roots causes demyelination, progressive axonal injury, and neuronal and axonal destruction. The prime focus of therapy is preservation of function in surviving neural tissue, which often requires surgical decompression and stabilization of skeletal elements to prevent further trauma, plus physiotherapy and rehabilitation. In some cases, especially those with minimal neurologic deficits, function can recover adequately with conservative therapy alone, by relying on the inherent stability of the vertebral column to prevent further trauma to the nervous system.

Because VFL commonly occur in animals that have incurred severe external trauma, there are frequently concomitant injuries to many other body systems. Injuries to the respiratory and circulatory systems can be more rapidly fatal than those affecting the vertebral column, so it is imperative that animals that have suffered multiple trauma should have their injuries rigorously prioritized using an emergency triage system.[3] Nevertheless, it is also essential that the possibility of a VFL is appreciated at an early stage so that physical maneuvers are carefully considered to avoid the risk of exacerbating neural damage. In many such cases it is prudent to secure the animal to an external splinting device such as a plank of wood or a stretcher.

Department of Veterinary Medicine, University of Cambridge, Madingley Road, Cambridge CB3 0ES, England, UK
E-mail address: knick.jeffery@gmail.com

Vet Clin Small Anim 40 (2010) 809–828
doi:10.1016/j.cvsm.2010.05.004 **vetsmall.theclinics.com**
0195-5616/10/$ – see front matter

ANATOMIC CONSIDERATIONS

Vertebral Column

Specific anatomic features of the vertebral column are important in understanding the relationship between the inciting trauma and the type of VFL, and also to determine optimal methods of fixation; they are well described in standard veterinary texts.[4,5] Points of particular interest are details of the intricate, and greatly varied, shape of the vertebrae themselves and the many ligamentous structures surrounding the vertebrae. Both these features contribute greatly to the balance between mobility and inherent stability of the vertebral column, because they permit constrained movement between vertebrae. Forced movement beyond these constraints can cause ligamentous rupture and vertebral facture.

The nature and extent of abnormal movement that causes VFL is variable between different regions of the vertebral column. For example, thoracic vertebrae have small articular facets that provide little resistance to torsional forces (see later discussion), but the ligamentous tissue associated with the extremely large spinous processes and the ribs very effectively limit motion between individual vertebral pairs in all 3 planes. Therefore fractures of articular facets are rare in this region, but rupture of ligaments between the spinous processes, or spinous process fracture, are relatively common. By contrast, mid-caudal lumbar vertebrae have large articular facets and accessory processes that limit motion to the sagittal plane, but are liable to fracture following excessive torsional load. A further aspect that has been relatively unexplored is possible susceptibility to fracture-luxation because of anomalies in vertebral development; careful anatomic studies of chondrodystrophic dogs have revealed numerous abnormalities, sometimes including aplasia of the articular facets of thoracolumbar vertebrae.[6] It is clear that such anomalies will predispose to VFL after relatively moderate trauma.

Not only do specific aspects of the anatomy of vertebrae and their ligaments cause susceptibility to definable types of force, but they can also be exploited in designing appropriate therapy. At its most basic level, the inherent stability of the mid-thoracic vertebral column means that surgical fixation is often not required in this area. More subtly, the large size of articular facets in the cervical region and their ability to prevent torsion can be exploited by incorporating them into internal fixation methods.

The histologic nature of various parts of the vertebrae themselves can be an important consideration. Fractures of the vertebral body will heal rapidly once reduced because they consist largely of well-vascularized cancellous bone; on the other hand, dense spinous processes may take many more weeks to heal satisfactorily, and sometimes form nonunions. Dense cortical bone also has greater resistance to fatigue failure associated with metallic implants.

Nervous System

Specific consequences of fracture-luxation at various regions

The significance of VFL rests almost entirely on their ability to disrupt neural tissue; therefore, although fractures of vertebral processes are common they are almost always of little significance. However, specific features of the anatomy of the spinal cord and the vertebral column in various regions imply differences in the significance of VFL at different sites. For instance, cranial cervical VFL often cause gross reduction of the size of the vertebral canal, but this is not always associated with severe injury to the spinal cord; it is not uncommon for animals with displaced atlantoaxial VFL to present with pain only.[7] The explanation is that the spinal cord occupies a relatively small proportion of the vertebral canal at this level. By contrast, within the cranial lumbar vertebrae (especially of chondrodystrophic dogs) the epidural space is small, meaning that even minimal vertebral displacement will commonly cause severe neural injury.

VFL that affect the spinal cord intumescences are of especial significance because these regions of the spinal cord contain the gray matter and nerves that supply the limbs, bladder, and anus. Injury to these regions (ie, vertebrae C4–T3 and L3–L5) carry a greater risk of permanent paralysis of the innervated regions because of the greater susceptibility of gray matter to injury (see the article by Natasha Olby elsewhere in this issue for further exploration of this topic) and also their larger diameter relative to the vertebral canal. Unfortunately, the ability of plastic responses to ameliorate the functional deficits that follow spinal cord injury is more restricted for gray matter lesions than white matter lesions.[8] It would seem that anecdotally, severe lesions of L5 vertebra are especially associated with poor prognosis for return of bladder function. Similarly, there is evidence to suggest that VFL at C2/3 are especially liable to be associated with failure of respiration.[9]

VFL can cause injuries to both the spinal cord and the associated nerves (ie, cauda equina and spinal nerves and roots), and the prognosis for recovery after injury to each varies a great deal (see the article by Natasha Olby elsewhere in this issue for further exploration of this topic). In general, spinal cord injuries are more severe because there is extremely limited regenerative potential. On the other hand, compression of peripheral nerves is often extremely painful to the patient and may require emergency surgical decompression on humane grounds.

ETIOLOGY

Trauma

Most commonly, VFL result from external force, such as that associated with road traffic accidents or falls, in which the normal structures are overwhelmed by the magnitude of the force. Road traffic accidents are the cause of approximately 40% to 60% of VFL in dogs and cats[7,10–13]; falls from great height (especially cats) and other external trauma such as gunshot, including airgun pellet injury in cats, make up the majority of other causes.

Pathologic Fracture

A significant proportion of VFL, especially in old animals, result from application of normal forces to an abnormal bone. There are many causes of pathologic bone weakening, including osteomyelitis (discospondylitis and spondylitis), primary or secondary tumor infiltration, and hyperparathyroidism. It is important to be aware of the high incidence of pathologic fractures in older, especially large, dogs; approximately 4% of osteosarcomas occur in the vertebral column[14] and there are many other tumor types that can weaken vertebral bone to cause pathologic fractures. Somewhat surprisingly, many vertebral tumors present with acute onset of clinical signs, presumably associated with catastrophic fracture, which can sometimes lead the unwary to suspect intervertebral disc disease. Fractures associated with vertebral tumors are rarely treated (because of the extreme pain and poor prognosis), although total excision is possible in selected cases[15]; pathologic fractures associated with osteomyelitis frequently require surgical intervention (see Ref.[16])

Iatrogenic and Idiopathic

Some surgical procedures that are carried out for other reasons can incur the risk of VFL, and such knowledge can be used to aid in planning both the procedure and aftercare. Of particular note is the risk of subluxation, often associated with fracture of the articular facets, following lumbosacral laminectomy.[17] This procedure has traditionally been carried out by excising bone of the lamina and a portion of the facets,[18] thereby increasing the susceptibility to torsional forces. More recently, several modifications of the procedure that reduce the extent of bone excision have been introduced to reduce this risk.[19] In his clinic the author has recently recognized what appear to be stress fractures of spinous processes, with similar characteristics of adjacent hyperostosis to those detected elsewhere in the skeleton of athletic animals.[20] In one dog this followed a partial corpectomy[21] but in the other appeared spontaneously (**Fig. 1**). In both cases simple exercise restriction alleviated the clinical signs.

Pathogenesis

The vertebral column is naturally subject to a variety of forces: compression, torsion, traction, and flexion-extension. Observed categories of VFL reflect the interaction between the nature of the inciting injury and the specific anatomy of the affected region of the vertebral column. As a consequence, certain types of fracture are more common at specific sites within the vertebral column. For instance, extreme flexion of the atlantoaxial articulation can lead to fracture of the dens, whereas flexion in the lumbar region often causes oblique fractures of the ventral aspect of the vertebral bodies (**Fig. 2**). Furthermore, young animals are susceptible to avulsion of the growth plates, especially following torsion (see **Fig. 2**). Torsion is also a common cause of luxations (**Fig. 3**), although frequently these cannot occur without concomitant fractures of restraining processes. In general, VFL occur with greatest frequency at junctions between relatively mobile and relatively immobile regions of the vertebral column.[22,23] Lastly, many vertebral fractures affect neither the vertebral canal nor the intervertebral foramina, and these rarely require surgical attention.

The remainder of this section focuses on VFL that cause neural dysfunction and outlines the regional susceptibility to VFL and their consequences.

- The cervical region (C1–C7) normally permits movement in all planes, including torsion. VFL are relatively uncommon in this region apart from those affecting the axis, which account for approximately 50% of all cervical fractures.[7] Dens fractures commonly result from an animal running at high speed into an obstacle, during which the neck is forcibly flexed. An important consideration is that severe displacement following VFL in the cervical region is often fatal and therefore such cases are rarely presented to the veterinarian. On the other hand, approximately 15% of animals presenting with cervical fractures exhibit pain only.[7]

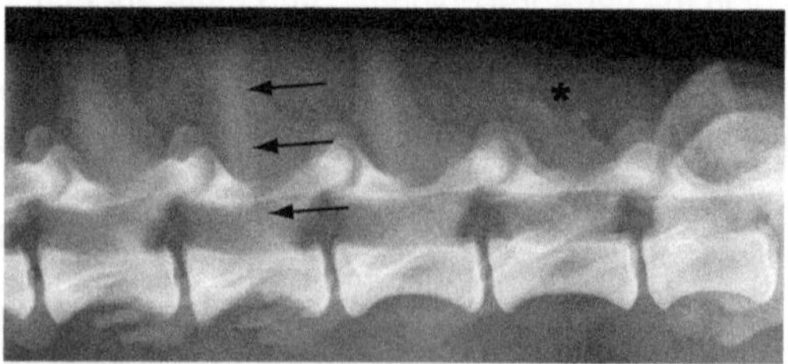

Fig. 1. Lateral radiograph of a 7-year-old dog with severe lumbar pain. Arrows indicate the radiolucent line coursing from dorsal to ventral through the spinous process of L4 vertebra. There is also apparent destruction of the L6 spinous process (*asterisk*). Neither lesion was associated with neoplasia or a traumatic event, and the L4 lesion was diagnosed as a stress fracture.

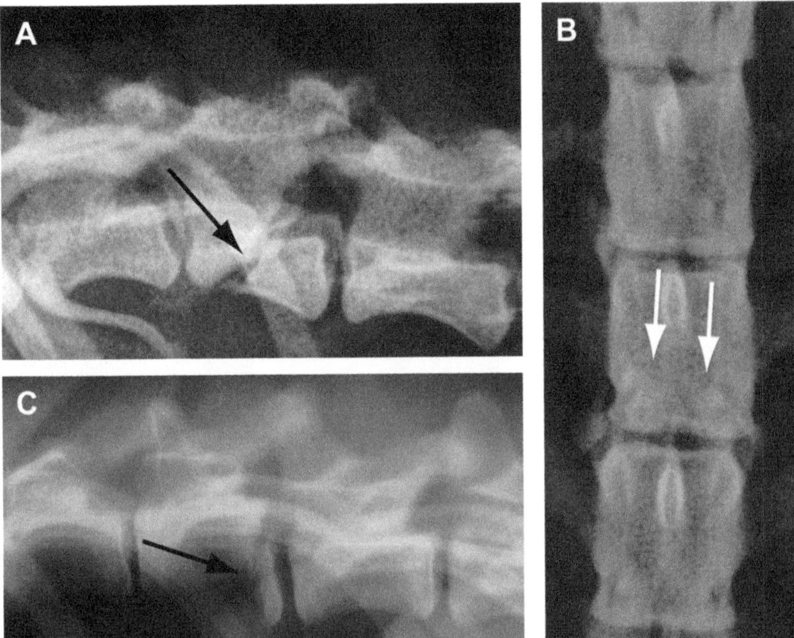

Fig. 2. Radiographs of VFL in the thoracolumbar region. (*A*) Lateral view of oblique fracture of L1 vertebral body. This fracture orientation (*arrow*) is associated with shearing forces generated by extreme flexion. (*B*) Ventrodorsal view of the same fracture illustrating lack of lateral displacement and apparent shortening of the affected vertebral body. The fracture line is faintly visible (*arrows*). (*C*) Lateral radiograph of a vertebral epiphyseal fracture (*arrow*) typical of those that occur in immature animals.

- The thoracic vertebral column (T1–T10) has considerable inherent rigidity, which permits little normal movement, except in the sagittal plane. VFL are relatively uncommon, often minor, and frequently require little additional stabilization.
- The thoracolumbar junction (T10–L2) is a very common site of VFL, constituting approximately 50% of all spinal fractures in both cats and dogs,[10,12] probably because of its location between the rigid thoracic spine and the well-muscled (and therefore relatively rigid) lumbar spine.[24] Many types of VFL are encountered within this region, depending on the magnitude and direction of the inciting force. Of importance is that the shape and orientation of the vertebral articular facets alter within this region, from ventrodorsal in the thoracic area to sagittal in the lumbar area, which is liable to increase the susceptibility to VFL. This susceptibility is exacerbated by the high frequency of congenital anomalies of the vertebral articular facets in this region.[6]
- VFL of the lumbar region constitute approximately 25% to 30% of all VFL.[10,12] Movement between vertebrae in the lumbar region (L3–L7) is restricted almost exclusively to the sagittal plane and there is also very strong associated musculature. Torsional forces are therefore strongly resisted but can lead to fracture of the accessory and articular processes when subject to overwhelming forces. The caudal lumbar area transmits propulsive forces from the pelvic limbs, which

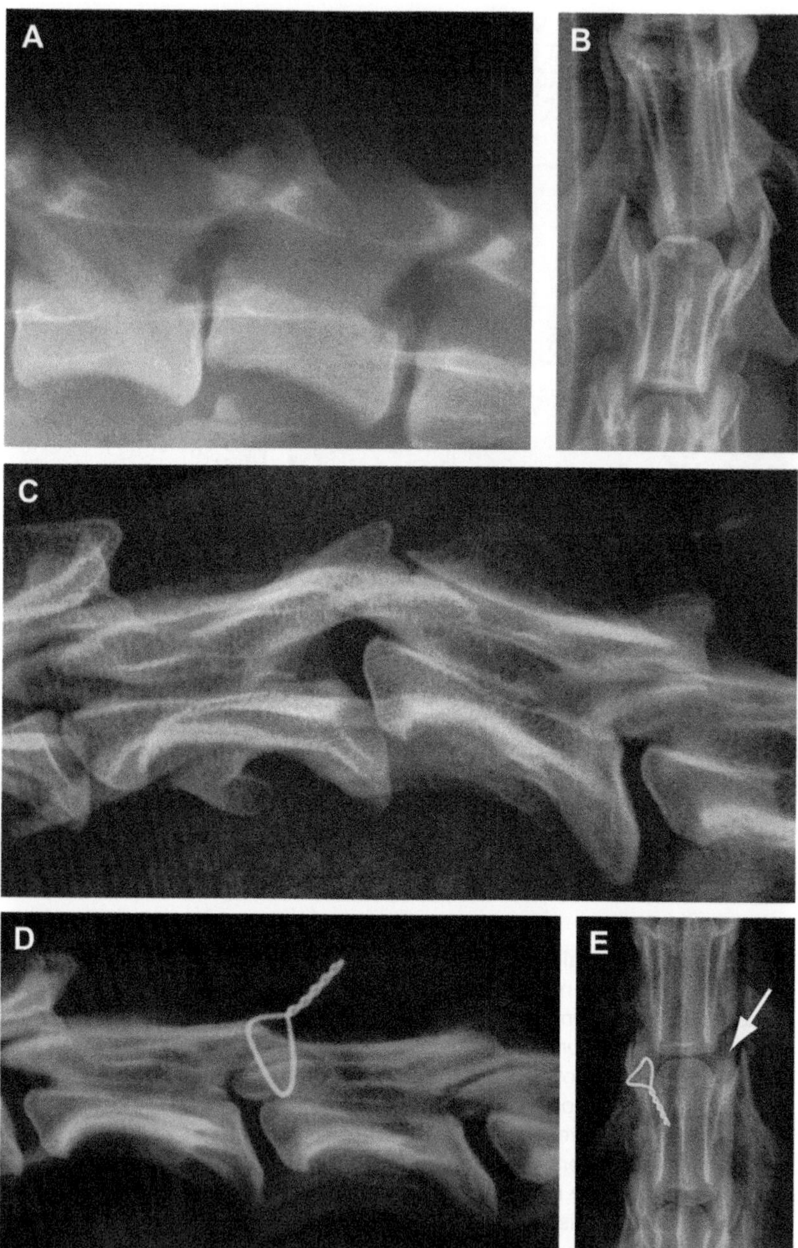

Fig. 3. Radiographs of typical vertebral luxations and subluxations. (*A*) Subluxation between L1 and L2 vertebrae. This lesion was associated with fracture of the articular processes. (*B*) Ventrodorsal, and (*C*) lateral views of luxation between C3 and C4 vertebrae in a greyhound that had run into a wall. The combination of compression and torsion had allowed the articular processes to luxate but they were not fractured. (*D*) Lateral, and (*E*) ventrodorsal views of the reduced luxation stabilized with a single wire suture through the right articular processes. Part of the left C4 articular process had to be removed (*arrow*) to accomplish reduction.

predominantly cause traction and compression of the vertebrae, reflected in the common types of VFL at this location (**Fig. 4**).

- Sacrococcygeal articulations allow movement in all planes, but the articular facets are small and there is little muscle support. This region often undergoes traction injury, especially in cats,[25] although it not always clear how this occurs; the most common explanation is that the tail gets trapped (for instance beneath an automobile wheel) when the animal is running.

DIAGNOSIS

Clinical Signs

Suspicion of VFL is usually straightforward: cases will typically present with spinal pain, neurologic deficits, or both, following obvious external trauma. However, affected animals will frequently have multiple injuries to other body systems, including some that may be rapidly fatal. It is of importance that these other injuries, which may not be immediately apparent (eg, dysrhythmias, tension pneumothorax) are not overlooked in favor of treating the obvious spinal injuries.[3]

Cases that have pathologic VFL typically exhibit a period of unexplained pain followed by catastrophic worsening with development of neurologic signs. Alternatively, neurologic signs develop acutely and are associated with vertebral fracture. At the time of presentation the best distinguishing feature is the lack of any known trauma, coupled with a typical signalment and history for each of the pathologic conditions, such as giant breed of advanced age or chronic polydipsia (suggesting, for example, the possibility of secondary renal hyperparathyroidism).

Neurologic Examination

In animals in which there are neurologic deficits the first step in diagnosis is the neurologic examination. The neurologic examination after spinal trauma is sometimes a little confusing initially because there are some unusual reactions that only occur immediately after spinal trauma. Thus, the Schiff-Sherrington phenomenon is common after severe injury to the thoracolumbar or lumbar region of the spine, and can initially suggest a lesion affecting the central nervous system cranial to the thoracic limbs. This impression is easily dispelled by finding normal thoracic limb gait and postural reactions during neurologic examination (should this be safe to perform). A second potentially confusing finding is the consequence of spinal shock. Immediately after a severe injury to the spinal cord there is loss or depression of the reflexes caudal to the lesion, including the myotatic reflexes, but more commonly observed in the flexor

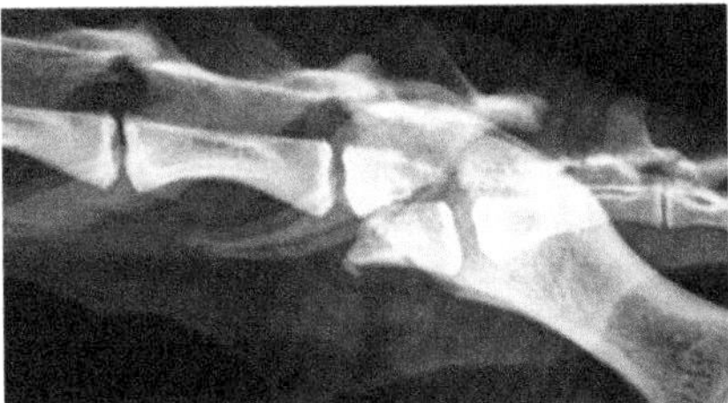

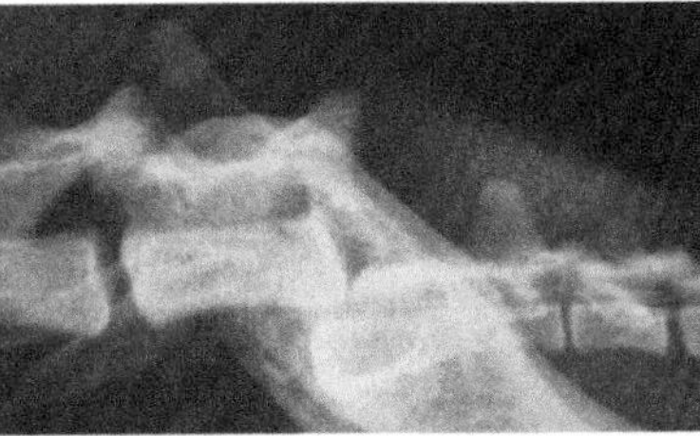

Fig. 4. Lateral radiographs of VFL of the lumbosacral junction to illustrate typical lesion orientation. (*Left*) An oblique fracture through the body of L7 vertebral body with cranioventral displacement of the caudal portion is typical of fractures at this location in both dogs and cats. (*Right*) In cats there is sometimes cranioventral luxation of the sacral portion without fractures of the vertebral body or articular processes.

and anal reflexes.[26] This finding can lead to the suspicion that the lesion is located within the lower motor neuron section of the spinal cord rather than more cranially. The panniculus reflex is often useful in discriminating between these possibilities because it will exhibit a "cutoff" level indicating a lesion within the T3 to L3 spinal cord segment. The signs of spinal shock are temporary and most will abate within 24 to 48 hours; this alteration is readily detected during serial neurologic examinations.

A further problem in neurologic localization is the possibility of multiple injuries: the "2-lesion problem" (**Fig. 5**). For instance, a lower motor neuron lesion will disguise the presence of an upper motor neuron lesion because the depressed postural reactions can be attributed to the lower motor neuron lesion. Similarly, lesions affecting the brain can inhibit the ability to detect spinal cord lesions within the C1 to C5 region because they provide an explanation for depressed postural reactions in the thoracic limbs. A useful distinguishing feature in this instance can be the frequency with which brain lesions are distinctly lateralized. In general, because of the risk of inadvertent injury through excessive movement, it is wise to assume that there are multiple neurologic injuries until proven otherwise.

Imaging

As a general rule, radiographs are sufficient to diagnose the majority of VFL.[23] Multiple VFL occur in approximately 5% to 10% of all affected animals[10,11] and therefore it is prudent to acquire lateral radiographs of the whole vertebral column (and the skull if appropriate). If sedation or anesthesia is required for radiography, extreme care must be exercised during movement and positioning of the animal for radiographs because of the associated loss of muscle tone. It is usually most convenient to obtain lateral radiographs as a survey, followed by ventrodorsal views of suspect regions if necessary. If at all possible, it is highly preferable to obtain the ventrodorsal views with the animal in lateral recumbency.

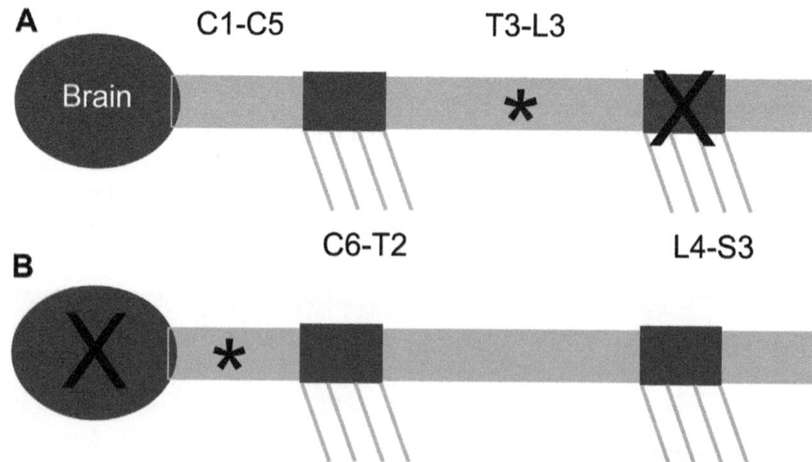

Fig. 5. Two examples of the "2-lesion problem"; there are many similar possibilities elsewhere in the nervous system. (*A*) A lesion affecting the lower motor neuron (LMN) component of limb control (*cross*) will obscure the presence of a second lesion within the T3-L3 segment of the spinal cord (*asterisk*) because the depressed postural reactions indicating a lesion at T3-L3 can be attributed to the LMN lesion only. (*B*) A lesion in the brain (*cross*), particularly one in the brainstem, may depress postural reactions in the limbs, thus obscuring the effect of a second lesion within the C1-C5 spinal cord segments (*asterisk*).

In cases in which a VFL is still suspected because of typical clinical signs and history, but which cannot be diagnosed with plain radiographs, the best subsequent choice is computed tomography (CT). This 3-dimensional imaging modality provides excellent definition of the vertebral bone (and with appropriate adjustment, ligamentous structures) and allows appreciation of impingement of disrupted material into the vertebral canal. If CT is not available, magnetic resonance imaging (MRI) provides an excellent method to identify regions of damage to the spinal cord, but images of bone are relatively poor. Contrast-enhanced imaging (myelography or CT myelography) is not usually justified because it will rarely produce additional useful information, and the necessary positioning (ie, flexion of the spine) may sometimes expose the animal to further risks. In addition, radiographic contrast material in the subarachnoid space can obscure clear visibility of bone fragments or other radiopaque material within the spinal canal.

TREATMENT

Options

The overriding objective of treatment of VFL is to provide an environment in which damaged neural tissues can recover optimal function. Therefore, the primary aims are to limit further damage (which could occur through persistent instability) and to relieve compression (by reestablishing normal dimensions and orientation to the vertebral canal and intervertebral foramina). In accordance with these aims, unstable and neurologically deteriorating animals (and, arguably, those with severe deficits) are usually optimally treated by surgery. An additional advantage is that it is often easier and less painful to care for VFL animals soon after surgical intervention than it is to provide optimal nursing care for animals that must be rested or retain external coaptation devices for prolonged periods. Nevertheless, many VFL do not require surgical intervention; such cases would usually exhibit minimal (or no) pain or neurologic deficit, minimal instability, or both. However, there is plentiful evidence that many other VFL can be satisfactorily managed nonoperatively.[7,13,27–29]

Thus, the critical factor in determining whether conservative or surgical therapy is most appropriate hinges on the issue of "instability." Instability in the context of VFL has traditionally been difficult to define, although appreciation of the forces acting on the vertebral column to create the lesion may lead to an understanding of whether it is likely or not. More recently, the application of analysis using the "3-column system" is very helpful in many cases. This scheme was originally developed for VFL treatment algorithms in human patients[30] and has since been adapted for use in dogs.[31] The concept is that there are 3 columns extending the length of the vertebral column and if 2 or more of these columns are disrupted, then there is instability (**Fig. 6**). A drawback to this approach is that it is necessary to appreciate that the position of the vertebrae on a single image does not necessarily reflect the full possible range of motion of the affected segment, nor the extent of movement that occurred at the time of the inciting incident.

Timing

It is surprising that there has long been controversy regarding how quickly to intervene in human VFL; however, this reflects to some extent the superior ability to instruct human patients to lie immobile for prolonged periods during which time their injuries can heal. The source of controversy is that many spinal cord injury patients have multiple organ trauma, and early intervention can risk the life of the patient if they are not suitably stabilized before anesthesia. Despite this controversy, there recently has been a developing consensus in favor of early intervention, which appears to be

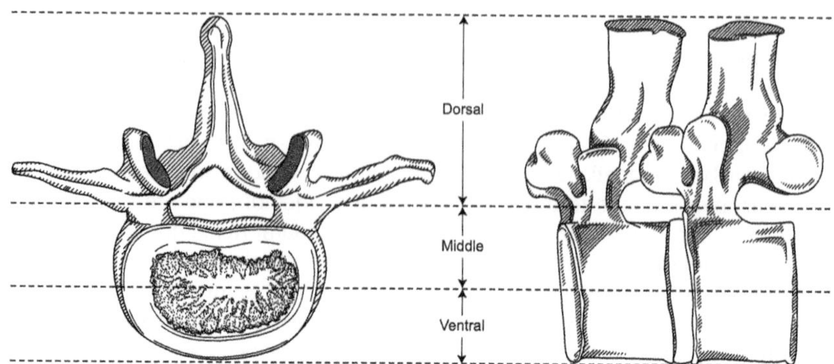

Fig. 6. The "3-column" system for assessing stability within the vertebral column. The dorsal column consists of the laminae, spinous processes, and their associated ligaments. The middle column consists of the dorsal longitudinal ligament, dorsal annulus, and dorsal cortex of the vertebral bodies. The ventral column consists of the ventral longitudinal ligament, ventral annulus, and ventral cortex of the vertebral bodies. (*Modified from* Shores A. Spinal trauma. Pathophysiology and management of traumatic spinal injuries. Vet Clin North Am Small Anim Pract 1992;22(4):875; with permission.)

associated with superior survival and neurologic outcome.[32–34] Nevertheless it is critical when translating this finding into veterinary patients to carefully consider the risks to life, or the risk of inducing a damaging reduction in blood pressure (which can worsen neural injuries) incurred through too hasty induction of anesthesia.

Application of Conservative Therapy

Although several types of external coaptation are available (see Refs.[7,28]), such as splinting and casting, experience with these options is often rather depressing because there are many possible complications, including loosening, skin abrasion sores, and pain. In addition, these external devices often increase the difficulties associated with bladder and bowel care. The easiest cases to handle nonoperatively are ambulatory cervical VFL patients, for instance those that have dens fractures.[7] For all cervical VFL it is often sufficient to simply wrap the cervical region in a padded dressing similar to how Robert Jones dressings are applied routinely applied to orthopedic patients. It is imperative to bear in mind the precise area that is being immobilized; mid-cervical VFL are the most straightforward because this area is easiest to immobilize, while those at the cranial and caudal limits of the cervical area are more difficult, because the bandage must be sufficiently tight to provide support but not so tight as to obstruct venous return. A bandage that is applied too loosely can increase motion at the cranial and caudal limits because the mid-section is immobilized.

Although splinting techniques for thoracic and lumbar VFL have been described,[29] they are frequently difficult to apply. Therefore, many conservatively treated VFL of this region are simply confined to a cage and taken out, on nonslip flooring, for toileting purposes only.

Application of Surgical Therapy

Decompression is usually attained simply by reducing the VFL; putting the bones back in their normal position will alleviate the compression in almost all cases. The possible—and rare—exceptions are those in which fractured pieces or bone remain within the vertebral canal. The need to remove small bone fragments is controversial and many studies suggest that it is unnecessary.[35–37] Instead it is thought that the small fragments are repulsed from the spinal cord by the rhythmic oscillations associated with respiratory movements and then are absorbed, perhaps because of loss of mechanical loading.[38] Studies in human patients show that what at first can be reasonably severe compression associated with bone fragments is gradually lost with time. Consequently, it would seem that there is a limited need for laminectomy or hemilaminectomy in the treatment of VFL. Exceptions might perhaps be made in cases in which transverse imaging defines portions of intervertebral disc annulus or nucleus within the canal and causing significant compression (ie, more than approximately 35%–50% of vertebral canal diameter).[39,40] Additional drawbacks to laminectomy or hemilaminectomy are the risks of causing further instability and increasing the difficulty in application of stabilizing implants. Occasionally, for instance in cases in which pain is the only clinical sign, simple removal of bone fragments may be all that is required (**Fig. 7**).

Stabilization is a key element of surgical treatment of VFL. After the bones have been replaced into the correct, or near-correct position, they must be fixed in place with orthopedic implants. During the reduction process, it is critical to realize that replacement of the bones into EXACTLY the correct position is very much secondary to the aim of preventing further injury to the spinal cord or risking iatrogenic further injury, because the spinal cord is able to tolerate considerable deformation in shape and size (ie, "compression") so long as it is static. Therefore, incomplete reduction without further trauma is greatly preferable to complete reduction that has caused additional neural injury. To decrease the risk of iatrogenic injury during reduction it is therefore important to have a reliable and tight grasp on the relevant fragments with appropriate instrumentation (towel clamps are frequently useful!) and to make the reduction in a simple, atraumatic movement and then hold the bones stably in position. It is almost always essential to have a surgical assistant.

Surgical Techniques

There are many surgical techniques by which the vertebrae can be stabilized in position once reduced. The variety of techniques required reflects the variation in shape of the vertebrae at different levels and the site and nature of adjacent anatomic structures, meaning that one technique cannot be universally applied to all VFL. Even when treating VFL within specific locations, there are no prospective trials to determine which technique is preferable in general or for specific VFL, and choice is often a personal preference. Furthermore, there is often a need to treat each VFL as a unique

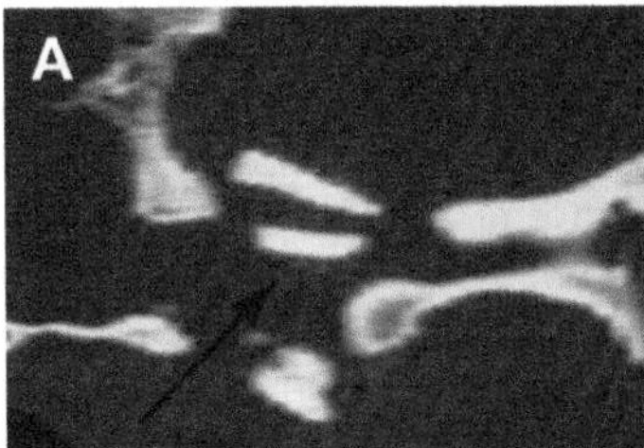

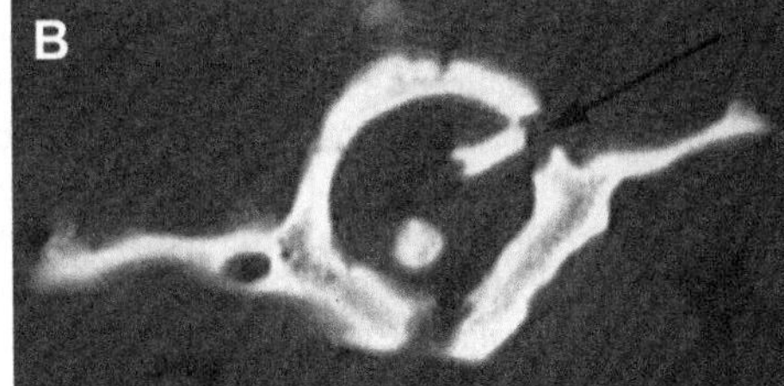

Fig. 7. CT scans of a fracture of the atlas from a dog with severe cervical pain but no neurologic deficits. (*A*) Sagittal reformatted image. (*B*) Transverse image, demonstrating loss of integrity of the arch of the atlas, with a detached bone fragment encroaching into the vertebral canal (*arrow*). The dog recovered uneventfully after removal of the loose fragment.

case and pragmatically adapt the well-described basic techniques to overcome specific problems that are encountered.

Any effective technique must permit stabilization by neutralizing the forces acting on the VFL, and be applicable without iatrogenic injury to neural tissue or neighboring structures. At each site it is often necessary to apply temporary fixation, such as interfacet wiring, that allows reduction while the definitive fixation is placed. The possible definitive techniques are now discussed with regard to applications at each location.

Atlantoaxial

Fractures of the dens are the most common VFL of the cervical spine in small animal patients, accounting for about one-third of all cervical fractures,[7] and are usually associated with dorsal displacement of the body of the axis relative to the atlas. Subluxation of the atlantoaxial joint is very common in small dogs, and can occur after minimal trauma if there is congenital hypoplasia of the dens. Several techniques have been used to stabilize the atlantoaxial junction after both fractures and subluxations, but these have not been compared against each other in controlled randomized trials, meaning that robust recommendations for preferred technique are not possible. Nevertheless, the following techniques have all been used successfully[41,42]: conservative,[43] dorsal wiring or modifications,[44,45] ventral cross-pinning or modifications,[46,47] dorsal pinning,[48] and ventral plating.[49]

Conservative therapy has been very successful in many cases with minimal clinical signs after fracture of the dens,[43] but would not usually be a first-choice option for a grossly displaced fracture or one in which the clinical signs are severe. Dorsal approaches that rely on passing a suture ventral to the dorsal arch of the axis carry the risk of iatrogenic injury to the medulla, either directly through contact, or indirectly through the flexion at the atlantoaxial junction that is required to pass the suture. Drilling away a part of the arch to facilitate passage of the suture can weaken the structure, increasing the risk of subsequent failure through bone tearing. Dorsal cross-pinning is designed to avoid these problems, but it can be difficult to place the pins appropriately. Ventral approaches carry the advantage that it is possible to promote fusion through bone grafting across the articular facets of axis and atlas, but carry the risk of failure though metallic implants tearing through the small mass of relatively soft bone.

Cervical

Fractures of the cervical spine usually involve concomitant luxation or subluxation, occasionally without any discernible fracture (see **Fig. 3**). Because of the shape of the bones in this region, simple, specifically tailored fixation[50] is frequently feasible (**Fig. 8**). The large vertebral bodies and convenient access via a ventral approach means that ventral application of pins (or screws) and polymethylmethacrylate (PMMA) is a common method of choice.[51,52] Conventional plating is difficult to apply, because it is not usually possible to ensure 2 cortical penetrations for each screw and difficult to place a sufficient number of screws to ensure sufficient holding to prevent loosening. Recently, the use of locking plates (eg, "ComPact" or "SOP" plates) has overcome these difficulties because their screws need penetrate only one cortex (see Ref.[53]) and, in the case of SOP plates, can more readily be contoured in all 3 planes to provide optimal screw placement. Fixation using the spinous processes is generally inappropriate because of their small size. Conservative therapy can be an attractive option for minimally displaced VFL.

Thoracic

Fractures in this region rarely require internal fixation, and usually simple cage rest will suffice to allow recovery. Fractures often involve portions of the vertebral body, such

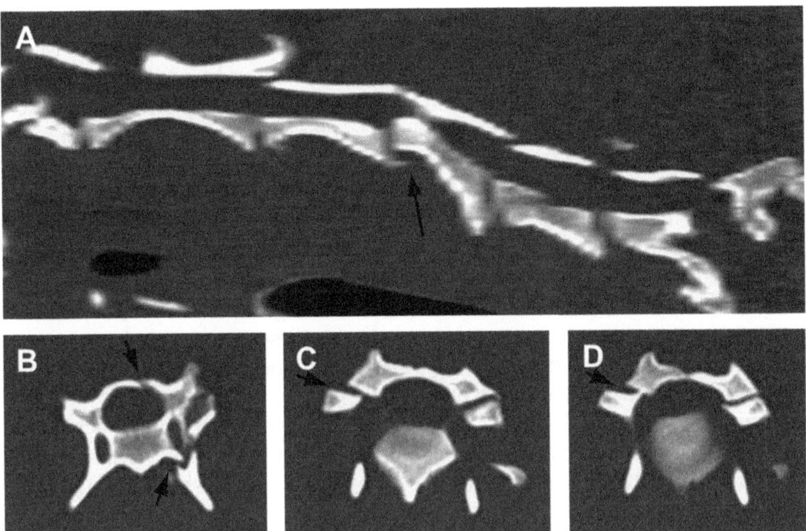

Fig. 8. CT scans of a cervical fracture-luxation in a dog with severe cervical pain. (*A*) sagittal reformatted image illustrating subluxation between C3 and C4 vertebrae (*arrow*). (*B*) Transverse image illustrating fractures of C4 lamina and transverse process (*arrows*). (*C, D*) Transverse images through C3/4 articulation demonstrating unilateral subluxation of the articular processes. This VFL was reduced and stabilized with a single wire suture similar to that shown in **Fig. 3**.

as the epiphyses or wedge fractures. The specific anatomic features of note here are the very large spinous processes, which provide good bone for fixation, the small vertebral bodies, and the limitations of access to the ventral aspect of the vertebrae posed by the sternum and rib cage.

The most easily applicable technique here is segmental pin-and-wire fixation (a modification of previous "spinal stapling" techniques), in which several K-wires or pins are applied parallel to the vertebral column and attached to the spinous processes and articular facets using wire[54]; a modified technique has also been reported,[55] by which tension can be applied to the VFL site. These techniques can provide very satisfactory fixation and neutralize forces in all 3 planes, and although relatively unstable in torsion this is not a particular problem in this region of the spine. The main drawback to this technique is the prolonged amount of time that can be required to expose and fix wires to 3 (or sometimes more) sites on each of at least 5 vertebrae. In the more caudal part of the thoracic spine vertebral bodies are larger and the ribs do not greatly obscure the operation site, so use of pins and PMMA[52] provides an acceptable alternative.

Thoracolumbar junction

The thoracolumbar junction is a very common site of VFL.[10,12] There are a variety of methods that can be used successfully, but the most popular are vertebral body plating,[56,57] pins and PMMA,[52] and segmental pin and wires.[54] The most popular during the past decade has been probably pins plus PMMA because it is a flexible method that can be applied to any vertebra with accessible (and relatively large) vertebral bodies, and the PMMA provides adequate fixation to allow eventual spinal stability and fusion. In some cases, in which the instability is relatively mild, unilateral application can be sufficient. The main drawbacks to PMMA use are the increased risk of persistent infection—which makes this a poor choice for open fractures—and the difficulties sometimes encountered with muscle and skin closure over a large mass of PMMA.

Conventional bone plating provides excellent stability when applied appropriately but can be technically difficult because of the size of the implants relative to the size of the vertebral bodies; it can be difficult to place a suitable number of screws. Use of corticocancellous 3.5-mm screws in a 2.7-mm dynamic compression plate can provide a very appropriate solution to this problem in many 10- to 35-kg dogs (**Fig. 9**). Impingement of a plate on the nerve root can be problematic, but the nerve roots can be sectioned in this area without severe deficits or further problems. As mentioned earlier, SOP plates provide another, more adaptable method to treat fractures or instability at this location.[58] These plates allow greater flexibility in placement, do not need to be contoured accurately to the bone surfaces, and lock into place without the need for double cortical penetration. Placement of 2 SOP plates provides the necessary number of screws for each vertebra.

Segmental pin and wires is another option, although limited by the drawbacks outlined (time considerations and excessive muscle dissection), but can be appropriate if there is a problem with integrity of the ventral portions of the vertebral bodies such that placement of fixation through the bodies would enhance instability or risk further fractures.

In the past, dorsal plastic (Lubra) plating has been used,[59] but this technique is dependent on intact spinous processes that are not always available. The ability of the plates to grip the spinous processes relies on friction.

Lumbar

The same techniques as used at the thoracolumbar junction are appropriate, although more caudally (ie, L5–L7) it can be difficult to gain sufficient access to the lateral aspect of the vertebral bodies to apply PMMA and pins, or more especially, plates. Furthermore, it is not an option to cut the roots at this level because these nerves innervate the pelvic limb musculature. Segmental pin and wires is therefore often a more useful option, especially because fractures at this level are often more oblique and difficult to stabilize before fixation.

Lumbosacral junction

This area presents several difficulties in fixation, most notably gaining access to the lateral aspect of the vertebral bodies that lie medial to the wings of the ilia. Fortunately a large proportion comprise oblique fractures of the caudal part of L7 with ventral

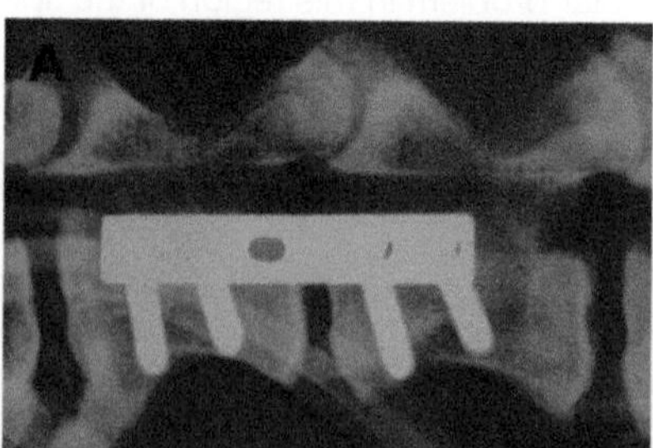

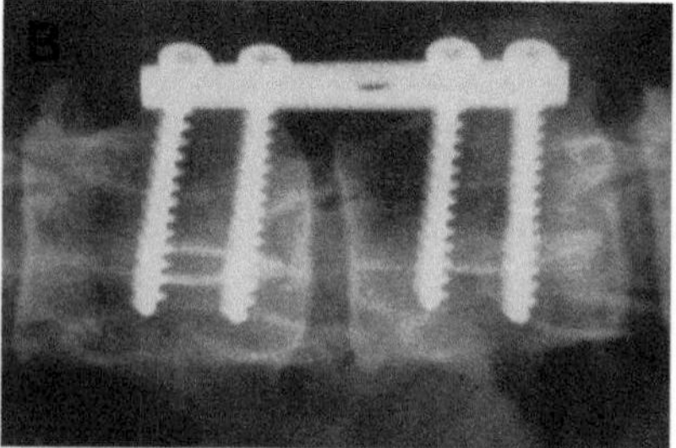

Fig. 9. Lateral (*A*) and ventrodorsal (*B*) radiographs of stabilized luxation between L1 and L2 vertebrae (resulting from discospondylitis) demonstrating the use of a 5-hole 2.7-mm dynamic compression plate combined with 4 3.5-mm diameter screws to take advantage of their superior bone gripping characteristics in vertebral body bone. Because the screws do not match the plate, their heads do not sink into the plate and give the appearance of being loose.

displacement of the sacrum. This VFL lends itself to stabilization with a simple transilial bar,[60] although sometimes additional support is also required (**Fig. 10**). Further approaches include extension of segmental pin and wires to include the ilia, and using pins and PMMA partly anchored into the ilia,[61,62] or combination with external fixators,[63] or with plastic plates.[64] One should realize that the vertebral canal of this region contains the cauda equina (spinal nerve) rather than the spinal cord. This configuration carries several implications: (a) recovery after spinal or peripheral nerve injury is usually much better than that after spinal cord injury; (b) loss of "deep pain sensation" does not carry the same grave prognosis as it would for spinal cord injury; and (c) nerve compression is often exceedingly painful and may require rapid decompression.

Sacral, sacrococcygeal, and intercoccygeal VFL

Sacrococcygeal and intercoccygeal fractures are very common injuries in cats and are thought to result from traction on the tail; they can cause lesions that affect urination as well as tail function. Prognosis is usually determined at the time of injury,[25] although it is possible that stabilization (or removal of the weight of the tail by amputation) may provide a more conducive environment in which the nerves can recover. Interfacet wiring (or use of nylon sutures) or adaptations of the spinal stapling techniques are most appropriate because the vertebral bodies are too small to allow fixation. Several different orientations of sacral fractures have been described,[65] which require individually tailored treatment depending on their stability and associated neurologic deficits.[66] Most commonly, reduction and stabilization have been assumed to occur during reduction of associated pelvic fractures.

CARE AND REHABILITATION OF ANIMALS THAT HAVE SUFFERED VFL

The intensity of care required for animals that have suffered VFL is variable, depending on the severity of the initial deficits and the type of intervention that has been used. In general, care for animals that have undergone surgery is more straightforward, because stability at the injury site allows for more vigorous handling without causing pain. The priorities in care are pain relief, reducing the risk of complications of

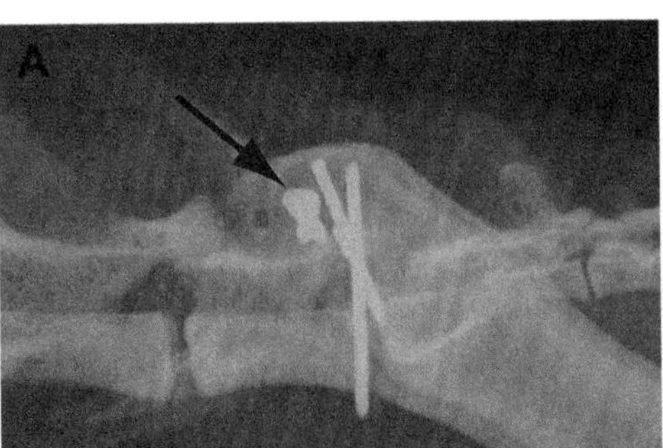

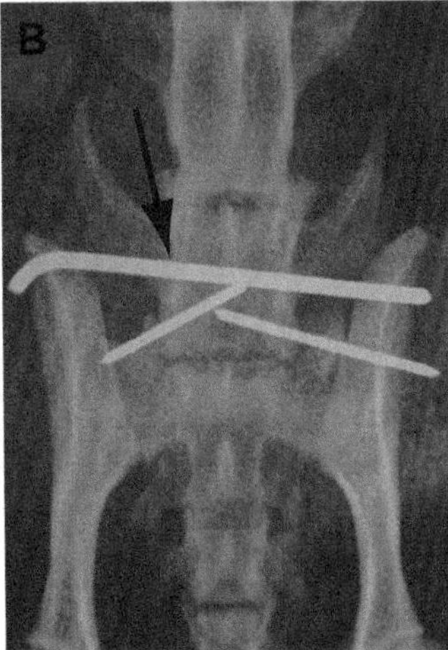

Fig. 10. Lateral (*A*) and ventrodorsal (*B*) radiographs of a stabilized L7/S1 luxation in a cat (see **Fig. 4**B). One transilial bar (*arrow*) is stabilizing the luxation but 2 K-wires were placed across the articular processes during surgery to provide interim stability and left in situ.

recumbency (especially pneumonia), emptying of the urinary bladder, and physiotherapy to promote limb use and reduce muscle atrophy.

Many drugs can be used for pain relief, extending from nonsteroidal anti-inflammatories to infusions of opiates. Many animals that have incurred VFL are in severe pain and opiate administration is mandatory; methadone and morphine are the most appropriate drugs for use in the early postinjury period in most instances, and pain relief can then be tapered through less potent drugs (such as buprenorphine and oral opiate drugs). Loss of appetite following opiate administration can be a problem, but is usually short lasting.

Prevention of complications of recumbency is best attended to by frequent moving of the animal, using slings and other support as necessary. Frequent (ie, every 2–4 hours) turning is also useful so that congestion of the lungs and pooling of blood in the extremities is discouraged. Coupage of the lungs may aid coughing to clear secretions from the airways and reduce the risk of pneumonia. Thick padded bedding is essential to prevent the development of bed sores, especially in large dogs.

There are several options for managing disorders of bladder emptying, including manual expression (or, more correctly in UMN lesions, "triggering" of urination), and intermittent and indwelling catheterization. There are complications with each method, and certain techniques are more appropriate for specific disorders. For instance, "lower motor neuron" bladder disorders, in which there is little resistance to bladder emptying, would be most easily treated by manual expression, whereas those animals with very high sphincter tone would be better treated by catheterization. Incomplete emptying (which is often a complication of manual expression of "upper motor neuron" bladders) and nonaseptic catheterization both carry the risk of urinary tract infections, which can be fatal. A recent study suggested that the infection rate following either method was similar and that infection risk was associated with duration of bladder dysfunction[67]; indiscriminate use of prophylactic antibiotics in animals with indwelling catheters should be avoided.[68]

Physiotherapy following spinal cord injury takes several forms depending on the stage after the injury. Initially, animals are frequently in a lot of pain when moved and so physiotherapy interventions must be gentle and can consist solely of massage of the limbs to promote better blood flow. As time progresses it is then useful to start simple range of motion exercises, with the affected paralyzed limbs being manipulated into "cycling" type movements simulating normal walking (often best in reverse). Later, as the animal becomes able to make more robust voluntary movements, swimming or partially submerged treadmill walking are widely used, although their efficacy in promoting recovery remains to be demonstrated.

It is imperative that a prolonged period of recovery is allowed for animals that have severe injuries. In human medicine it is well established that full recovery from a spinal cord injury may take up to (and sometimes even longer) than 12 months, and quadriplegic human patients are commonly hospitalized for up to 9 months. Recovery appears to take place more quickly in dogs and cats; most recovery of function will occur by 3 months after the injury. The author's own observations suggest that severely injured patients often do not exhibit any change in function within up to 2 to 3 weeks, yet will ultimately recover satisfactory function. It is important not to euthanize such cases prematurely!

COMPLICATIONS

Complications following VFL are reasonably common and are often associated with limb disuse and bladder dysfunction. Implants can become loosened in situ, which commonly presents as pain, and postoperative infection can be a problem, especially in association with PMMA implants. Revision surgery is occasionally required to remove or replace implants.

SUMMARY

Few new techniques for the treatment of VFL have emerged during the past decade, but the increasingly widespread availability of advanced imaging facilities has enabled veterinarians to diagnose VFL with greater reliability and appreciate in detail the exact nature of the vertebral column injuries. This advance has permitted a more "tailored" approach to treatment, such that the specific anomalies associated with each VFL can be attended to specifically. For this reason, unilateral pins and bone cement fixation in the thoracolumbar segment and unilateral facet wiring in the cervical area have been recognized as feasible, and have become prominent methods of treating VFL in small animals. Future improvement in outcome after VFL is most likely to arise from new developments in the treatment of spinal cord injury.

REFERENCES

1. Marioni-Henry K, Vite CH, Newton AL, et al. Prevalence of diseases of the spinal cord of cats. J Vet Intern Med 2004;18(6):851–8.
2. Fluehmann G, Doherr MG, Jaggy A. Canine neurological diseases in a referral hospital population between 1989 and 2000 in Switzerland. J Small Anim Pract 2006;47(10):582–7.
3. Crowe DT. Patient triage. In: Siverstein DC, Hopper K, editors. Small animal critical care medicine. 1st edition. Missouri: Elsevier; 2009. p. 5–9.
4. Evans HE. The skeleton. In: Evans HE, editor. Miller's anatomy of the dog. 3rd edition. Philadelphia: WB Saunders; 1993. p. 122–218.
5. Evans HE. Arthrology. In: Evans HE, editor. Miller's anatomy of the dog. 3rd edition. Philadelphia: WB Saunders; 1993. p. 219–57.
6. Breit S. Osteological and morphometric observations on intervertebral joints in the canine pre-diaphragmatic thoracic spine (Th1-Th9). Vet J 2002;164(3): 216–23.
7. Hawthorne JC, Blevins WE, Wallace LJ, et al. Cervical vertebral fractures in 56 dogs: a retrospective study. J Am Anim Hosp Assoc 1999;35(2):135–46.
8. Jeffery ND, Blakemore WF. Spinal cord injury in small animals. 1. Mechanisms of spontaneous recovery. Vet Rec 1999;144(15):407–13.
9. Beal MW, Paglia DT, Griffin GM, et al. Ventilatory failure, ventilator management, and outcome in dogs with cervical spinal disorders: 14 cases (1991–1999). J Am Vet Med Assoc 2001;218(10):1598–602.
10. Bali MS, Lang J, Jaggy A, et al. Comparative study of vertebral fractures and luxations in dogs and cats. Vet Comp Orthop Traumatol 2009;22(1): 47–53.
11. Feeney DA, Oliver JE. Blunt spinal trauma in the dog and cat: insight into radiographic lesions. J Am Anim Hosp Assoc 1980;16(6):885–90.
12. Bruce CW, Brisson BA, Gyselinck K. Spinal fracture and luxation in dogs and cats: a retrospective evaluation of 95 cases. Vet Comp Orthop Traumatol 2008; 21(3):280–4.
13. Selcer RR, Bubb WJ, Walker TL. Management of vertebral column fractures in dogs and cats: 211 cases (1977-1985). J Am Vet Med Assoc 1991;198(11): 1965–8.

14. Heyman SJ, Diefenderfer DL, Goldschmidt MH, et al. Canine axial skeletal osteosarcoma. A retrospective study of 116 cases (1986 to 1989). Vet Surg 1992; 21(4):304–10.
15. Chauvet AE, Hogge GS, Sandin JA, et al. Vertebrectomy, bone allograft fusion, and antitumor vaccination for the treatment of vertebral fibrosarcoma in a dog. Vet Surg 1999;28(6):480–8.
16. Cabassu J, Moissonnier P. Surgical treatment of a vertebral fracture associated with a haematogenous osteomyelitis in a dog. Vet Comp Orthop Traumatol 2007;20(3):227–30.
17. Moens NM, Runyon CL. Fracture of L7 vertebral articular facets and pedicles following dorsal laminectomy in a dog. J Am Vet Med Assoc 2002;6:807–10.
18. Oliver J, Selcer R, Simpson S. Cauda equina compression from lumbosacral malarticulation and malformation in the dog. J Am Vet Med Assoc 1978;173: 207–14.
19. Kinzel S, Koch J, Stopinski T, et al. Cauda equina compression syndrome: retrospective study of surgical treatment with partial dorsal laminectomy in 86 dogs with lumbosacral stenosis. Berl Munch Tierartzl Wochenschr 2004;117:334–40.
20. Pleasant RS, Baker GJ, Muhlbauer MC, et al. Stress reactions and stress fractures of the proximal palmar aspect of the third metacarpal bone in horses: 58 cases (1980–1990). J Am Vet Med Assoc 1992;201(12):1918–23.
21. Moissonnier P, Meheust P, Carozzo C. Thoracolumbar lateral corpectomy for treatment of chronic disk herniation: technique description and use in 15 dogs. Vet Surg 2004;33(6):620–8.
22. Bruecker KA. Principles of vertebral fracture management. Semin Vet Med Surg (Small Anim) 1996;11(4):259–72.
23. Kinns J, Mai W, Seiler G, et al. Radiographic sensitivity and negative predictive value for acute canine spinal trauma. Vet Radiol Ultrasound 2006;47(6):563–70.
24. Hansen HJ. A pathologic-anatomical study on disc degeneration in dog, with special reference to the so-called enchondrosis intervertebralis. Acta Orthop Scand Suppl 1952;11:1–117.
25. Smeak DD, Olmstead ML. Fracture/luxation if the sacrococcygeal area in the cat: a retrospective study of 51 cases. Vet Surg 1985;14(4):319–24.
26. Smith PM, Jeffery ND. Spinal shock–comparative aspects and clinical relevance. J Vet Intern Med 2005;19(6):788–93.
27. Bagley RS. Spinal fracture or luxation. Vet Clin North Am Small Anim Pract 2000; 30(1):133–53.
28. Carberry CA, Flanders JA, Dietz AE, et al. Nonsurgical management of thoracic and lumbar spinal fractures and fracture/luxations in the dog and cat: a review of 17 cases. J Am Anim Hosp Assoc 1989;25(1):43–5.
29. Patterson RH, Smith GK. Backsplinting for treatment of thoracic and lumbar fracture/luxation in the dog: principles of application and case series. Vet Comp Orthop Traumatol 1992;4:179–87.
30. Denis F. Spinal instability as defined by the three-column spine concept in acute spinal trauma. Clin Orthop Relat Res 1984;189:65–76.
31. Shores A. Spinal trauma. Pathophysiology and management of traumatic spinal injuries. Vet Clin North Am Small Anim Pract 1992;22(4):859–88.
32. La Rosa G, Conti A, Cardali S, et al. Does early decompression improve neurological outcome of spinal cord injured patients? Appraisal of the literature using a meta-analytical approach. Spinal Cord 2004;42(9):503–12.
33. Croce MA, Bee TK, Pritchard E, et al. Does optimal timing for spine fracture fixation exist? Ann Surg 2001;233(6):851–8.

34. Fehlings MG, Perrin RG. The timing of surgical intervention in the treatment of spinal cord injury: a systematic review of recent clinical evidence. Spine 2006; 31(Suppl 11):S28–35.
35. Leferink VJ, Nijboer JM, Zimmerman KW, et al. Burst fractures of the thoracolumbar spine: changes of the spinal canal during operative treatment and follow-up. Eur Spine J 2003;12(3):255–60.
36. Chakera TM, Bedbrook G, Bradley CM. Spontaneous resolution of spinal canal deformity after burst-dispersion fracture. AJNR Am J Neuroradiol 1988;9(4):779–85.
37. Dai LY. Remodeling of the spinal canal after thoracolumbar burst fractures. Clin Orthop Relat Res 2001;382:119–23.
38. Scapinelli R, Candiotto S. Spontaneous remodeling of the spinal canal after burst fractures of the low thoracic and lumbar region. J Spinal Disord 1995;8(6): 486–93.
39. Hashimoto T, Kaneda K, Abumi K. Relationship between traumatic spinal canal stenosis and neurologic deficits in thoracolumbar burst fractures. Spine 1988; 13(11):1268–72.
40. Dimar JR 2nd, Glassman SD, Raque GH, et al. The influence of spinal canal narrowing and timing of decompression on neurologic recovery after spinal cord contusion in a rat model. Spine 1999;24(16):1623–33.
41. Thomas WB, Sorjonen DC, Simpson ST. Surgical management of atlantoaxial subluxation in 23 dogs. Vet Surg 1991;20(6):409–12.
42. Beaver DP, Ellison GW, Lewis DD, et al. Risk factors affecting the outcome of surgery for atlantoaxial subluxation in dogs: 46 cases (1978–1998). J Am Vet Med Assoc 2000;216(7):1104–9.
43. Havig ME, Cornell KK, Hawthorne JC, et al. Evaluation of nonsurgical treatment of atlantoaxial subluxation in dogs: 19 cases (1992–2001). J Am Vet Med Assoc 2005;227(2):257–62.
44. Chambers JN, Betts CW, Oliver JE. The use of non-metallic suture material for stabilization of atlantoaxial subluxation. J Am Anim Hosp 1977;13:602–4.
45. LeCouteur RA, McKeown D, Johnson J, et al. Stabilization of atlantoaxial subluxation in the dog, using the nuchal ligament. J Am Vet Med Assoc 1980;177(10): 1011–7.
46. Sorjonen DC, Shires PK. Atlanto-axial instability: a ventral surgical technique for decompression, fixation and fusion. Vet Surg 1981;10:22–9.
47. Denny HR, Gibbs C, Waterman A. Atlantoaxial subluxation in the dog: a review of 30 cases and an evaluation of treatment by lag screw fixation. J Small Anim Pract 1988;29:37–47.
48. Jeffery ND. Dorsal cross pinning of the atlantoaxial joint: new surgical technique for atlantoaxial subluxation. J Small Anim Pract 1996;37(1):26–9.
49. Stead AC, Anderson AA, Coughlan A. Bone plating to stabilize atlanto-axial subluxation in four dogs. J Small Anim Pract 1993;34:462–5.
50. Seim HB. Surgery of the cervical spine. In: Fossum TW, editor. Small animal surgery. 3rd edition. Missouri (Iowa): Mosby; 2007. p. 1402–59.
51. Blass CE, Waldron DR, van Ee RT. Cervical stabilization in three dogs using Steinman pins and methylmethacrylate. J Am Anim Hosp Assoc 1988;24:61.
52. Blass CE, Seim HB. Spinal fixation in dogs using Sreinman pins and methylmethacrylate. Vet Surg 1984;13:203–10.
53. Trotter EJ. Cervical spine locking plate fixation for treatment of cervical spondylotic myelopathy in large breed dogs. Vet Surg 2009;38(6):705–18.
54. McAnulty JF, Lenehan TM, Maletz LM. Modified segmental spinal stabilisation in repair of spinal fractures and luxations in dogs. Vet Surg 1986;15:143–9.

55. Voss K, Montavon PM. Tension band stabilization of fractures and luxations of the thoracolumbar vertebrae in dogs and cats: 38 cases (1993–2002). J Am Vet Med Assoc 2004;225(1):78–83.
56. Swaim SF. Vertebral body plating for spinal immobilization. J Am Vet Med Assoc 1971;158:1683–95.
57. McKee WM. Spinal trauma in dogs and cats: a review of 51 cases. Vet Rec 1990; 126(12):285–9.
58. McKee WM, Downes CJ. Vertebral stabilisation and selective decompression for the management of triple thoracolumbar disc protrusions. J Small Anim Pract 2008;49(10):536–9.
59. Yturraspe DJ, Lumb WV. The use of plastic spinal plates for internal fixation of the canine spine. J Am Vet Med Assoc 1972;161(12):1651–7.
60. Slocum B, Rudy RL. Fractures of the seventh lumbar vertebra in the dog. J Am Anim Hosp Assoc 1975;11:167–74.
61. Beaver DP, MacPherson GC, Muir P, et al. Methylmethacrylate and bone screw repair of seventh lumbar vertebral fracture-luxations in dogs. J Small Anim Pract 1996;37(8):381–6.
62. Weh JM, Kraus KH. Use of a four pin and methylmethacrylate fixation in L7 and the iliac body to stabilize lumbosacral fracture-luxations: a clinical and anatomic study. Vet Surg 2007;36(8):775–82.
63. Ullman SL, Boudrieau RJ. Internal skeletal fixation using a Kirschner apparatus for stabilization of fracture/luxations of the lumbosacral joint in six dogs. A modification of the transilial pin technique. Vet Surg 1993;22(1):11–7.
64. Lewis DD, Stampley A, Bellah JR, et al. Repair of sixth lumbar vertebral fracture-luxations, using transilial pins and plastic spinous-process plates in six dogs. J Am Vet Med Assoc 1989;194(4):538–42.
65. Anderson A, Coughlan AR. Sacral fractures in dogs and cats: a classification scheme and review of 51 cases. J Small Anim Pract 1997;38(9):404–9.
66. Kuntz CA, Waldron D, Martin RA, et al. Sacral fractures in dogs: a review of 32 cases. J Am Anim Hosp Assoc 1995;31(2):142–50.
67. Bubenik L, Hosgood G. Urinary tract infection in dogs with thoracolumbar intervertebral disc herniation and urinary bladder dysfunction managed by manual expression, indwelling catheterization or intermittent catheterization. Vet Surg 2008;37(8):791–800.
68. Bubenik LJ, Hosgood GL, Waldron DR, et al. Frequency of urinary tract infection in catheterized dogs and comparison of bacterial culture and susceptibility testing results for catheterized and noncatheterized dogs with urinary tract infections. J Am Vet Med Assoc 2007;231(6):893–9.

Intervertebral Disc Disease in Dogs

Brigitte A. Brisson, DMV, DVSc

KEYWORDS

- Intervertebral • Disc • Disk • Herniation • Fenestration
- Neurosurgery

Intervertebral disc (IVD) herniation is a common cause of neurologic dysfunction in dogs. During the last 60 years, IVD herniation has been the focus of significant research aiming to describe and understand this debilitating condition and to improve imaging and therapeutic options for clinical patients. This article is a summary of the clinically relevant literature that aims to guide clinicians in their decision making when diagnosing and treating canine IVD disease.

PATHOPHYSIOLOGY

Anatomy of the IVD

The IVDs are interposed between each vertebral body except the first and second cervical vertebrae (C1-C2) and each of the fused sacral vertebrae.[1,2] In a craniocaudal view, the cervical discs are nearly circular in shape, the thoracic discs are more oval, and the lumbar discs are bean shaped.[1] Thoracic discs are narrower than cervical and lumbar discs.[1,3] The caudal cervical discs (C4-C5 and C5-C6) along with the L2 to L3 disc space are the widest, whereas C2 to C3 and L4 to L5 are the narrowest.[4] Dachshunds are reported to have wider IVDs than other breeds.[4] The IVD is composed of an outer fibrous ring, the annulus fibrosus (AF), which surrounds an eccentric amorphous gelatinous center, the nucleus pulposus (NP).[1] Each disc is bound cranially and caudally by hyaline cartilaginous vertebral end plates,[1–3] and dorsally and ventrally by dorsal and ventral longitudinal ligaments.[1] The intercapital (conjugal) ligaments connect the rib heads from T2 to T10 crossing over each IVD and course between the AF and the dorsal longitudinal ligament.[1,2] This additional dorsal constraint is believed to reduce the rate of disc herniations between T2 to T3 and T10 to T11.[3,5–7] In contrast to King's findings,[1] Hansen[3] reported that the intercapital ligament at T10 is thin or nonexistent.

The AF is 1.5 to 2.8 times thicker ventrally than it is dorsally (**Figs. 1** and **2**), which results in the eccentric localization of the NP within the IVD and is believed to increase the risk for extrusion or herniation dorsally toward the vertebral canal.[1,2] Histologically,

Department of Clinical Studies, Ontario Veterinary College, University of Guelph, Guelph, Ontario N1G 2W1, Canada
E-mail address: bbrisson@uoguelph.ca

Vet Clin Small Anim 40 (2010) 829–858
doi:10.1016/j.cvsm.2010.06.001 **vetsmall.theclinics.com**
0195-5616/10/$ – see front matter

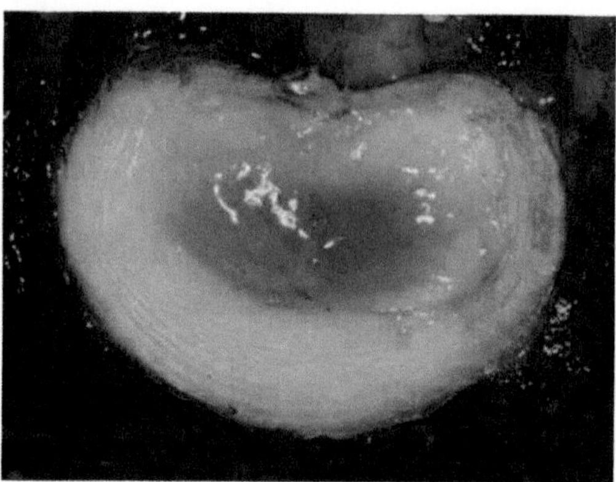

Fig. 1. Transverse section of a normal IVD. The AF bands surround the globoid and gelatinous NP. The ventral annulus is significantly thicker than the dorsal AF.

the AF is composed of an outer layer of densely packed collagen fibers in a fibrous matrix with a narrow inner layer of fibrocartilage located adjacent to the NP.[3,8] Seventy percent of the AF dry weight is from collagen.[9]

The NP is a remnant of the notochord that forms the central region of the IVD. Young, healthy discs contain a NP that is globoid and gelatinous with a high water content, allowing the disc to function as a hydroelastic cushion that maintains its width during loading (see **Fig. 1**).[9] Histologically, the NP is separated from the AF by a transitional or perinuclear zone (TZ).[3,8] Nonchondrodystrophic dogs have a narrow TZ, which consists of fibrocartilage, whereas the TZ of beagles and dachshunds is 3 to 4 times wider than that of greyhounds, is disorganized, and occupies the major portion of the AF.[3,8]

Only the outer layers of the AF are supplied by blood vessels.[3,10] The remainder of the AF and the NP are believed to receive their nutrition by diffusion through the cartilaginous end plates.[3,11,12] The peripheral third of the AF may be sparsely innervated,

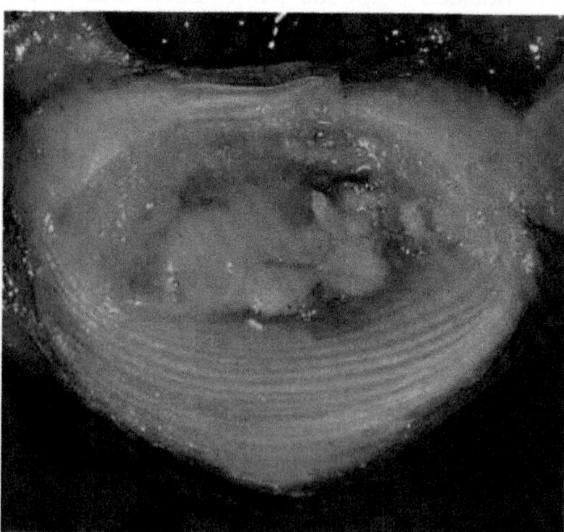

Fig. 2. Transverse section of a degenerate IVD from a chondrodystrophic dog. The gelatinous NP has been replaced by mineralized and chondroid material.

whereas the inner layers of the AF and NP are not innervated.[3,10] The dorsal longitudinal ligament overlying the IVD is extensively innervated and stretching and tearing of the outer AF and dorsal longitudinal ligament are proposed as a cause of discogenic pain in dogs.[10]

IVD Degeneration

IVD degeneration is a normal process that occurs with aging.[5,13] Degenerative changes in chondrodystrophic and nonchondrodystrophic IVD are generally referred to as chondroid metaplasia and fibrous metaplasia, respectively.[3,5,14]

Chondroid metaplasia is characterized by a loss of glycosaminoglycans, an increase in collagen content, and a decrease in water content, resulting in a general loss of the hydroelastic properties of the disc and its ability to withstand pressure.[9,14] The progressive transformation of the gelatinous NP to hyaline cartilage can begin as early as 2 months of age in dachshunds and involves the replacement of mesenchymal cells of the NP with chondrocyte-type cells.[3] The process begins in the TZ but eventually spreads to most of the NP and inner AF.[3,8] Grossly, the transparent gelatinous NP is transformed to a gray-white to yellow fibrocartilaginous tissue (see **Fig. 2**).[1,3] Chondrodystrophic dogs have 75% to 90% of their gelatinous NP transformed to a more hyaline and cartilaginous tissue by 1 year of age, whereas nonchondrodystrophic greyhound discs maintain high noncollagenous protein levels into old age.[3,9,14–17] Chondroid metaplasia occurs along the entire vertebral column. A total of 24% to 90% of dachshunds develop mineralization of one or more IVD, with a mean of 2.3 calcified discs per dog.[3,14,18–20] Calcifications have been reported in all discs,[3,18–20] but the discs of the thoracic region, especially between T10 and T13, are most frequently calcified radiographically.[18–21]

Fibrous metaplasia is an age-related degenerative process that occurs independently of breed but is documented more commonly in nonchondrodystrophic dogs 7 years and older.[3,5,14] It is characterized by a fibrous collagenization of the NP with concurrent degeneration of the AF and can occur anywhere along the vertebral column.[3,14] This degenerative process leads to bulging of the NP within the weakened AF and ultimately dorsal IVD protrusion.[3,14] Unlike its chondroid counterpart, fibrous metaplasia affects only a small number of discs and mineralization is infrequent.[3] A total of 40% to 60% of dogs aged 7 years or older show biochemical evidence of NP degeneration and 10% to 30% exhibit macroscopic IVD protrusion.[14]

IVD Extrusion and Protrusion

IVD extrusion (also known as Hansen type I) is typically associated with chondroid degeneration and involves the herniation of nuclear material through all layers of the ruptured AF into the vertebral canal.[3,5] The abnormal forces generated by the degenerate and mineralized NP cause tears to develop within the AF; as each break aligns, they form a channel through which the abnormal NP can eventually extrude.[3,5] Extruded disc material can be dispersed, showing no clear association with the parent disc space (sometimes classified as Funkquist type III), or nondispersed and located in close proximity to the affected disc space (Hansen type I).[22–24] Gross descriptions of Hansen type I IVD extrusion suggest that the rupture can be through, or lateral to, the dorsal longitudinal ligament[3,5,14,25] and that it may extrude in an irregular, flat, raised, circular, or conical pattern.[25] On gross sagittal section, the remaining NP appears yellow and is often mineralized.[3] Occasionally, tracts from this material through the inner and outer AF are seen at post mortem but they are rarely straight and are generally difficult to follow.[3,25] The extruded disc material is irregular, brittle, grainy, sometimes plasterlike, and varies from white-yellow to gray-yellow or even gray-red if blood from a damaged venous sinus mixes with it.[3,26] In chronic extrusions, the nuclear material may adhere fibrinously or fibrously to the dura mater or it can be resorbed.[3,25,26] The chemical composition of acute Hansen type I extradural material and of the remaining intervertebral NP are identical, confirming the migration of the NP through the AF.[25] With time, fibrous tissue develops at the edge of the extruded NP and can become interspersed with collagen fibers from the dorsal longitudinal ligament.[25] The cytologic and histopathologic appearance of extruded degenerate disc material was recently compared to determine if cytology was a reliable intraoperative tool to differentiate between degenerate disc material and a neoplastic process.[27] The variability in cytologic findings and frequent presence of dysplastic spindloid cells displaying cytologic criteria of malignancy suggest that impression smears from extruded disc material are cytologically indistinguishable from a mesenchymal neoplasm.[27]

IVD protrusion (also known as Hansen type II) is typically associated with fibroid degeneration and is characterized by a shift of the NP secondary to a partial rupture and weakening of the AF, causing a focal extension of the AF and NP into the vertebral canal either ventral or ventrolateral to the dorsal longitudinal ligament.[3,5,14,25] Protrusions are usually smooth, firm, and round and are rarely adhered to the dura mater.[3,25] On transverse section, the outer AF and the dorsal longitudinal ligament are intact, there is no evidence of hemorrhage, and nuclear mineralization is rare.[3,25]

Although Hansen's[3,5,14] postmortem studies suggested that type I extrusions occur more commonly in chondrodystrophic breeds and that type II protrusions occur more commonly in nonchondrodystrophic breeds,[3,5,14] more recent studies have shown that 62% to 92% of nonchondrodystrophic dogs weighing more than 20 kg with thoracolumbar (TL) IVD herniation experience nuclear extrusion as opposed to annular protrusion.[28,29] Chondrodystrophic dogs can also develop Hansen type II annular protrusions but do so less commonly.[14,24,30]

Incidence and Patient Predisposition

The overall prevalence of disc herniation in the dog has been reported as 2%.[31] A total of 19% to 24% of dachshunds (up to 62% within certain lineages)[32,33] are expected to display clinical signs relating to IVD herniation in their lifetime and account for 45% to 73% of all cases of acute disc extrusion in dogs.[3,6,32–38] Dachshunds are 12.6 times more likely to develop IVD herniation than other breeds[34] followed by the Pekingese, beagle and cocker spaniel, which are reportedly 10.3, 6.4, and 2.6 times more likely to develop IVD herniation, respectively, than other breeds.[34] Beagles reportedly have a 10-times-higher incidence of cervical disc herniation than TL herniation.[6] A few studies[39,40] reported the beagle as the breed most commonly treated for cervical IVD herniation, but dachshunds still predominate in most studies.[6,41–44]

Chondrodystrophic canine breeds include the dachshund, Pekingese, French bulldog, and beagle.[5,8] The American cocker spaniel is often included in the chondrodystrophic classification because of its predisposition for IVD herniation but this has not been confirmed.[14,26,34] Other small breeds reported to be at increased risk of developing IVD herniation include the Lhasa apso, Jack Russell terrier, bichon frisé, Maltese, miniature poodle, and shih tzu.[33–36,45,46] The most common large-breed dogs reported to develop type I IVD are mixed breeds, German shepherd dogs, Labrador retrievers, rottweilers, dalmatians, and Doberman pinschers.[28,29,42] Hansen type II IVD protrusion develops most commonly in German shepherd dogs.[29]

IVD herniation is rare before 2 years of age; it peaks between 3 and 7 years of age in chondrodystrophic patients and generally develops in nonchondrodystrophic patients at a mean of 6 to 8 years of age.[6,28,29,35,37] Older dogs reportedly have a higher incidence of cervical disc disease.[6] A strong sex predilection has not been reported[5,6,26,37] although some reports found that males and spayed females were at higher risk of developing IVD herniation than females.[33,35,40,47] The risk of extrusion is not related to parameters such as body weight, condition score, or activity level.[26,30,48,49]

DIAGNOSTIC TECHNIQUES FOR IVD HERNIATION

Survey Radiography

Lateral and ventrodorsal survey radiography should be performed under general anesthesia to decrease motion and to ensure proper positioning.[50] Radiographic evidence of IVD mineralization is supportive of degeneration but not disc herniation.[18–21] Calcification of the affected IVD space is rarely noted at the time of diagnosis.[51] An increased prevalence of disc mineralization exists in dachshunds, with an average of 2.3 mineralized discs per dog.[20] Disc calcification was a significant predictor of disc herniation[21] and also a risk factor for recurrent herniation following surgery.[52,53] Radiographic mineralization of thoracic discs has been reported to disappear without signs of extrusion and is believed to result from progressive disc degeneration rather than disc regeneration.[18,19,21]

Other radiographic changes supportive of IVD herniation include narrowing or wedging of the IVD space, narrowing of the articular facets, narrowing or increased opacity of the intervertebral foramen, presence of mineralized disc material within the vertebral canal, and vacuum phenomenon.[50,54,55] Narrowing of the IVD space is considered to be the most useful radiographic sign but it has only a moderate sensitivity and predictive value, whereas the vacuum phenomenon is rare but accurate in identifying the herniated disc.[54] Survey radiographs have a reported accuracy of 51% to 94.7% for the correct identification of the herniated disc space for surgical decompression.[35,54,56–61] Despite the high reported sensitivity of radiography for localizing the lesion in some studies, this modality cannot be used alone for diagnosing IVD herniation because it does not provide information on lateralization of the extrusion, extent, and degree of spinal cord compression and presence of other lesions.[61] Although spondylosis deformans is not associated with Hansen type I IVD herniation, an association between radiographically visible spondylosis deformans and Hansen type II IVD herniation may exist.[62]

Myelography

Myelography has been the standard imaging modality for diagnosing IVD extrusion in dogs. The reported accuracy of myelography for lesion localization ranges from 72% to 97% and its accuracy for lateralization of the lesion ranges from 53% to 100%.[46,55,57–61,63–69]

Lumbar myelography is more technically demanding than cervical myelography but it is more likely to show TL lesions because the injection can be performed under pressure with a reduced risk of seizure.[58] Punctures up to T13 to L1 can reportedly produce a diagnostic myelogram, with no side effects.[64] However, injections cranial to L5 to L6 lead to a canalogram in 4.4% to 20% of cases, potentially worsening the neurologic deficits.[57,64] Fluoroscopy can be used to direct needle placement, confirm subarachnoid contrast flow, and localize the site of herniation during injection. Ventrodorsal and lateral radiographic projections of the area of concern are obtained immediately after contrast injection.[55,57] Attenuation, thinning, or deviation of the contrast column suggesting an extradural compression is considered diagnostic for IVD herniation but axial deviation of the contrast column in the ventrodorsal or oblique projections is required to determine lateralization of the lesion and guide the surgical approach (**Fig. 3**).[46,55,57,64] Eight ventrodorsal myelographic contrast patterns have been reported in small-breed dogs with confirmed TL IVD extrusion.[46] Six of the 8 patterns were consistent with a lateralized or ventrolateral extrusion, whereas 2 were consistent with ventrally located disc extrusions.[46] The reported overall accuracy of the ventrodorsal projection in this study was 89%.[46] In 83% of dogs with unequal gaps in the contrast column, disc material was found on the side with the shorter gap; this phenomenon was termed paradoxic contrast obstruction.[46] Oblique myelographic projections are reportedly of greater benefit than the ventrodorsal projection for circumferential localization and have been recommended for all cases.[55,57,69] Combined oblique and ventrodorsal projections are considered more useful than either projection alone.[69]

Loss of the myelographic contrast in an area 5 times the length of the second lumbar vertebra has been associated with a negative outcome in dogs with TL IVD extrusion that have lost deep pain perception (DPP).[70] In this study, dogs with spinal cord swelling/L2 ratios less than 5.0 had a recovery rate of 61%, whereas dogs with a ratio greater than or equal to 5.0 had a recovery rate of 26%.[70] In contrast, the extent of spinal cord swelling determined by myelography was not found to be a useful prognostic indicator in another study.[71]

The reported incidence of postmyelographic seizures following iohexol myelography ranges from 0% to 10% and has been associated with patient weight (larger

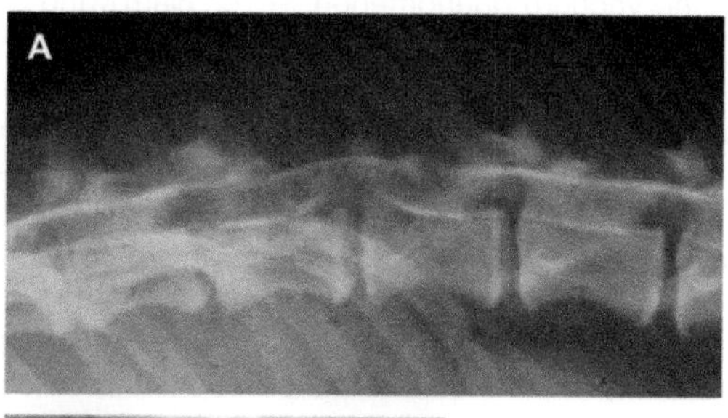

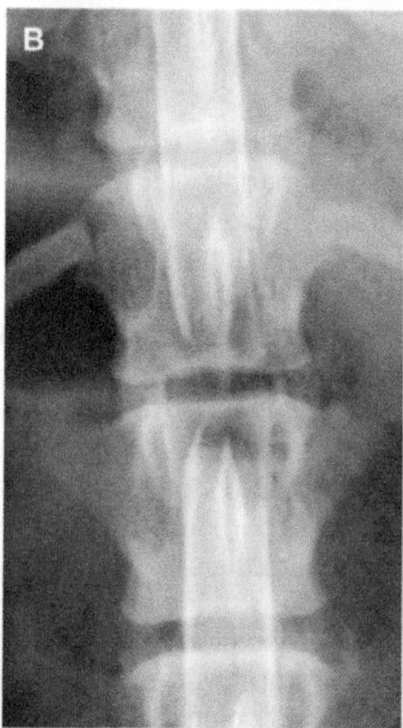

Fig. 3. Lateral (*A*) and ventrodorsal (*B*) myelographic projections showing deviation of the contrast column at T13 to L1 on the right side.

patients), volume of contrast injected (higher volumes), cerebellomedullary injection, lesion location (cervical more likely), sex (higher risk in males), and breed (higher risk in Doberman pinschers).[58,68,72–76] Injection at L5 to L6 and myelography in dogs lighter than 20 kg are associated with lower rates of postmyelographic seizures.[68,73] Supporting this finding, a recent study found a 1.61% and 9.29% rate of postmyelographic seizure in dogs weighing 9 to 20 kg and more than 20 kg, respectively, with an overall rate of 2.98%.[76] Although it has been suggested that surgical intervention and prolonged anesthesia may be protective after iohexol myelography,[72,74] surgery did not independently lower the prevalence of seizures in a more recent study.[73]

Cerebrospinal Fluid Analysis

Cerebrospinal fluid (CSF) is sometimes collected before myelography. Based on previously published results, it is recommended to collect the fluid caudal to the suspected lesion to maximize the yield of diagnostic information from CSF analysis.[77] A recent report on lumbar CSF analysis in dogs with type I IVD revealed pleocytosis in 51% of dogs, including 23% with cervical lesions and 61% with TL lesions.[78] Increase in protein concentration was more common in dogs with cervical (60%) than TL (16%) IVD extrusion, and a predominance of lymphocytes was significantly more common in dogs examined more than 7 days from the onset of signs, which might suggest an immune-mediated response to chronically herniated disc material.[78]

Computed Tomography Imaging

Computed tomography (CT) is a sensitive and noninvasive diagnostic tool that can be used as an adjunct to myelography or as the sole diagnostic procedure to avoid the potential side effects of myelography.[79] CT is quick, has no known side effects (other than exposure to radiation), provides information about lesion lateralization, and has the potential for the images to be reformatted into other imaging planes and three-dimensional images to improve their diagnostic value.[61,68,79,80] Median examination times for myelography, CT, and helical CT were 32 minutes, 8 minutes, and 4 minutes, respectively, in one study, making CT an attractive imaging method.[61] Failure to include the entire spine and inability to identify transitional TL vertebra on the lateral CT scout view can limit the ability to determine accurate vertebral anatomy and complicate lesion localization at surgery.[61] CT generates high-quality bone imaging but is not considered the modality of choice to image soft tissues. A recent study comparing CT and myelography revealed similar diagnostic sensitivities (83.6% and 81.8%, respectively) for localizing the site of disc herniation; however, CT was more sensitive than myelography (80% vs 38%) in detecting chronic lesions because of disc mineralization, and myelography was more sensitive in dogs weighing less than 5 kg (100% vs 50%).[68] Similarly, another study reported that the agreement of myelography, CT, and helical CT with surgical findings was 94.7%, 100%, and 94.7%, respectively, for lesion localization and 78.9%, 87.4%, and 85.3%, respectively, for lesion localization and lateralization.[61] The accuracy of CT and myelography to determine lateralization of the lesion were also comparable at 95.6% and 91.7%, respectively, in an earlier study.[63] Olby and colleagues[79] reported that extruded disc material can be visualized as a heterogeneous hyperattenuating extradural mass using CT without contrast enhancement; these findings are supported by those of Israel and colleagues.[68] In this study, it was possible to differentiate hemorrhage from extruded disc and the spinal cord.[79] Attenuation also increased as mineralization of the IVD material increased, allowing differentiation between acute and chronic extrusions (**Fig. 4**A, B).[79] Intrathecal contrast injection (**Fig. 4**C) has been recommended if the

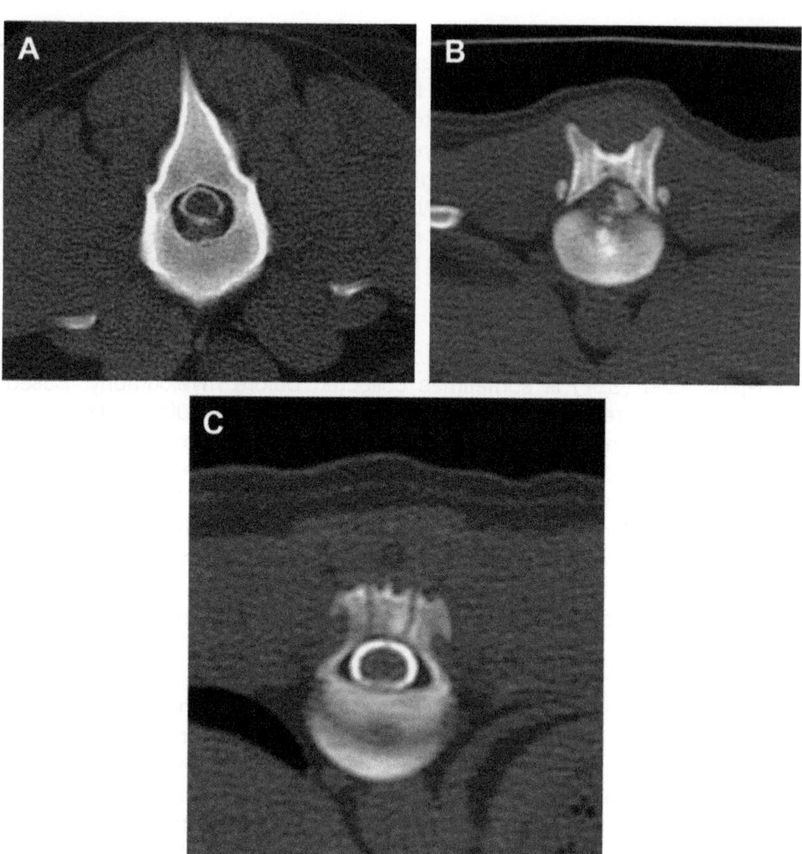

Fig. 4. CT image of a soft (nonmineralized) disc extrusion (*A*), mineralized disc extrusion (*B*), and a normal CT myelogram (*C*).

scan is not definitive but some investigators recommend that it be performed in all cases because contrast enhancement can delineate lesions that were not visible before contrast injection.[68,81] A 3% to 11% increase in certainty score for correct diagnoses was reported when surgeons read multiplanar (MPR) CT images compared with two-dimensional CT images to diagnose TL IVD extrusions in dogs.[80] In addition, the MPR CT images subjectively required less time to interpret.[80] The oblique transverse and curved dorsal MPR views were considered most helpful.[80]

Magnetic Resonance Imaging

Magnetic resonance imaging (MRI) is considered the best diagnostic method for early detection of disc degeneration in dogs[82] and for imaging the cervical spinal cord, discs, and associated structures (**Fig. 5**).[83] Complete agreement between MRI and surgical findings was reported with regard to the affected TL IVD and lesion lateralization in 2 studies.[23,84] Besalti and colleagues[23] reported complete agreement between dispersion pattern predicted on MRI and the surgical findings, whereas Naude and colleagues[84] found complete agreement with regard to craniocaudal distribution in 69% of cases. A study comparing consecutive MRI and myelography in 24 small-breed dogs admitted for first-time TL IVD extrusion confirmed that MRI is consistently

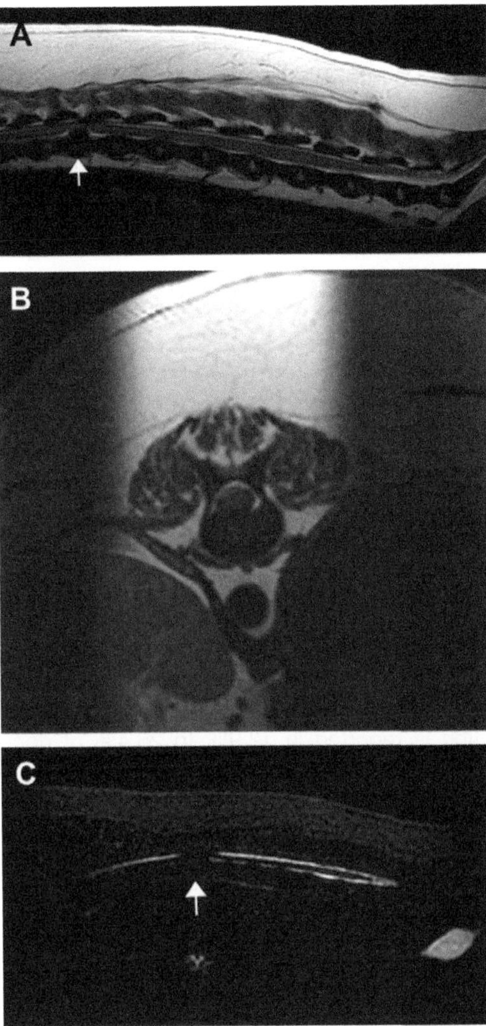

Fig. 5. Sagittal (*A*) and transverse (*B*) T2-weighted MR images of an extruded disc at T12 to T13 (*arrow*) with evidence of disc degeneration at T10 to T11, T11 to T12, T12 to T13 and T13 to L1. Heavily weighted T2 sequence (MR myelogram) showing the absence of CSF signal ventrally and dorsally at T12 to T13 (*arrow*) (*C*).

more accurate than myelography for determining the site and side of the lesion.[51] Compared with T1-weighted and short time inversion recovery images, T2-weighted images are reportedly more accurate and precise, and therefore potentially more reliable for determining the length of extruded disc material.[84] Overall, MRI is considered a good tool to guide surgical decision making with regard to the size and location of TL laminectomy but because MR images tend to underestimate the size of the extruded material, a slightly larger surgical window than that indicated on MRI is recommended to ensure that all extruded disc material is removed.[23,84]

Although dispersed extruded IVD material is believed to be associated with more concussive lesions than nondispersed extrusions, an association was not found between the MRI dispersion pattern and the preoperative and postoperative neurologic status or outcome and should therefore not be used to make treatment or prognostic recommendations.[23] Increased MRI signal intensity in the TL spinal cord has been associated with a poor prognosis for recovery in paraplegic dogs.[23,38,85] Successful recovery of dogs with no DPP that had a hyperintense lesion on T2-weighted images was only 31%.[85] In contrast, the absence of hyperintensity within the spinal cord on T2-weighted images was associated with a successful recovery for all paraplegic dogs regardless of DPP.[85] Similar to what has been reported with myelography,[86] the degree of spinal cord compression seen on MRI in dogs with IVD extrusion was not associated with the rate of onset, duration of clinical signs, or postoperative outcome.[87,88] Although the degree of spinal cord compression noted on MRI was not associated with the severity of neurologic signs at presentation for TL lesions,[87] it was for cervical lesions.[88]

Although MRI is considered superior to myelography for diagnosing unilateral single compressions, in an older study, myelography was the modality of choice to accurately determine the active lesion in 12 of 53 human patients with multilevel disease.[89] MRI is considered superior to myelography for diagnosing extradural compressions caused by hemorrhage.[90,91] Vertebral sinus hemorrhage can result in a filling defect that extends over several vertebral bodies and cannot be differentiated from an extensive extradural compression or spinal cord swelling on myelography.[29,79,90,91] By identifying varying signal intensities, MRI sequences such as the gradient-echo sequence can enable the differentiation between disc material and hemorrhage.[90,91]

CERVICAL IVD DISEASE

Clinical Presentation

Cervical disc herniation is reported in 12.9% to 25.4% of dogs with IVD herniation.[5,6,34] A total of 15% to 61% of cervical IVD herniation cases present with signs of cervical hyperpathia, guarding of the neck, and muscle fasciculations without neurologic deficits.[40,88,92–94] The lower rate of neurologic deficits compared with patients with TL IVD herniation is believed to be related to the large vertebral canal/spinal cord ratio of the cervical vertebral column. Thus, larger disc extrusions can occur without severely compromising the spinal cord. Unilateral or bilateral lameness caused by lower cervical nerve root compression (nerve root signature) has been reported in 15% to 50% of cases.[41,88,92,93] Results of a recent study suggest that the withdrawal reflex in dogs with cervical disc herniation is not reliable for differentiating C1 to C5 or C6 to T2 lesions because a decreased withdrawal reflex does not always indicate a lesion from C6 to T2.[95] Although infrequent, ataxia with tetraparesis or even tetraplegia can develop and has been reported in 9.1% to 17.6% of patients undergoing surgery for cervical disc disease.[39,40,42,44,96] Nonambulatory tetraparesis is reported less frequently in dachshunds than in other breeds.[96] Loss of DPP and respiratory difficulty is possible in extreme cases but is rarely reported.[44] Small-breed dogs, especially dachshunds and beagles, are most commonly affected, but recent studies show that 24% to 50% of cases involve nonchondrodystrophic, large breeds, with Labrador retrievers and rottweilers being most commonly affected.[39,40,42–44,88,92,93] The mean age at the time of diagnosis is 6 to 8 years.[42–44,88,92,93]

Diagnosis

Although both Hansen type I and II disc herniations occur in the cervical region, Hansen type I extrusions are most common in both small- and large-breed dogs.[42] C2 to C3 is the most commonly affected disc space in the cervical spine of small-breed dogs,[6,42,88,92,93] whereas C6 to C7 is the most commonly affected disc space in large-breed dogs.[42] Recent studies have reported C5 to C6[44] and C6 to C7[88] as the most commonly affected disc spaces among all dog breeds presenting for cervical IVD herniation.

Diagnosis of cervical disc herniation is based on lesion localization from the neurologic examination, radiography, and myelography $\pm$ CT or MRI. Disc calcification and narrowing of the affected disc space are commonly noted on survey radiography and are generally believed to correlate with the myelographic findings.[93,97] However, a study evaluating the accuracy of localization of cervical IVD herniation using survey radiographs alone found an overall accuracy of only 35%.[98] In cases in which multiple sites of extrusion were confirmed myelographically, the active lesion was incorrectly identified in 16% to 31% of cases using survey radiographs alone.[98] Of 50 dogs with neck pain but with no evidence of neurologic deficits, 94% showed a deviation of the ventral contrast column at myelography, with 60% of 50 dogs having a moderate to severe deviation of the spinal cord.[93] Based on these findings, it has been recommended that all dogs presenting with neck pain and a suspicion of cervical IVD herniation undergo diagnostic imaging regardless of their neurologic status.[93] Most studies report a single cervical disc herniation on myelography.[92–94] Nondiagnostic myelography has been reported in dogs with lateral or intraforaminal cervical disc extrusions.[97] For this reason, oblique radiographic views should be performed in all patients with clinical signs supportive of cervical IVD that do not have a compressive lesion on lateral and ventrodorsal myelographic projections.[97] Oblique projections allow the visualization of mineralized disc material within the affected foramina.[97] MRI would also allow its visualization and would represent the only diagnostic tool capable of identifying nonmineralized foraminal or lateral extrusions.[83,99] MRI findings of cervical IVD herniation include narrowing of the IVD, displacement or loss of the epidural fat, and a change in the shape of the spinal cord.[83] A recent MRI study found that the degree of cervical spinal cord compression was significantly associated with the presurgical neurologic status but not with speed of onset, duration of signs, postoperative neurologic status, or outcome.[88] A moderate agreement was found between lateralization of cervical lesions from clinical signs and MRI findings, with 9 of 33 cases having lateralization noted on MRI but not clinically.[88]

Conservative Treatment

Conservative treatment focuses on exercise restriction, typically confining the patient to a small cage for 2 to 6 weeks to reduce the risk of continued extrusion while the ruptured AF heals.[43,100] Physical therapy, administration of analgesics, muscle relaxants, and antiinflammatory drugs have also been advocated but are of unknown benefit. The use of a harness instead of a neck collar and leash is important.

Of 32 clinical cases treated conservatively with various medications and acupuncture, 69% were assessed as having recovered in one study, but 37% of cases developed signs of recurrence.[101] A more recent study[43] retrospectively assessed 88 dogs with presumptive cervical disease and reported that 48.9% of dogs were managed successfully, 33% had recurrence, and 18.1% were deemed to have failed conservative treatment. Of the dogs included in this study, 97% were ambulatory at the time of presentation.[43] Less severe neurologic status and administration of a nonsteroidal antiinflammatory drug (NSAID) were associated with a successful outcome but steroid use and the duration of cage rest were not.[43] These results are in agreement with an older study that reported a 36.3% recurrence rate in dogs treated conservatively, which is higher than the 5.6% recurrence rate noted in surgically treated dogs.[39]

Most clinicians agree that medical management of cervical IVD herniation is best suited for mildly affected patients with an acute history.[39,43,92]

Surgical Treatment

Surgical treatment of cervical IVD herniation is typically recommended in dogs that display severe neck pain, neurologic deficits, or recurrence or deterioration of clinical signs after medical management or dogs that have a chronic history at the time of presentation.[42,44,92] Although fenestration alone has been reported to yield acceptable recovery rates,[40] it does not provide spinal cord decompression and is not considered a satisfactory therapeutic modality for cervical IVD extrusion.[92] A study of 111 ambulatory dogs with cervical IVD herniation revealed that ventral decompression was significantly superior to cervical fenestration with regard to improved neurologic status (87% vs 73%) and speed of recovery.[41] Decompressive procedures currently used to treat cervical IVD herniation include ventral slot decompression and less commonly dorsal laminectomy or hemilaminectomy.[92,94,97,102,103] Lateral approaches to the midcervical spine (C3-C6) have also been described to address lateralized or foraminal lesions.[97,104,105] A retrospective study showed no difference in outcome after ventral or dorsal cervical decompression techniques used in small- and large-breed dogs.[42]

The ventral slot procedure is performed through a ventral approach to the cervical spine and provides access for removal of ventrally located disc material but does not allow significant spinal cord decompression or removal of lateralized or dorsally located IVD material. Identification of the IVD space of interest is based on palpation of landmarks such as the ventral process of C1 and the large transverse processes of C6. A bony slot of approximately one-third the width and one-third the length of the vertebrae has been recommended to prevent postoperative instability.[106] Slots of excessive dimensions, especially in the caudal cervical spine, can lead to subluxation and postoperative neurologic deterioration.[92,107] If intact, the dorsal longitudinal ligament must be excised to access the vertebral canal for removal of the extruded disc material.[108] Prophylactic fenestration of adjacent discs can be accomplished through the ventral approach if deemed appropriate, but prophylactic fenestration of the cervical discs is currently less in favor. Resection of the cranial aspect of the manubrium to facilitate ventral access to the C7 to T1 disc space was recently described in one dog without complication.[109]

The dorsal laminectomy procedure does not allow the removal of ventrally located herniated disc material but achieves spinal cord decompression by removing the roof of the vertebral canal.[94] Some investigators believe that this approach is advantageous in small dogs, in which adequate ventral slot size may be difficult to achieve.[94] Cervical hemilaminectomy is more technically demanding and results in more tissue trauma but is reportedly the only approach that allows removal of foraminal or lateral disc extrusions.[97]

Complications associated with surgical procedures used to treat cervical IVD include worsening of the neurologic status,[41] persistent neck pain,[40] hemorrhage,[41,92,97,110] respiratory acidosis and cardiac arrhythmias,[41] hypotension and bradycardia resulting in death,[110] vertebral instability and subluxation,[92,107] and recurrence of IVD extrusion.[39,40,96] In a study evaluating intra- and postoperative mortality, an overall death rate of 8% was reported but was significantly higher in dogs treated with dorsal decompression (12%) than with ventral decompression (5%).[110] Deaths were related to intraoperative hemorrhage, respiratory arrest 3 to 10 hours postoperatively, and cardiovascular decompensation.[110] Postoperative cervical instability and subluxation are presumably related to the dimensions of the ventral slot (slot/vertebral body ratio of 0.5 or greater in most cases) and seems to affect most commonly the caudal cervical spine (C4-C7) of small-breed dogs.[107] Modifications of the ventral slot have been reported in an attempt to reduce the potential for cervical instability and subluxation.[103]

Prognosis for Surgically Managed Cervical IVD Herniation

Prognosis for dogs that present with neck pain alone or mild neurologic deficits and that retain an ambulatory status is good.[42,43,92] Ambulatory dogs undergoing surgical decompression typically remain ambulatory postoperatively.[42,92] A recent retrospective evaluation of 144 small-breed dogs and 46 medium- to large-breed dogs with confirmed cervical IVD extrusion documented resolution of signs in 99% of cases that underwent surgical decompression; only 22% of dogs in this study were nonambulatory before surgery.[42] All dogs that were nonambulatory with DPP before surgery regained the ability to walk within a mean of 6 days postoperatively in one study,[42] whereas studies focused on nonambulatory tetraparetic dogs report full recovery rates of 58% to 62%.[44,96] Of patients undergoing dorsal laminectomy with various neurologic grades, 67% recovered normal ambulation 2 weeks postoperatively and 100% were ambulatory at final recheck 5 to 44 months postoperatively.[94] Similar results were reported with ventral slot decompression, all cases of which were eventually reported to have an excellent outcome regardless of neurologic status before surgery.[92] Dogs with peracute histories had more severe neurologic dysfunction before surgery in one study[88] and took longer to return to function in another[92] but their overall neurologic status improved more as a result of surgery compared with dogs with slower clinical progression.[88] Small-breed dogs regained ambulatory status sooner than large-breed dogs (4.5 vs 7 days) in one report[42] and were as much as 5 times more likely to recover than large-breed dogs in another.[44] Dogs that regained the ability to walk within 96 hours after surgery were more than 6 times more likely to have complete recovery, compared with dogs that remained nonambulatory at 96 hours postoperatively.[44,96] Although a previous study[96] suggested that lesion localization (cranial cervical better than caudal cervical) and neurologic status were prognostic indicators of outcome, larger and more recent studies do not support these findings.[42,44] One study recently reported an 83% recovery rate for patients presenting with tetraplegia.[44] Residual deficits are reported in 17% of dogs presenting with nonambulatory tetraparesis.[96] Recurrence of cervical hyperpathia and/or tetraparesis was reported in 0% to 17% of cases after surgical decompression.[42,44,92]

TL IVD DISEASE

TL IVD herniation is reported in 66% to 87% of dogs with IVD herniation.[5,6,34] The discs located between T12 and L3 have been shown to be at higher risk of herniation but the most commonly affected disc spaces in chondrodystrophic dogs are T12 to T13 and T13 to L1.[3,6,26,35,37,38,45,55,56,111–113] Although chondrodystrophic breeds, especially the dachshund, are affected most frequently, large-breed dogs such as the German shepherd dog also develop acute Hansen type I TL IVD extrusions.[28] In large-breed dogs, L1 to L2[28,29] and T13 to L1[29] followed by L2 to L3[28,29] are most frequently affected. Although rare, IVD herniation does occur in the upper thoracic region. T9 to T10 IVD herniation has been reported in dachshunds,[7] and a recent report documented IVD herniation at T2 to T3 in 3 German shepherd dogs.[114]

Clinical Presentation

TL disc herniation can cause varying degrees of back pain and neurologic deficits that range from mild paraparesis to paraplegia with or without loss of DPP. Upper motor neuron (UMN) signs are associated with most IVD extrusions but lower motor neuron (LMN) signs are possible and indicate a lower lumbar lesion. Large-breed dogs with annular protrusions tend to be significantly older and have a significantly more chronic onset of neurologic signs and milder neurologic dysfunction than large-breed dogs with nuclear extrusions.[29]

Diagnosis

Diagnosis of TL IVD and lesion localization is based on the results of the neurologic examination, radiography, myelography, CT or MRI. Although 24% to 80% of dogs with TL IVD herniation reportedly present with clinical signs that are lateralized to the right or left side, [35,46,55,56,58–60] clinical lateralization is reported as the least reliable factor in determining the side on which to perform surgery.[60] Asymmetrical clinical signs contralateral to the myelographic or surgically confirmed lesion occur frequently in dogs with type I IVD extrusion,[35,59,60,115] with 2 studies reporting that surgical lateralization corresponded to the neurologic lateralization in only 48.1% and 61% of cases.[35,59] In a study that specifically examined lateralization, 35% of dogs presenting acutely had a myelographic lesion contralateral to their clinical lateralization compared with only 11% of chronic cases.[115] Other studies report that 14% to 25% of cases had myelographic and surgical lateralization contralateral to the clinical lateralization, respectively.[46,55,60] The discrepancy between the clinical, diagnostic, and surgical findings may result from a ventral or bilateral disc extrusion that causes asymmetric clinical signs in which disc material could be retrieved from either side of the vertebral canal, from an asymmetrical extrusion that leads to more spinal cord trauma on the opposite site as a result of compression of the spinal cord against the vertebral canal (contrecoup injury), or because of contralateral inflammation, hemorrhage, or spinal cord swelling.[46,58,60] The absence of clinical lateralization does not negate the possibility of myelographic lateralization.[55,60]

Reported correlation between myelographic localization and surgical findings ranges greatly and depends on the quality of the myelogram and whether there is any evidence of myelographic lateralization on the ventrodorsal or oblique projections. The results of recent studies indicate that the side of spinal cord decompression corresponds with the myelographic findings in all dogs showing myelographic lateralization.[46,69] Similarly, correlation between MRI and surgical findings is reportedly 100% for lesion localization and lateralization.[23,84] A recent study of 24 dogs receiving consecutive MRI and myelography showed that MRI was consistently superior to myelography for determining lesion localization and lateralization.[51] Although small-breed dogs with a history of several episodes of back pain tend to have a single lesion on myelography,[35] 47% of large-breed dogs with Hansen type II protrusions had multiple annular protrusions at myelography.[29] MR myelography or conventional myelography may be superior to conventional MRI sequences (eg, T2 weighted) in identifying the active lesion in dogs with multiple TL disc herniations.[51,57,89]

A total of 15.8% and 30.5% of dogs were reported to have anatomic vertebral variations such as TL transitional vertebrae, abnormal ribs, or transverse processes that could complicate surgical localization and warrant preoperative radiographs to guide surgery.[57,61] Radiographs and myelography (97.9%) were more accurate than CT (87.4%) or helical CT (88.4%) to determine vertebral numbers and anatomic variations in 19 chondrodystrophic dogs.[61]

Conservative Treatment

Conservative management of TL IVD herniation typically consists of strict confined rest, antiinflammatory drugs, muscle relaxants, analgesics, and physical therapy.[116–118] Although cage rest is the most important aspect of conservative management to prevent continued nuclear extrusion through the ruptured AF and to reduce the risk of self-trauma as a result of incoordination,[116,117] a retrospective evaluation revealed that the duration of cage rest did not affect the success of medical therapy.[117] Although conservative therapy was reportedly successful in 100% of dogs presenting with hyperpathia ± mild neurologic deficits, 50% of patients showed signs consistent with a recurrence 1 to 36 months after the first episode.[118] Other studies have reported success rates of approximately 50% in dogs suspected of TL IVD herniation, with recurrence rates of approximately 30%.[117,119] A 13% rate of residual ataxia was reported for conservatively managed dogs.[119]

A study of 78 dogs suspected of TL IVD extrusion showed that dogs treated with an NSAID or methylprednisolone had lower recurrence rates than dogs treated with other corticosteroids.[118] However, the use of corticosteroids for treating TL IVD remains controversial. Corticosteroid administration has been associated with lower quality of life score and decreased odds of successful outcome in conservatively managed patients.[117] In this study, dogs with suspected TL IVD that received an NSAID were more likely to have higher quality of life scores compared with dogs that did not receive an NSAID.[117] Electroacupuncture used in conjunction with Western medical treatments such as corticosteroids and rest was recently reported to increase neurologic recovery from 58.3% to 88.5% and to reduce the time to recovery of ambulation and DPP.[120] It is well accepted that conservative management is not appropriate for dogs that have lost DPP.[119]

Surgical Treatment

IVD fenestration was initially described as a treatment modality for disc extrusion,[121–123] but its therapeutic efficacy was later questioned because it does not provide spinal cord decompression.[124,125] Furthermore, patients presenting with neurologic deficits that were treated with fenestration alone reportedly had prolonged recovery times similar to those of patients treated conservatively[125,126] and were less likely to recover than if treated with decompressive surgery.[123,126] A more recent study described a technique for partial percutaneous discectomy and reported an 88.8% recovery rate for patients that still had DPP with a mean time for first improvement of 8.3 days.[127] Poor success was reported for dogs without DPP that were treated with percutaneous discectomy.[127] Similarly, other studies do not recommend disc fenestration alone for dogs with paralysis or loss of DPP.[126,128]

Surgical decompression with removal of extruded disc material is a well-accepted treatment modality for patients with severe or progressive neurologic deficits[22,35,56,124,129–136] and has also been recommended for patients with minimal neurologic deficits or back pain alone.[86,118,124] Positive clinical outcome has been associated with complete removal of the offending disc material rather than simple vertebral canal decompression.[56,137] Early decompression using atraumatic surgical technique is optimal for functional recovery to occur. Decompression without removal of extruded disc material does not restore normal arterial and venous hemodynamics and is not considered adequate.[56,137] Although delays before surgery did not seem to affect outcome in dogs with mild to severe neurologic deficits in some studies,[71,85,86,113,138] they are believed to be detrimental in patients with rapidly progressing neurologic dysfunction,[35,71,138] and have been shown to significantly affect the rate of recovery in dogs that have lost DPP.[70,71,111,113]

Traditional surgical decompression of TL IVD extrusion can be accomplished by dorsal laminectomy[130,131,139] and hemilaminectomy.[124] Procedures such as the pediculectomy, minihemilaminectomy, extended pediculectomy, and partial pediculectomy have aimed to achieve spinal cord decompression through less invasive approaches and by removing less vertebral bone. [65,66,135,140,141] These procedures are reportedly quicker, they provide access to the ventral and lateral aspects of the vertebral canal for removal of the extruded disc material, create less tissue trauma and less vertebral instability, and lead to a more rapid postoperative recovery.[66,133,140–142] The corpectomy procedure is described as a less invasive approach to treat chronic Hansen type I or type II disc herniations because it limits manipulation of the spinal cord during disc removal and avoids the temporary clinical worsening noted with other procedures.[143]

Hemilaminectomy is the most popular approach to the TL spinal cord. It was associated with a more satisfactory decompression by removal of disc material,[144] significantly higher rate of postoperative neurologic improvement,[145] decreased risk of laminectomy membrane formation,[144] and less postoperative biomechanical instability[146] compared with dorsal laminectomy. This procedure provides direct access to the lateral and ventral aspects of the vertebral canal, facilitating removal of the extruded material for complete spinal cord decompression and providing access to the disc space for fenestration.[144] However, it has an increased risk of venous sinus hemorrhage compared with the dorsal laminectomy procedure.[144] The dorsal approach to the spine for hemilaminectomy allows access to the contralateral side without repositioning the patient in cases in which a bilateral procedure is necessary. The hemilaminectomy procedure involves the removal of the articular facets and may therefore lead to some degree of vertebral instability. Although bilateral hemilaminectomy did not result in clinical evidence of vertebral instability in normal dogs,[147] the additional instability resulting from disc herniation may warrant some form of vertebral stabilization for bilateral or extensively long approaches. Delayed recovery or clinical deterioration noted 1 to 10 days postoperatively was recently reported in 5.8% of patients undergoing hemilaminectomy and was most commonly associated with residual spinal cord compression caused by an incorrect surgical approach, failure to remove all the extruded disc material, or recurrent disc extrusion.[148]

The window provided by the pediculectomy or minihemilaminectomy is adequate for visualizing the ventrolateral aspect of the vertebral canal and provides excellent access for retrieval of ventral or lateralized disc material, yet limiting intraoperative spinal cord manipulation.[135] Preservation of the articular facets reduces postoperative vertebral instability compared with the hemilaminectomy procedure.[142] The approach used for pediculectomy or minihemilaminectomy also allows direct access to the IVD for fenestration.[135,141] Like the hemilaminectomy procedure, the pediculectomy window is performed close to the vertebral sinus and foraminal structures, requiring care to prevent hemorrhage and nerve root damage. The partial pediculectomy may provide too small a window to decompress extensive lesions or ensure that all the extruded disc material is removed and has the added disadvantage that it requires blind probing of the vertebral canal, which can increase the risk of venous sinus bleeding.[141] A pediculectomy can easily be converted into a hemilaminectomy or be extended over several adjacent vertebrae if required. I have performed continuous pediculectomies over as many as 5 contiguous vertebrae without complication. Because the pediculectomy does not invade the articular facets, it can also be performed bilaterally without causing vertebral instability, assuming that a portion of the pedicle remains intact cranial and/or caudal to the pediculectomy window to prevent disconnecting the dorsal lamina from the vertebral body. A recent report has documented dorsal laminar subluxation in a dog following bilateral minihemilaminectomy and fenestration of T12 to T13 and bilateral pediculectomy at T13.[149]

The corpectomy procedure has been recommended for Hansen type II IVD protrusions and for chronic cases of type I IVD extrusions in which removal of disc material is likely to be incomplete or result in significant worsening of the neurologic status because of disc encapsulation and adhesion to the spinal cord, nerve root, and venous sinuses.[143] This technique is performed through a lateral approach to the spine and involves the removal of a portion of the adjacent vertebral bodies on either side of the affected disc.[143] This ventral access to the vertebral canal allows removal of disc material and avoids trauma to the overlying spinal cord.[143] An initial report of 15 small- and large-breed clinical cases treated by corpectomy revealed excellent results, with none of the cases showing a worsening of their clinical signs and all dogs improving neurologically after the procedure.[143]

Durotomy is no longer recommended as a therapeutic procedure for spinal cord trauma but it retains some value as a diagnostic tool for myelomalacia and as a possible prognostic indicator in patients that have lost DPP.[70,71,112,150,151] Although the potential for durotomy to cause significant morbidity has been raised,[152] it did not significantly affect postoperative recovery in cases presenting without DPP that underwent hemilaminectomy with durotomy compared with those that underwent hemilaminectomy alone.[151] The presence of extensive myelomalacia is typically associated with a poor prognosis but focal myelomalacia does not preclude neurologic recovery.[70,151] Moreover, the absence of visual evidence of myelomalacia does not ensure neurologic recovery.[70,151] A diffuse and progressive form of myelomalacia called ascending-descending myelomalacia has been reported to occur in 1% to 3.2% of patients admitted for IVD herniation,[119,153] and in 10.9% to 32.6% of those presenting without DPP.[26,70,71,138,154–156] This generalized form of myelomalacia progresses cranially and caudally within the spinal cord parenchyma within hours to days, leading to respiratory paralysis within 5 to 10 days.[119] Ascending-descending myelomalacia has been associated with Funkquist type III disc extrusions.[22,155]

Prophylactic IVD Fenestration and Recurrent Disc Herniation

IVD fenestration typically involves the mechanical removal of the NP through a window created in the lateral AF using an air drill and burr (power-assisted fenestration) or a scalpel blade (blade fenestration) (**Fig. 6**).[106,157] The effectiveness of fenestration is governed by the amount of NP removed.[158] A study comparing blade and power-assisted fenestration revealed that power-assisted fenestration removed on average 65% of the NP compared with approximately 41% of the NP being removed with blade fenestration.[157] I believe that either technique can remove large amounts of disc material as long as the surgeon is comfortable with the technique chosen. Another study determined that using the lateral approach for IVD fenestration may increase the efficiency of the procedure compared with the dorsal or dorsolateral surgical approaches by providing a better angle and working depth for fenestration.[159] Other reported techniques for prophylactic ablation of the IVD include percutaneous laser fenestration[160] and chemonucleolysis.[161]

In 1970, Funkquist[131] reported that recurrent disc herniation was at least as frequent in patients that had undergone a laminectomy alone as in patients that had been treated conservatively. Fenestration of the herniated disc space has since been encouraged to prevent further extrusion of disc material through the ruptured AF in the early postoperative period.[112,131,162] A recent study[162] that performed repeat MRI immediately and 6 weeks postoperatively confirmed recurrent disc herniation in 6 of 10 patients that did not undergo fenestration of the affected disc space at the time of surgical decompression. Three of these 6 patients displayed clinical signs (pain and/or paresis) compatible with the recurrent herniation noted on MRI.[162] Early

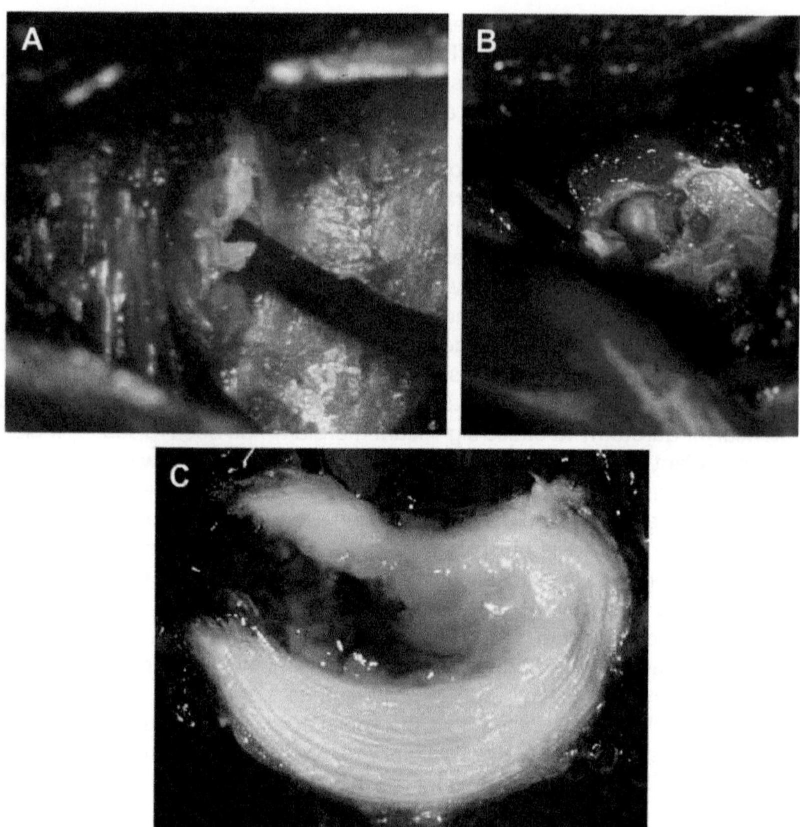

Fig. 6. Disc space during (*A*) and after (*B*) surgical fenestration through a dorsolateral approach to the spine. Transverse section of a disc space after fenestration was performed (*C*).

recurrences reportedly occur within 4 to 6 weeks of surgery and are generally related to nuclear extrusion at the site of initial IVD extrusion. [45,162,163]

All IVDs are subject to degeneration and chondrodystrophic breeds have been reported to develop on average 2.5 IVD herniations per dog.[3,5] Fenestration of IVD spaces adjacent to the surgical lesion has been advocated as a prophylactic measure to future disc herniation.[65,119,121,122,124–126,131–133,164] Recurrence rates of 0% to 24.4% with prophylactic fenestration[65,119,125,126,128,164] and 2.67% to 41.7% without prophylactic fenestration[35,112,119,131,134,163–165] have been reported. The most recent retrospective studies report unconfirmed recurrence rates of 19.2% without prophylactic fenestration[52] and confirmed recurrence rates of 4.4% in a population of dogs that frequently underwent prophylactic fenestration.[45] The latter study also revealed that 15.8% of dog owners reached by telephone follow-up reported their dog developed signs compatible with recurrent IVD herniation and that 44% of these dogs were euthanized elsewhere for suspected recurrence.[45] A recent prospective study randomized 207 small-breed dogs undergoing surgical decompression for TL IVD extrusion to either receive single-site fenestration at the site of decompression (n = 103) or multiple-site prophylactic fenestration of all disc spaces between T11 and L4 (n = 104) with a median follow-up for recurrence of 3.4 years.[53] The surgically confirmed recurrence rate in this study was 12.7% with a significantly lower recurrence rate for dogs in the multiple-site fenestration group (7.45%) compared to dogs in the single-site fenestration group (17.89%).[53] In addition, only dogs from the single-site fenestration group developed more than one recurrence in this study.[53] The reported rate of recurrent IVD herniation for large-breed dogs is 11% to 12%.[28,29]

Although in some studies dachshunds were more likely to develop recurrent TL IVD herniation compared with other breeds,[45,163] this was not found to be the case in others.[52,53] Disc mineralization at the time of first surgery has been associated with recurrent IVD herniation in dogs.[52,53] Late recurrent IVD herniation occurs at a mean time of 8 to 14 months after the first surgery and typically within 36 months of the first event.[45,52,53,125,163,165] Recurrences occur at a new disc space in 88% to 100% of cases,[45,53,163,165] and more than 70% of recurrences occur in a region that could have been readily fenestrated at the first surgery.[163] Most recurrences occur at a site immediately adjacent to or one disc space away from the first lesion or from a fenestrated disc space, suggesting that disc herniation and fenestration may have a biomechanical effect on adjacent disc spaces.[45,52,53,163] This finding is supported by the fact that the AF has been shown to be an important stabilizing structure and that fenestration significantly contributes to vertebral instability.[142] The incidence of recurrence at L4 to L5 and L5 to L6 in dogs prophylactically fenestrated between T11 to T12 and L3 to L4 is reportedly 45.5% to 57.1%[45,53]; this is considered high because the reported rates of spontaneous disc extrusion at these disc space are between 3.7% and 7%.[5,6,35,45]

Reported complications associated with fenestration include increased anesthetic and surgical times,[112] displacement of disc material into the vertebral canal and/or spinal cord trauma causing worsening of neurologic grade,[166,167] hemorrhage,[45,53] pneumothorax,[45,166] soft-tissue and nerve-root trauma leading to postoperative pain, scoliosis and abdominal wall weakness,[53,65,166] diskospondylitis,[125,168] and difficulty identifying one or more disc spaces for fenestration.[45,53] Most reported complications are minor and have no long-term negative effects.[45,53,65,166]

Laminectomy Membrane Formation

Laminectomy membrane formation is believed to result in an 8% failure rate after vertebral surgery in humans.[169,170] Three of 187 (1.6%) dogs were surgically confirmed as having complications that responded to removal of a laminectomy membrane in one report.[35] Although this condition is suspected in clinical patients displaying signs of spinal cord compression following a laminectomy procedure, an actual rate of occurrence has not been reported in veterinary patients.[129,139] A variety of materials have been implanted in an effort to reduce the occurrence of laminectomy membrane formation but several remain of questionable value. Although free fat grafts have been most popular, these have been reported to lead to significant spinal cord compression, especially in the first few weeks after implantation.[152,171] No advantage has been reported to support the use of a pedicled fat graft rather than a free fat graft.[152] Free fat grafts and cellulose membrane are somewhat effective at reducing laminectomy membrane formation but experimentally the free fat grafts are associated with a high rate of significant neurologic complications that seem to resolve within 3 to 10 days after implantation.[171] Neither the free fat graft nor the cellulose membrane is recommended to cover a modified dorsal laminectomy.[171]

Prognosis for Surgically Managed TL IVD Herniation

Reported recovery rates for nonambulatory chondrodystrophic or small-breed dogs that retain DPP before decompressive surgery vary between 86% and 96%.[45,47,49,111,112,165,172,173] The overall recovery rate for nonchondrodystrophic large-breed dogs with Hansen type I IVD extrusions is slightly lower at 78% to 85%,[28,29] whereas the overall recovery rate for nonchondrodystrophic large-breed dogs with Hansen type II IVD protrusions is between 22% and 52%.[29]

The presence of DPP has been reported by many as the most important prognostic factor for return to function.[28,37,49,70,111,112] A recent study showed that dogs with preoperative DPP had a 1.7-times-better chance of becoming ambulatory than those without.[49] Although duration of clinical signs and severity of neurologic dysfunction were not associated with outcome in some studies,[85,112,174] peracute (<an hour) loss of motor function in dogs with no DPP has been associated with a poorer prognosis compared with dogs with a slow, progressive loss of ambulatory function.[71] This finding is likely related to the significant spinal cord injury caused by a sudden, high-velocity IVD extrusion compared with a slow, gradual IVD extrusion.[71] Other studies state that speed of onset and duration of clinical signs should not be used to advise owners about prognosis.[85,138]

The overall reported recovery rates for dogs undergoing TL decompressive surgery with questionable or absent DPP range between 0% and 76%.[35,37,45,49,59,62,70,111–113,119,126,138,145,151,165,175,176] In contrast, only 25% of large-breed dogs with Hansen type I TL IVD extrusion having lost DPP are reported to recover after undergoing decompressive surgery.[28] Although recovery has been reported in dogs that lost DPP more than 72 hours preoperatively,[59,71,175] functional recovery is rare in patients that are treated conservatively or that undergo decompressive surgery more than 48 hours after losing DPP.[37,70] Dogs undergoing surgery within 12 hours of losing DPP have a higher recovery rate.[37,70,71,111] One study[111] reported a 55.6% rate of recovery for dogs that underwent surgery within 12 hours of losing DPP, whereas only 25% of dogs treated 12 to 36 hours after losing DPP recovered. Similarly, Duval and colleagues[70] reported a 53% recovery rate if surgery occurred less than 12 hours after losing DPP and 38% and 43% recovery rates between 12 and 24 hours and 24 and 48 hours, respectively. The prognosis for recovering function is poor if DPP does not return within 2 to 4 weeks.[71,138,176]

Time to ambulation after decompressive surgery is important to owners wishing to pursue surgical treatment. The mean time required to recover ambulatory status in dogs that lose purposeful movement but retain DPP reportedly varies between 6.7 and 12.9 days.[47,172,173] However, a more recent study noted that many patients return to ambulatory function only 2 to 4 weeks postoperatively.[49] Olby and colleagues[138] reported a mean time to ambulation of 7.5 weeks for 87 dogs with severe spinal cord injury, with 62% of dogs walking within 4 weeks of surgery. In contrast, large-breed dogs that were ambulatory before surgery took on average 5.6 weeks to recover and those that were nonambulatory but retained DPP before surgery took 7 weeks to recover.[28] Residual deficits are reported in 20% to 25% of chondrodystrophic dogs presenting with severe neurologic deficits.[112,141] The fecal and urinary incontinence rates for dogs presenting without DPP and undergoing surgery were 41% and 32%, respectively.[138] A 40% rate of residual neurologic and gait deficits was reported in larger-breed dogs and should be discussed with owners.[28]

Administration of dexamethasone or methylprednisolone sodium succinate did not reveal an improved outcome in dogs with surgically treated TL IVD but was associated with a higher rate of gastrointestinal and urinary tract complications as well as longer hospital stay and increased cost to the owners.[177,178] In contrast, postoperative physical therapy seems to have a positive effect on return to ambulatory status.[49]

Lower motor neuron lesions have historically been associated with a poorer prognosis compared with UMN lesions. Although LMN lesions may be associated with a slower return to function compared with UMN lesions,[179] lesion localization does not seem to affect the rate of recovery.[138,179] A more recent study looking at outcome and prognostic factors in 308 cases of TL IVD herniation supported this finding by showing that the affected IVD space did not have an effect on the ability to ambulate or the time to ambulation.[49] This study showed that patients presenting with LMN lesions were 2 times more likely to regain strong ambulatory status sooner than patients presenting with UMN lesions.[49]

Functional recovery after repeat surgery for recurrent TL IVD extrusion is generally identical to that of first-time extrusion.[45,49,53,179]

SUMMARY

Despite the large body of knowledge gained in the last 60 years, canine IVD disease remains a common and challenging condition. MRI has improved our ability to diagnose IVD herniation more accurately and a variety of medical and surgical options allow clinicians to customize the treatment plan specifically to each patient. Although it is difficult to predict, the prognosis for many patients affected by IVD herniation is positive. The significance of recurrent IVD herniation and the role of fenestration are still questionable.

ACKNOWLEDGMENTS

I am grateful to Dr Alexandra Squires Bos for the work she performed under my supervision during her graduate training and for her permission to use a portion of this work in this article.

REFERENCES

1. King AS, Smith RN. A comparison of the anatomy of the intervertebral disc in dog and man: with reference to herniation of the nucleus pulposus. Br Vet J 1955;3:135–49.
2. Evans HE. Miller's anatomy of the dog. 3rd edition. Philadelphia: WB Saunders; 1993.
3. Hansen HJ. A pathologic-anatomical study on disc degeneration in dog, with special reference to the so-called enchondrosis intervertebralis. Acta Orthop Scand Suppl 1952;11:1–117.
4. Dallman MJ, Moon ML, Giovannitti-Jensen A. Comparison of the width of the intervertebral disc space and radiographic changes before and after intervertebral fenestration in dogs. Am J Vet Res 1991;52:140–5.
5. Hansen HJ. A pathologic-anatomical interpretation of disc degeneration in dogs. Acta Orthop Scand 1951;20:280–93.
6. Gage ED. Incidence of clinical disc disease in the dog. J Am Anim Hosp Assoc 1975;11:135–8.
7. Wilkens BE, Selcer R, Adams WH, et al. T9-T10 intervertebral disc herniation in three dogs. Vet Comp Orthop Traumatol 1996;9:177–8.
8. Braund KG, Ghosh P, Taylor TK, et al. Morphological studies of the canine intervertebral disc. The assignment of the beagle to the achondroplastic classification. Res Vet Sci 1975;19:167–72.
9. Ghosh P, Taylor TK, Braund KG. The variation of the glycosaminoglycans of the canine intervertebral disc with ageing. I. chondrodystrophoid breed. Gerontology 1977;23:87–98.
10. Forsythe WB, Ghoshal NG. Innervation of the canine thoracolumbar vertebral column. Anat Rec 1984;208:57–63.

11. Maroudas A, Stockwell RA, Nachemson A, et al. Factors involved in the nutrition of the human lumbar intervertebral disc. Cellularity and diffusion of glucose in vitro. J Anat 1975;120:113–30.
12. Nachemson A, Lewin T, Maroudas A, et al. In vitro diffusion of dye through the end-plates and the annulus fibrosus of human lumbar intervertebral disks. Acta Orthop Scand 1970;41:589–607.
13. Modic MT, Masaryk TJ, Ross JS, et al. Imaging of degenerative disk disease. Radiology 1988;168:177–86.
14. Hansen HJ. Comparative views of the pathology of disk degeneration in animals. Lab Invest 1959;8:1242–65.
15. Gosh P, Taylor TK, Braund KG, et al. A comparative chemical and histological study of the chondrodystrophoid and nonchondrodystrophoid canine intervertebral disc. Vet Pathol 1976;13:414–27.
16. Ghosh P, Taylor TK, Braund KG, et al. The collagenous and non-collagenous protein of the canine intervertebral disc and their variation with age, spinal level and breed. Gerontology 1976;22:124–34.
17. Ghosh P, Taylor TK, Braund KG. Variation of the glycosaminoglycans of the intervertebral disc with ageing. II. Non-chondrodystrophoid breed. Gerontology 1977;23:99–109.
18. Jensen VF. Asymptomatic radiographic disappearance of calcified intervertebral disc material in the dachshund. Vet Radiol Ultrasound 2001;42: 141–8.
19. Jensen VF, Arnbjerg J. Development of intervertebral disk calcification in the dachshund: a prospective longitudinal radiographic study. J Am Anim Hosp Assoc 2001;37:274–82.
20. Stigen O. Calcification of intervertebral discs in the dachshund. A radiographic study of 327 young dogs. Acta Vet Scand 1991;32:197–203.
21. Jensen VF, Beck S, Christensen KA, et al. Quantification of the association between intervertebral disk calcification and disk herniation in dachshunds. J Am Vet Med Assoc 2008;233:1090–5.
22. Funkquist B. Thoraco-lumbar disk protrusion with severe cord compression in the dog I. Clinical and patho-anatomic observations with special reference to the rate of development of the symptoms of motor loss. Acta Vet Scand 1962; 3:256–74.
23. Besalti O, Ozak A, Pekcan Z, et al. The role of extruded disk material in thoracolumbar intervertebral disk disease: a retrospective study in 40 dogs. Can Vet J 2005;46:814–20.
24. Besalti O, Pekcan Z, Sirin YS, et al. Magnetic resonance imaging findings in dogs with thoracolumbar intervertebral disk disease: 69 cases (1997–2005). J Am Vet Med Assoc 2006;228:902–8.
25. Vaughan LC. Studies on intervertebral disc protrusion in the dog. 3. Pathological features. Br Vet J 1958;114:350–5.
26. Hoerlein BF. Intervertebral disc protrusions in the dog. Incidence and pathological lesions. Am J Vet Res 1953;14:260–9.
27. Royal AB, Chigerwe M, Coates JR, et al. Cytologic and histopathologic evaluation of extruded canine degenerate disks. Vet Surg 2009;38:798–802.
28. Cudia SP, Duval JM. Thoracolumbar intervertebral disk disease in large, nonchondrodystrophic dogs: a retrospective study. J Am Anim Hosp Assoc 1997; 33:456–60.
29. Macias C, McKee WM, May C, et al. Thoracolumbar disc disease in large dogs: a study of 99 cases. J Small Anim Pract 2002;43:439–46.

30. Levine JM, Levine GJ, Kerwin SC, et al. Association between various physical factors and acute thoracolumbar intervertebral disk extrusion or protrusion in dachshunds. J Am Vet Med Assoc 2006;229:370–5.
31. Bray JP, Burbidge HM. The canine intervertebral disk: part one: structure and function. J Am Anim Hosp Assoc 1998;34:55–63.
32. Ball MU, McGuire JA, Swaim SF, et al. Patterns of occurrence of disk disease among registered dachshunds. J Am Vet Med Assoc 1982;180:519–22.
33. Priester WA. Canine intervertebral disc disease - occurrence by age, breed, and sex among 8,117 cases. Theriogenology 1976;6:293–303.
34. Goggin JE, Li AS, Franti CE. Canine intervertebral disk disease: characterization by age, sex, breed, and anatomic site of involvement. Am J Vet Res 1970;31: 1687–92.
35. Brown NO, Helphrey ML, Prata RG. Thoracolumbar disk disease in the dog: a retrospective analysis of 187 cases. J Am Anim Hosp Assoc 1977;13:665–72.
36. Olby NJ, Harris T, Burr J, et al. Recovery of pelvic limb function in dogs following acute intervertebral disc herniations. J Neurotrauma 2004;21:49–59.
37. Knecht CD. Results of surgical treatment for thoracolumbar disc protrusion. J Small Anim Pract 1972;13:449–53.
38. Levine JM, Fosgate AV, Rushing CR, et al. Magnetic resonance imaging in dogs with neurological impairment due to acute thoracic and lumbar intervertebral disc herniation. J Vet Intern Med 2009;23:1220–6.
39. Russell SW, Griffiths RC. Recurrence of cervical disc syndrome in surgically and conservatively treated dogs. J Am Vet Med Assoc 1968;153:1412–7.
40. Denny HR. The surgical management of cervical disc protrusions in the dog: a review of 40 cases. J Small Anim Pract 1978;19:251–7.
41. Fry JR, Johnson AL, Hungerford L, et al. Surgical treatment of cervical disc herniations in ambulatory dogs. Ventral decompression vs fenestration, 111 cases (1980–1988). Prog Vet Neurol 1991;2:165–73.
42. Cherrone KL, Dewey CW, Coates JR, et al. A retrospective comparison of cervical intervertebral disk disease in nonchondrodystrophic large dogs vs small dogs. J Am Anim Hosp Assoc 2004;40:316–20.
43. Levine JM, Levine GJ, Johnson SI, et al. Evaluation of success of medical management for presumptive cervical intervertebral disk herniation in dogs. Vet Surg 2007;36:492–9.
44. Hillman RB, Kengeri SS, Waters DJ. Reevaluation of predictive factors for complete recovery in dogs with nonambulatory tetraparesis secondary to cervical disk herniation. J Am Anim Hosp Assoc 2009;45:155–63.
45. Brisson BA, Moffatt SL, Swayne SL, et al. Recurrence of thoracolumbar intervertebral disk extrusion in chondrodystrophic dogs after surgical decompression with or without prophylactic fenestration: 265 cases (1995–1999). J Am Vet Med Assoc 2004;224:1808–14.
46. Bos AS, Brisson BA, Holmberg DL, et al. Use of the ventrodorsal myelographic view to predict lateralization of extruded disk material in small-breed dogs with thoracolumbar intervertebral disk extrusion: 104 cases (2004–2005). J Am Vet Med Assoc 2007;230:1860–5.
47. Ferreira AJ, Correia JH, Jaggy A. Thoracolumbar disc disease in 71 paraplegic dogs: influence of rate of onset and duration of clinical signs on treatment results. J Small Anim Pract 2002;43:158–63.
48. Cimino Brown D, Conzemius MG, Shofer FS. Body weight as a predisposing factor for humeral condylar fractures, cranial cruciate rupture and intervertebral disc disease in cocker spaniels. Vet Comp Orthop Traumatol 1996;9:75–8.

49. Ruddle TL, Allen DA, Schertel ER, et al. Outcome and prognostic factors in non-ambulatory Hansen type I intervertebral disc extrusions: 308 cases. Vet Comp Orthop Traumatol 2006;19:29–34.
50. Burk RL. Problems in the radiographic interpretation of intervertebral disc disease in the dog. Probl Vet Med 1989;1:381–401.
51. Bos AS. Clinical usefulness of MRI and myelography in the diagnosis of intervertebral disc extrusion in dogs [DVSc thesis]. University of Guelph. Guelph, Canada; 2008. p. 113–49.
52. Mayhew PD, McLear RC, Ziemer LS, et al. Risk factors for recurrence of clinical signs associated with thoracolumbar intervertebral disk herniation in dogs: 229 cases (1994–2000). J Am Vet Med Assoc 2004;225:1231–6.
53. Brisson BA, Holmberg DL, Parent J, et al. Comparison of the effect of single-site and multiple-site disc fenestration on the rate of recurrence of thoracolumbar intervertebral disc extrusion in dogs: a prospective, randomized, controlled study. J Am Vet Med Assoc, submitted for publication.
54. Lamb CR, Nichols A, Targett M, et al. Accuracy of survey radiographic diagnosis of intervertebral disc protrusion in dogs. Vet Radiol Ultrasound 2002;3:222–8.
55. Tanaka H, Nakayama M, Takase K. Usefulness of myelography with multiple views in diagnosis of circumferential location of disc material in dogs with thoracolumbar intervertebral disc herniation. J Vet Med Sci 2004;66:827–33.
56. McKee WM. A comparison of hemilaminectomy (with concomitant disk fenestration) and dorsal laminectomy for the treatment of thoracolumbar disk protrusion in dogs. Vet Rec 1992;130:296–300.
57. Kirberger RM, Roos CJ, Lubbe AM. The radiological diagnosis of thoracolumbar disc disease in the dachshund. Vet Radiol Ultrasound 1992;33:255–61.
58. Olby NJ, Houlton JE. Correlation of plain radiographic and lumbar myelographic findings with surgical findings in thoracolumbar disc disease. J Small Anim Pract 1994;35:345–50.
59. Yovich JC, Read R, Eger C. Modified lateral spinal decompression in 61 dogs with thoracolumbar disc protrusion. J Small Anim Pract 1994;35:351–6.
60. Schulz KS, Walker M, Moon M, et al. Correlation of clinical, radiographic, and surgical localization of intervertebral disc extrusion in small-breed dogs: a prospective study of 50 cases. Vet Surg 1998;27:105–11.
61. Hecht S, Thomas WB, Marioni-Henry K, et al. Myelography vs. computed tomography in the evaluation of acute thoracolumbar intervertebral disk extrusion in chondrodystrophic dogs. Vet Radiol Ultrasound 2009;50:353–9.
62. Levine GJ, Levine JM, Walker MA, et al. Evaluation of the association between spondylosis deformans and clinical signs of intervertebral disk disease in dogs: 172 cases (1999–2000). J Am Vet Med Assoc 2006;228:96–100.
63. Olby NJ, Muñana KR, Sharp NJ, et al. A comparison of computed tomography and myelography in the diagnosis of acute intervertebral disc protrusions in dogs. Proc ACVIM 1999;17:705.
64. McCartney WT. Lumbar myelography in 79 dogs, using different puncture sites. Vet Rec 1997;141:417–9.
65. Black AP. Lateral spinal decompression in the dog: a review of 39 cases. J Small Anim Pract 1988;29:581–8.
66. Lubbe AM, Kirberger RM, Verstraete FJM. Pediculectomy for thoracolumbar spinal decompression in the dachshund. J Am Anim Hosp Assoc 1994;30:233–8.
67. De Risio L, Sharp NJ, Olby NJ, et al. Predictors of outcome after dorsal decompressive laminectomy for degenerative lumbosacral stenosis in dogs: 69 cases (1987–1997). J Am Vet Med Assoc 2001;219:624–8.

68. Israel SK, Levine JM, Kerwin SC, et al. The relative sensitivity of computed tomography and myelography for identification of thoracolumbar intervertebral disk herniations in dogs. Vet Radiol Ultrasound 2009;50:247–52.
69. Gibbons SE, Macias C, De Stefani A, et al. The value of oblique versus ventrodorsal myelographic views for lesion lateralization in canine thoracolumbar disc disease. J Small Anim Pract 2006;47:658–62.
70. Duval J, Dewey C, Roberts R, et al. Spinal cord swelling as a myelographic indicator of prognosis: a retrospective study in dogs with intervertebral disc disease and loss of deep pain perception. Vet Surg 1996;25:6–12.
71. Scott HW, McKee WM. Laminectomy for 34 dogs with thoracolumbar intervertebral disc disease and loss of deep pain perception. J Small Anim Pract 1999;40:417–22.
72. Allan GS, Wood AK. Iohexol myelography in the dog. Vet Radiol 1988;29:78–82.
73. Barone G, Ziemer LS, Shofer FS, et al. Risk factors associated with development of seizures after use of iohexol for myelography in dogs: 182 cases (1998). J Am Vet Med Assoc 2002;220:1499–502.
74. Lewis DD, Hosgood G. Complications associated with the use of iohexol for myelography of the cervical vertebral column in dogs: 66 cases (1988–1990). J Am Vet Med Assoc 1992;200:1381–4.
75. Wheeler SJ, Davies JV. Iohexol myelography in the dog and cat: a series of one hundred cases, and a comparison with metrizamide and iopamidol. J Small Anim Pract 1985;26:247–56.
76. da Costa RC, Dobson H, Lusk A, et al. Risk factors for post-myelographic seizures in dogs–503 cases. J Vet Intern Med 2009;23:707–8.
77. Thomson CE, Kornegay JN, Stevens JB. Analysis of cerebrospinal fluid from the cerebellomedullary and lumbar cisterns of dogs with focal neurologic disease: 145 cases (1985–1987). J Am Vet Med Assoc 1990;196:1841–4.
78. Windsor RC, Vernau KM, Sturges BK, et al. Lumbar cerebrospinal fluid in dogs with type I intervertebral disc herniation. J Vet Intern Med 2008;22:954–60.
79. Olby NJ, Muñana KR, Sharp NJ, et al. The computed tomographic appearance of acute thoracolumbar intervertebral disc herniations in dogs. Vet Radiol Ultrasound 2000;41:396–402.
80. King JB, Jones JC, Rossmeisl JH Jr, et al. Effect of multi-planar CT image reformatting on surgeon diagnostic performance for localizing thoracolumbar disc extrusions in dogs. J Vet Sci 2009;10:225–32.
81. Shimizu J, Yamada K, Mochida K, et al. Comparison of the diagnosis of intervertebral disc herniation in dogs by CT before and after contrast enhancement of the subarachnoid space. Vet Rec 2009;165:200–2.
82. Sether LA, Yu S, Haughton VM, et al. Intervertebral disk: normal age-related changes in MR signal intensity. Radiology 1990;177:385–8.
83. Levitski RE, Lipsitz D, Chauvet AE. Magnetic resonance imaging of the cervical spine in 27 dogs. Vet Radiol Ultrasound 1999;40:332–41.
84. Naude SH, Lambrechts NE, Wagner WM, et al. Association of preoperative magnetic resonance imaging findings with surgical features in dachshunds with thoracolumbar intervertebral disk extrusion. J Am Vet Med Assoc 2008;232:702–8.
85. Ito D, Matsunaga S, Jeffery ND, et al. Prognostic value of magnetic resonance imaging in dogs with paraplegia caused by thoracolumbar intervertebral disk extrusion: 77 cases (2000–2003). J Am Vet Med Assoc 2005;227:1454–60.
86. Sukhiani HR, Parent JM, Atilola MA, et al. Intervertebral disk disease in dogs with signs of back pain alone: 25 cases (1986–1993). J Am Vet Med Assoc 1996;209:1275–9.

87. Penning V, Platt SR, Dennis R, et al. Association of spinal cord compression seen on magnetic resonance imaging with clinical outcome in 67 dogs with thoracolumbar intervertebral disc extrusion. J Small Anim Pract 2006;47:644–50.
88. Ryan TM, Platt SR, Llabres-Diaz FJ, et al. Detection of spinal cord compression in dogs with cervical intervertebral disc disease by magnetic resonance imaging. Vet Rec 2008;163:11–5.
89. Hashimoto K, Akahori O, Kitano K, et al. Magnetic resonance imaging of lumbar disc herniation: comparison with myelography. Spine 1990;15:1166–9.
90. Tidwell AS, Specht A, Blaeser L, et al. Magnetic resonance imaging features of extradural hematomas associated with intervertebral disc herniation in a dog. Vet Radiol Ultrasound 2002;43:319–24.
91. Tartarelli CL, Baroni M, Borghi M. Thoracolumbar disc extrusion associated with extensive epidural haemorrhage: a retrospective study of 23 dogs. J Small Anim Pract 2005;46:485–90.
92. Seim HB 3rd, Prata RG. Ventral decompression for the treatment of cervical disk disease in the dog: a review of 54 cases. J Am Anim Hosp Assoc 1982;18: 233–40.
93. Morgan PW, Parent J, Holmberg DL. Cervical pain secondary to intervertebral disc disease in dogs; radiographic findings and surgical implications. Prog Vet Neurol 1993;4:76–80.
94. Gill PJ, Lippincott CL, Anderson SM. Dorsal laminectomy in the treatment of cervical intervertebral disk disease in small dogs: a retrospective study of 30 cases. J Am Anim Hosp Assoc 1996;32:77–80.
95. Forterre F, Konar M, Tomek A, et al. Accuracy of the withdrawal reflex for localization of the site of cervical disk herniation in dogs: 35 cases (2004–2007). J Am Vet Med Assoc 2008;232:559–63.
96. Waters DJ. Nonambulatory tetraparesis secondary to cervical disk disease in the dog. J Am Anim Hosp Assoc 1989;25:647–53.
97. Felts JF, Prata RG. Cervical disk disease in the dog: intraforaminal and lateral extrusions. J Am Anim Hosp Assoc 1983;19:755–60.
98. Somerville ME, Anderson SM, Gill PJ, et al. Accuracy of localization of cervical intervertebral disk extrusion or protrusion using survey radiography in dogs. J Am Anim Hosp Assoc 2001;37:563–72.
99. Chambers JN, Selcer BA, Sullivan SA, et al. Diagnosis of lateralized lumbosacral disc herniation with magnetic resonance imaging. J Am Anim Hosp Assoc 1997;33:296–9.
100. Coates JR. Intervertebral disk disease. Vet Clin North Am Small Anim Pract 2000;30:77–110.
101. Janssens LA. The treatment of canine cervical disc disease by acupuncture: a review of thirty-two cases. J Small Anim Pract 1985;26:203–12.
102. Tanaka H, Nakayama M, Takase K. Usefulness of hemilaminectomy for cervical intervertebral disk disease in small dogs. J Vet Med Sci 2005;67:679–83.
103. McCartney W. Comparison of recovery times and complication rates between a modified slanted slot and the standard ventral slot for the treatment of cervical disc disease in 20 dogs. J Small Anim Pract 2007;48:498–501.
104. Lipsitz D, Bailey CS. Lateral approach for cervical spinal cord decompression. Prog Vet Neurol 1992;3:39–44.
105. Rossmeisl JH, Lanz OI, Inzana KD, et al. A modified lateral approach to the canine cervical spine: procedural description and clinical application in 16 dogs with lateralized compressive myelopathy or radiculopathy. Vet Surg 2005;34:436–44.

106. Sharp NJ, Wheeler SJ. Small animal spinal disorders: diagnosis and surgery. 2nd edition. Philadelphia: Elsevier Mosby; 2005.
107. Lemarié RJ, Kerwim SC, Partington BP, et al. Vertebral subluxation following ventral cervical decompression in the dog. J Am Anim Hosp Assoc 2000;36:348–58.
108. Prata RG, Stroll SG. Ventral decompression and fusion for the treatment of cervical disc disease in the dog. J Am Anim Hosp Assoc 1973;9:462–72.
109. Bush MA, Owen MR. Modification of the ventral approach to the caudal cervical spine by resection of the manubrium in a dog. Vet Comp Orthop Traumatol 2009;22:514–6.
110. Clark DM. An analysis of intraoperative and early postoperative mortality associated with cervical spinal decompressive surgery in the dog. J Am Anim Hosp Assoc 1986;22:739–44.
111. Gambardella PC. Dorsal decompressive laminectomy for treatment of thoracolumbar disc disease in dogs: a retrospective study of 98 cases. Vet Surg 1980;9:24–6.
112. Scott HW. Hemilaminectomy for the treatment of thoracolumbar disc disease in the dog: a follow-up study of 40 cases. J Small Anim Pract 1997;38:488–94.
113. Knecht CD. The effect of delayed hemilaminectomy in the treatment of intervertebral disc protrusion in dogs. J Am Anim Hosp Assoc 1970;13:71–7.
114. Gaitero L, Añor S. Cranial thoracic disc protrusions in three German Shepherd dogs. Vet J 2009;182:349–51.
115. Smith JD, Newell SM, Budsberg SC, et al. Incidence of contralateral versus ipsilateral neurological signs associated with lateralised Hansen type I disc extrusion. J Small Anim Pract 1997;38:495–7.
116. Wilcox KR. Conservative treatment of thoracolumbar intervertebral disc disease in the dog. J Am Vet Med Assoc 1965;147:1458–60.
117. Levine JM, Levine GJ, Johnson SI, et al. Evaluation of the success of medical management for presumptive thoracolumbar intervertebral disk herniation in dogs. Vet Surg 2007;36:482–91.
118. Mann FA, Wagner-Mann CC, Dunphy ED, et al. Recurrence rate of presumed thoracolumbar intervertebral disc disease in ambulatory dogs with spinal hyperpathia treated with anti-inflammatory drugs: 78 cases (1997–2000). J Vet Emerg Crit Care 2007;17:53–60.
119. Davies JV, Sharp NJ. A comparison of conservative treatment and fenestration for thoracolumbar intervertebral disc disease in the dog. J Small Anim Pract 1983;24:721–9.
120. Hayashi AM, Matera JM, Fonseca Pinto AC. Evaluation of electroacupuncture treatment for thoracolumbar intervertebral disk disease in dogs. J Am Vet Med Assoc 2007;231:913–8.
121. Olsson SE. Observations concerning disc fenestration in dogs. Acta Orthop Scand 1951;20:349–56.
122. Olsson SE. Surgical treatment with special reference to the value of disc fenestration. Acta Orthop Scand Suppl 1951;8:51–70.
123. Flo GL, Brinker WO. Lateral fenestration of thoracolumbar discs. J Am Anim Hosp Assoc 1975;11:619–26.
124. Hoerlein BF. The status of the various intervertebral disc surgeries for the dog in 1978. J Am Anim Hosp Assoc 1978;14:563–70.
125. Funkquist B. Investigations of the therapeutic and prophylactic effects of disc evacuation in cases of thoraco-lumbar herniated discs in dogs. Acta Vet Scand 1978;19:441–57.

126. Butterworth SJ, Denny HR. Follow-up study of 100 cases with thoracolumbar disc protrusions treated by lateral fenestration. J Small Anim Pract 1991;32: 443–7.
127. Kinzel S, Wolff M, Buecker A, et al. Partial percutaneous discectomy for treatment of thoracolumbar disc protrusion: retrospective study of 331 dogs. J Small Anim Pract 2005;46:479–84.
128. Knapp DW, Pope ER, Hewett JE, et al. A retrospective study of thoracolumbar fenestration in dogs using a ventral approach: 160 cases (1976 to 1986). J Am Anim Hosp Assoc 1990;26:543–9.
129. Funkquist B, Schantz B. Influence of extensive laminectomy on the shape of the spinal canal. Acta Orthop Scand Suppl 1962;56:7–50.
130. Funkquist B. Thoracolumbar disk protrusion with severe cord compression in the dog; III. Treatment by decompressive laminectomy. Acta Vet Scand 1962; 3:344–66.
131. Funkquist B. Decompressive laminectomy in thoraco-lumbar disc protrusion with paraplegia in the dog. J Small Anim Pract 1970;11:445–51.
132. Gage ED. Modifications in dorsolateral hemilaminectomy and disc fenestration in the dog. J Am Anim Hosp Assoc 1975;11:407–11.
133. Braund KG, Taylor TK, Ghosh P, et al. Lateral spinal decompression in the dog. J Small Anim Pract 1976;17:583–92.
134. Prata RG. Neurosurgical treatment of thoracolumbar disks: the rationale and value of laminectomy with concomitant disk removal. J Am Anim Hosp Assoc 1981;17:17–26.
135. Bitetto WV, Thacher C. A modified lateral decompression technique for treatment of canine intervertebral disk disease. J Am Anim Hosp Assoc 1986;23: 409–13.
136. Bitetto WV, Kapatkin AS. Intraoperative problems associated with intervertebral disc disease. Probl Vet Med 1989;1:434–44.
137. Doppman JL, Girtow M. Angiographic study of the effect of laminectomy in the presence of acute anterior epidural masses. J Neurosurg 1976;45:195–202.
138. Olby NJ, Levine J, Harris T, et al. Long-term functional outcome of dogs with severe injuries of the thoracolumbar spinal cord: 87 cases (1996–2001). J Am Vet Med Assoc 2003;222:762–9.
139. Trotter EJ, Brashmer TH, deLahunta A. Modified deep dorsal laminectomy in the dog. Cornell Vet 1975;65:402–27.
140. Jeffery ND. Treatment of acute and chronic thoracolumbar disc disease by 'mini hemilaminectomy'. J Small Anim Pract 1988;29:611–6.
141. McCartney W. Partial pediculectomy for the treatment of thoracolumbar disc disease. Vet Comp Orthop Traumatol 1997;10:117–21.
142. Hill TP, Lubbe AM, Guthrie AJ. Lumbar spine stability following hemilaminectomy, pediculectomy, and fenestration. Vet Comp Orthop Traumatol 2000;13: 165–71.
143. Moissonnier P, Meheust P, Carozzo C. Thoracolumbar lateral corpectomy for treatment of chronic disk herniation: technique description and use in 15 dogs. Vet Surg 2004;33:620–8.
144. Gage ED, Hoerlein BF. Hemilaminectomy and dorsal laminectomy for relieving compressions of the spinal cord in the dog. J Am Vet Med Assoc 1968;152: 351–9.
145. Muir P, Johnson KA, Manley PA, et al. Comparison of hemilaminectomy and dorsal laminectomy for thoracolumbar intervertebral disc extrusion in dachshunds. J Small Anim Pract 1995;36:360–7.

146. Smith GK, Walter MC. Spinal decompressive procedures and dorsal compartment injuries: comparative biomechanical study in canine cadavers. Am J Vet Res 1988;49:266–73.
147. Swaim SF, Vandevelde M. Clinical and histologic evaluation of bilateral hemilaminectomy and deep dorsal laminectomy for extensive spinal cord decompression in the dog. J Am Vet Med Assoc 1977;170:407–13.
148. Forterre F, Gorgas D, Dickomeit M, et al. Incidence of spinal compressive lesions in chondrodystrophic dogs with abnormal recovery after hemilaminectomy for treatment of thoracolumbar disc disease: a prospective magnetic resonance imaging study. Vet Surg 2010;39:165–72.
149. Arthurs G. Spinal instability resulting from bilateral mini-hemilaminectomy and pediculectomy. Vet Comp Orthop Traumatol 2009;22:422–6.
150. Parker AJ. Durotomy and saline perfusion in spinal cord trauma. J Am Anim Hosp Assoc 1975;11:412–3.
151. Loughin CA, Dewey CW, Ringwood PB, et al. Effect of durotomy on functional outcome of dogs with type I thoracolumbar disc extrusion and absent deep pain perception. Vet Comp Orthop Traumatol 2005;18:141–6.
152. Trevor PB, Martin RA, Saunders GK, et al. Healing characteristics of free and pedicle fat grafts after dorsal laminectomy and durotomy in dogs. Vet Surg 1991;30:282–90.
153. Lu D, Lamb CR, Targett MP. Results of myelography in seven dogs with myelomalacia. Vet Radiol Ultrasound 2002;43:326–30.
154. Griffiths IR. Some aspects of the pathology and pathogenesis of the myelopathy caused by disc protrusions in the dog. J Neurol Neurosurg Psychiatry 1972;35:403–13.
155. Griffiths IR. The extensive myelopathy of intervertebral disc protrusions in dogs ('the ascending syndrome'). J Small Anim Pract 1972;13:425–38.
156. Griffiths IR. Some aspects of the pathogenesis and diagnosis of lumbar disc protrusion in the dog. J Small Anim Pract 1972;13:439–47.
157. Holmberg DL, Palmer NC, Van Pelt D, et al. A comparison of manual and power-assisted thoracolumbar disc fenestration in dogs. Vet Surg 1990;19:323–7.
158. Shores A, Cechner PE, Cantwell HD, et al. Structural changes in thoracolumbar disks following lateral fenestration. A study of radiographic, histologic and histochemical changes in the chondrodystrophic dog. Vet Surg 1985;14:117–23.
159. Morelius M, Bergadano D, Schawalder P, et al. Influence of surgical approach on the efficacy of the intervertebral disk fenestration: a cadaveric study. J Small Anim Pract 2007;48:87–92.
160. Dickey DT, Bartels KE, Henry GA, et al. Use of the holmium yttrium aluminum garnet laser for percutaneous thoracolumbar intervertebral disc ablation in dogs. J Am Vet Med Assoc 1996;208:1263–7.
161. Miyabayashi T, Lord PF, Bubielzig RR, et al. Chemonucleolysis with collagenase. A radiographic and pathologic study in dogs. Vet Surg 1992;21:189–94.
162. Forterre F, Konar M, Spreng D, et al. Influence of intervertebral disc fenestration at the herniation site in association with hemilaminectomy on recurrence in chondrodystrophic dogs with thoracolumbar disc disease: a prospective MRI study. Vet Surg 2008;37:399–405.
163. Dhupa S, Glickman N, Waters DJ. Reoperative neurosurgery in dogs with thoracolumbar disc disease. Vet Surg 1999;28:421–8.
164. Levine SH, Caywood DD. Recurrence of neurological deficits in dogs treated for thoracolumbar disk disease. J Am Anim Hosp Assoc 1984;20:889–94.

165. Necas A. Clinical aspects of surgical treatment of thoracolumbar disc disease in dogs. A retrospective study of 300 cases. Acta Vet Brno 1999;68:121–30.
166. Bartels KE, Creed JE, Yturraspe DJ. Complications associated with the dorsolateral muscle-separating approach for thoracolumbar disk fenestration in the dog. J Am Vet Med Assoc 1983;183:1081–3.
167. Tomlinson J. Tetraparesis following cervical disc fenestration in two dogs. J Am Vet Med Assoc 1985;14:240–6.
168. Hoerlein BF. The treatment of intervertebral disc protrusion in the dog. Proceedings of the American Veterinary Medical Association 1952;89:206–12.
169. Burton CV, Kirkaldy-Willis WH, Yong-Hing K, et al. Causes of failure of surgery on the lumbar spine. Clin Orthop Relat Res 1981;157:191–9.
170. Burton CV. Causes of failure of surgery on the lumbar spine: ten-year follow-up. Mt Sinai J Med 1991;58:183–7.
171. da Costa RC, Pippi NL, Graça DL, et al. The effects of free fat graft or cellulose membrane implants on laminectomy membrane formation in dogs. Vet J 2006; 171:491–9.
172. Davis GJ, Brown DC. Prognostic indicators for time to ambulation after surgical decompression in non-ambulatory dogs with acute thoracolumbar disc extrusions: 112 cases. Vet Surg 2002;31:513–8.
173. Bush WW, Tiches DM, Kamprad C, et al. Functional outcome following hemilaminectomy without methylprednisolone sodium succinate for acute thoracolumbar disk disease in 51 non-ambulatory dogs. J Vet Emerg Crit Care 2007;17:72–6.
174. Kazakos G, Polixopoulou SZ, Patsikas MN, et al. Duration and severity of clinical signs as prognostic indicators in 30 dogs with thoracolumbar disk disease after surgical decompression. J Vet Med A Physiol Pathol Clin Med 2005;52:147–52.
175. Anderson SM, Lippincott CL, Gill PJ. Hemilaminectomy in dogs without deep pain perception. A retrospective study of 32 cases. Calif Vet 1991;45:24–8.
176. Laitinen OM, Puerto DA. Surgical decompression in dogs with thoracolumbar intervertebral disc disease and loss of deep pain perception: a retrospective study of 46 cases. Acta Vet Scand 2005;46:79–85.
177. Boag AK, Otto CM, Drobatz KJ. Complications of methylprednisolone sodium succinate in dachshunds with surgically treated intervertebral disc disease. J Vet Emerg Crit Care 2001;11:105–10.
178. Levine JM, Levine GJ, Boozer L, et al. Adverse effects and outcome associated with dexamethasone administration in dogs with acute thoracolumbar intervertebral disk herniation: 161 cases (2000–2006). J Am Vet Med Assoc 2008;232:411–7.
179. Dhupa S, Glickman N, Waters DJ. Functional outcome in dogs after surgical treatment of caudal lumbar intervertebral disk herniation. J Am Anim Hosp Assoc 1999;35:323–31.

Fibrocartilaginous Embolic Myelopathy in Small Animals

Luisa De Risio, DVM, MRCVS, PhD[a,*], Simon R. Platt, BVM&S, MRCVS[b]

KEYWORDS

- Fibrocartilaginous embolic myelopathy • Ischemic myelopathy
- Dog • Cat

Fibrocartilaginous embolic myelopathy (FCEM) has been reported commonly in dogs[1–9] and sporadically in several other species, including humans,[10] cats,[11,12] horses,[13] pigs,[14] turkeys,[15] a lamb,[16] a calf,[17] a tiger,[18] a tayra,[19] and a pigtail macaque.[20] FCEM occurs when fibrocartilaginous material histologically and histochemically identical to the nucleus pulposus of the intervertebral disc occludes the spinal vasculature, causing ischemic necrosis of dependent regions of spinal cord parenchyma. Neurologic signs are peracute in onset and have distribution and severity referable to the site and extent of the spinal cord infarction. Neurologic signs usually stabilize within 24 hours, and subsequently remain static or improve depending on the severity and extent of the ischemic insult.

PATHOPHYSIOLOGY

The various hypotheses on the pathogenesis of FCEM are best understood after reviewing the vascular anatomy of the spinal cord.

Vascular Anatomy of the Spinal Cord

The arterial supply of the spinal cord originates from spinal branches of the paired vertebral arteries in the cervical spine, intercostal arteries in the thoracic spine, and lumbar and sacral arteries in the lumbar and sacral spine, respectively.[21,22] The paired spinal branches enter the vertebral canal through the intervertebral foramina, penetrate the dura mater, and divide into dorsal and ventral radicular arteries. Some of these supply only the nerve roots, whereas others also contribute to the anastomotic

[a] Neurology/Neurosurgery Unit, Centre for Small Animal Studies, Animal Health Trust, Lanwades Park, Kentford, Newmarket, Suffolk, CB8 7UU, UK
[b] Department of Small Animal Medicine and Surgery, College of Veterinary Medicine, University of Georgia, 501 DW Brooks Drive, Athens, GA 30602, USA
* Corresponding author.
E-mail address: luisa.derisio@aht.org.uk

Vet Clin Small Anim 40 (2010) 859–869
doi:10.1016/j.cvsm.2010.05.003
vetsmall.theclinics.com

plexus on the surface of the spinal cord and to the dorsal and ventral spinal arteries (**Fig. 1**A).

The percentage of ventral radicular arteries contributing to the unpaired ventral spinal artery has been reported to be 88.8% in the cervical region, 31.2% in the thoracic region, and 45.0% in the lumbar region of the spinal cord.[23] The ventral spinal artery extends the entire length of the spinal cord along the ventral median fissure, is larger in diameter at the cervical and lumbar regions than in the thoracic region, and gives rise to the central arteries.[23]

The central arteries supply most of the gray matter and part of the lateral and ventral white matter of the spinal cord, sending branches to each side, or alternatively and irregularly to the left or right side of the spinal cord. The mean percentage of central arteries that send branches bilaterally has been reported to be 21% in the cervical region, 42% in the thoracic region, and 63% in the lumbar region of the spinal cord.[23] The asymmetric distribution of the central artery at several spinal cord segments explains why its embolization can result in unilateral ischemia/infarction and lateralized neurologic deficits.

The percentage of dorsal radicular arteries contributing to the paired dorsal spinal arteries has been reported to be 88.1% in the cervical region, 49.6% in the thoracic region, and 60.0% in the lumbar region of the spinal cord.[23] The dorsal spinal arteries are continuous throughout the spinal cord, have a larger diameter in the cervical and lumbar regions than in the thoracic region, and supply the dorsal white and gray matter.[23] The anastomotic plexus on the surface of the spinal cord gives rise to radial arteries that enter the spinal cord and supply the lateral and ventral white matter.[22]

The venous drainage of the spinal cord consists of several intraparenchymal little veins distributed in a radial pattern to a network of veins on the surface of the spinal

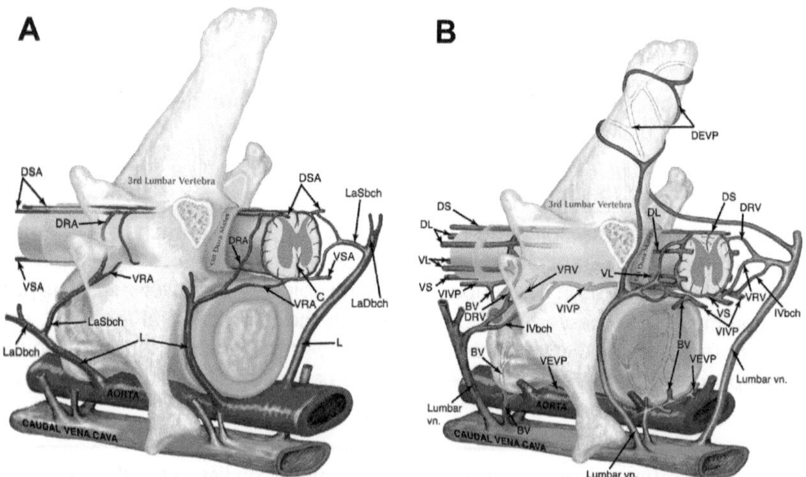

Fig. 1. (*A*) Arterial supply to the lumbar spinal cord. C, central artery; DRA, dorsal radicular artery; DSA, dorsal spinal artery (paired); L, lumbar artery; LaDbch, lumbar artery dorsal branch; LaSbch, lumbar artery spinal branch; VSA, ventral spinal artery; VR, ventral radicular artery. (*B*) Venous drainage of the lumbar spinal cord. BV, basivertebral vein; DEVP, dorsal external vertebral venous plexus; DL, dorsolateral vein (paired); DRV, dorsal radicular vein; DS, dorsal spinal vein; IVbch, intervertebral vein branch; VEVP, ventral external vertebral venous plexus; VIVP, ventral internal vertebral venous plexus; VL, ventrolateral vein (paired); VRV, ventral radicular vein; VS, ventral spinal vein.

cord (see **Fig. 1**B).[22,24] These veins drain into the ventral internal vertebral venous plexus, which mainly consists of two valveless large veins on the floor of the vertebral canal. These veins converge at mid-vertebral body level, occasionally anastomose, and diverge over the intervertebral disc. They are connected with the basivertebral veins that drain the vertebral bodies. The ventral internal vertebral venous plexus drains at the level of the intervertebral foramina via branches of the intervertebral veins into the major veins of each region of the spine (vertebral, azygos, and caudal vena cava in the cervical, thoracic, and lumbar region, respectively).[24]

Pathophysiology Hypotheses

The intraparenchymal (intrinsic) spinal cord arteries are functional end arteries and their occlusion results in ischemia of the territory supplied. In patients with FCEM, the embolizing material has been identified as fibrocartilage histologically and histochemically identical to the nucleus pulposus of the intervertebral disc. Several hypotheses have been proposed to explain how the fibrocartilaginous material, originating from the intervertebral disc nucleus pulposus, enters the spinal vascular system.

Hypothesis 1

Direct penetration of nucleus pulposus fragments into spinal cord or vertebral vessels. Direct penetration into the venous system, which is more likely than into the arterial system because arteries have relatively thick muscular walls. However, an injection type of entrance through the arterial wall has been proposed.[3] Arteriovenous anastomoses have been shown in the epidural and periradicular space in dogs and humans and could explain the presence of emboli on either side of the circulation, regardless of whether the entry point is arterial or venous. In dogs with histologically confirmed FCEM, extruded degenerated disc material has been identified into the internal vertebral venous plexus adjacent to the affected spinal cord segment.[1,25,26] Increased intrathoracic and intraabdominal pressure during coughing, straining, exercise, or trauma (Valsalva's maneuver) could generate retrograde venous propulsion of the fibrocartilage into the intrinsic spinal arteries and veins.

Hypothesis 2

Chronic inflammatory neovascularization (arterial and venous) of the degenerated intervertebral disc. In-growth of blood vessels within the degenerated annulus fibrosus has been documented in humans and in nonchondrodystrophic dogs with disc degeneration. A sudden rise in intervertebral disc pressure exceeding arterial blood pressure may result in penetration of nucleus pulposus fibrocartilage into the newly formed intervertebral disc blood vessels and progression into the intrinsic spinal cord vasculature. Fibrocartilage, histochemically identical to the nucleus pulposus, has been identified within newly formed blood vessels in the degenerated intervertebral disc of two dogs with histologically confirmed FCEM.[26]

Hypothesis 3

Presence of embryonic remnant vessels within the nucleus pulposus (which is normally avascular in adults). The hypothesized mechanism of entrance of the fibrocartilage into the intrinsic spinal cord vasculature is similar to the one described earlier.

Hypothesis 4

Mechanical herniation of nucleus pulposus into the vertebral bone marrow sinusoidal venous channels, with subsequent retrograde entrance into the basivertebral vein and internal vertebral venous plexus. This hypothesis also may apply to human beings because Schmorl's nodules (focal masses of fibrocartilage within the vertebral body cancellous bone) are not uncommon. However, Schmorl's nodules are extremely rare in dogs and have never been reported in dogs with histologically confirmed FCEM.

In addition, it has been hypothesized that fibrocartilage may arise from vertebral growth-plate cartilage in immature dogs or metaplasia of the vascular endothelium, which later ruptures into the lumen and embolizes within the intrinsic spinal cord vasculature.

The ischemic injury caused by the arterial obstruction initiates a series of biochemical and metabolic changes that result in neuronal and glial cell death (secondary spinal cord injury).[27] The gray matter is affected more severely than the white matter because of its greater metabolic demand.

CLINICAL PRESENTATION

FCEM has been reported most commonly in large and giant breed dogs. However, it has been described also in small breed dogs (particularly miniature schnauzers)[1–8] and has been confirmed histologically in two chondrodystrophic breed dogs.[6,28] Approximately 80% of dogs with FCEM diagnosed antemortem or confirmed histologically had a body weight greater than 20 kg.[1,2,5,8] The reported male-to-female ratio has ranged from 1:1[2] to approximately 2.5:1[4,8] in different studies. The age at diagnosis in dogs has ranged from 2 months[29] to 11 years and 11 months,[8] with a median of 5 or 6 years in most studies.[1,2,5,8]

The typical clinical presentation is characterized by peracute (<6 hours) onset of nonprogressive and nonpainful (after the first 24 hours), and often asymmetric myelopathy. In 29%[8] to 80%[2] of dogs with an antemortem diagnosis of FCEM, and in 43%[5] to 61%[2] of dogs with histologic diagnosis of FCEM, the owner reported that the dog was performing some type of physical activity, such as walking, running, or playing, at onset of neurologic signs. Signs of sudden and transient hyperalgesia (eg, yelping as in pain) were observed by the owners at the onset of neurologic signs in approximately 50% of dogs in one study[2] and in only 12% of dogs in another study.[5] Most commonly, maximal neurologic deterioration occurs within the first 6 to 24 hours and is followed by gradual improvement or stabilization of signs, depending on the extent and severity of the ischemic injury.[2,5,8] Rarely, neurologic dysfunction can progress for longer than 24 hours, possibly from additional embolizations or secondary spinal cord injury.

Neurologic deficits vary depending on the location and severity of the spinal cord ischemic injury, and are asymmetric in 53% to 86% of dogs.[1,2,5,8] The most commonly affected spinal cord segments have been L4-S3 (43%–47%) and C6-T2 (30%–33%) in dogs with a histologic diagnosis of FCEM,[2,5] and L4-S3 (44%–50%) and T3-L3 (27%–42%) in dogs with an antemortem diagnosis of FCEM.[2,5,8] Commonly, neurologic deficits refer to the affected spinal cord segment (eg, C1-5, C6-T2, T3-L3, or L4-S3). However, in the acute stages of the disease, a decreased withdrawal reflex has been observed in severely paraparetic and paraplegic dogs, with MRI changes consistent with FCEM within the T3-L3 spinal cord segment.[8] Most of these dogs had an interruption of the cutaneous trunci reflex consistent with the site of FCEM on MRI.[8]

Experts have suggested that the transient depression or abolition of pelvic limb spinal reflexes in dogs with acute thoracolumbar spinal cord injury results from sudden interruption of descending supraspinal input on motor neurons and interneurons, fusimotor depression, and increased segmental inhibition.[30] Focal mild to moderate hyperesthesia can sometimes be elicited on palpation of the affected spinal segments in dogs examined within the first few hours after onset of neurologic signs, although this rapidly resolves.

Most cats reported with FCEM have been domestic short hairs. Males and females were nearly equally represented. The age at onset of FCEM ranged from 4 to 12 years and most affected cats were older than 7 years.[11,12] Onset was acute in all reported cats, and nonprogressive after the first 24 hours of disease in most of them. However, clinical deterioration was observed over 2 to 5 days in a few cats with histologically confirmed FCEM. None of the reported cats had a history of trauma or exercise at the onset of disease and none had discomfort or hyperesthesia on spinal palpation. The most commonly affected spinal cord segments have been C6-T2; however, any spinal cord segment can be affected. All reported cats had asymmetric neurologic signs.

DIFFERENTIAL DIAGNOSES

Material other than fibrocartilage, such as thrombi or bacterial, parasitic, neoplastic, or fat emboli, can obstruct the intrinsic spinal blood vessels and result in spinal cord ischemia and necrosis. The clinical presentation and MRI findings are very similar or identical to the ones that characterize FCEM. Underlying medical conditions that may predispose to embolization or thrombosis, including cardiomyopathy, hypothyroidism, hyperthyroidism, hyperadrenocorticism, chronic renal failure, and hypertension, should be considered and investigated, particularly in cats.

Another condition that results in peracute onset of nonprogressive (after the first 24 hours), and often asymmetric, myelopathy is the so-called acute noncompressive nucleus pulposus extrusion[31] or traumatic intervertebral disc extrusion.[32] This condition occurs when nondegenerated nucleus pulposus extrudes during strenuous exercise or trauma, contuses the spinal cord, and dissipates within the epidural space, causing minimal to no spinal cord compression. Discomfort or hyperesthesia during palpation of the affected spinal segments has been reported in 57% of dogs with acute noncompressive nucleus pulposus extrusion,[31] and represents the main clinical finding to differentiate this condition from FCEM because it generally persists for more than 24 hours. High-field MRI and experience in neuroimaging help differentiate these two diseases.[7,8,31,32] The MRI features of acute noncompressive nucleus pulposus extrusion include the presence of a focal intramedullary hyperintensity overlying a narrowed intervertebral disc, with reduced volume and signal intensity of the nucleus pulposus on T2-weighted fast spin echo (FSE) images, and extraneous material or signal change within the epidural space dorsal to the affected disc, with absent or minimal spinal cord compression.[31,32]

Other differential diagnoses include compressive intervertebral disc extrusion, infectious and immune-mediated focal myelitis, neoplasia, and intra- and extramedullary hemorrhage (eg, secondary to coagulopathy). History, clinical signs, disease progression, and diagnostic findings (particularly MRI and cerebrospinal fluid [CSF] analysis) allow these disorders to be differentiated from FCEM.

For patients with unknown or incomplete history, exogenous traumatic spinal injury (resulting in vertebral fracture, subluxation/luxation, spinal cord contusion, or hemorrhage) should be considered in the differential diagnoses list. Patients with exogenous traumatic spinal injury generally present with severe spinal hyperesthesia and should be manipulated minimally and carefully until survey spinal radiographs rule out an unstable lesion.

DIAGNOSIS

The definitive diagnosis of FCEM can be reached only through histologic examination of the affected spinal cord segments. The antemortem diagnosis of FCEM is based on the typical clinical presentation (peracute nonprogressive after 24 hours, nonpainful, usually asymmetric myelopathy) and exclusion of other causes of peracute/acute focal myelopathy (through diagnostic imaging and CSF analysis). In addition, complete blood cell count, serum biochemistry, coagulation profile, and echocardiography can help rule out diseases that can predispose to thromboembolism, such as vasculitis and endocarditis.

Plain Radiographs

Plain radiographs of the spine help rule out vertebral fracture, subluxation/luxation, neoplasia, and osteomyelitis/discospondylitis.

Myelography

The main value of myelography in the antemortem diagnosis of FCEM is the exclusion of other causes of peracute/acute focal myelopathy, particularly those resulting in spinal cord compression, such as intervertebral disc extrusion. In dogs and cats with FCEM, myelography may be normal or may show an intramedullary pattern suggesting focal spinal cord swelling in the acute stage of the disease. This pattern has been observed in 39% to 47% of dogs with a histologic diagnosis of FCEM and in approximately 26% of dogs with an antemortem diagnosis of FCEM.[2,5] However, an intramedullary pattern may also be observed with other causes of myelopathy, including focal myelitis, intramedullary neoplasia, intraparenchymal hemorrhage, and acute noncompressive nucleus pulposus extrusion. Acute noncompressive nucleus pulposus extrusion should be suspected when the area of spinal cord swelling is above a collapsed intervertebral disc space (on good-quality radiographs with optimal patient positioning) and focal spinal hyperesthesia persists for more than 24 hours.

CT

CT can also help to rule out other causes of peracute/acute myelopathy. CT–myelogram may show an intramedullary pattern of spinal cord swelling in the acute stage of FCEM.

MRI

MRI of the affected spinal region is the preferred diagnostic imaging modality for the antemortem diagnosis of FCEM. In addition to excluding other causes of myelopathy, it allows visualization of signal intensity changes suggestive of ischemic infarction of the spinal cord. These changes include a focal, relatively sharply demarcated, and often asymmetric intramedullary lesion (oedematous infarcted tissue), predominantly involving the gray matter that appears hyperintense to normal spinal cord gray matter on T2-weighted FSE images, and iso- or hypointense to normal spinal cord gray matter on T1-weighted FSE images (**Fig. 2**).[7–11] Focal spinal cord swelling is a common finding.[8] Postcontrast T1-weighted FSE images may show various degrees of enhancement of the affected area, generally on the fifth to seventh day of disease.[7–10] Sometimes no intraparenchymal signal intensity changes are observed on MRI performed within 24 to 72 hours after onset of FCEM.[8,33] The degree and extent of the ischemic injury and the availability of high contrast resolution MRI influence the ability to detect signal intensity changes in the early stage of FCEM.[8,34] Dogs that are ambulatory on presentation are more likely to have a normal MRI than nonambulatory dogs.[8]

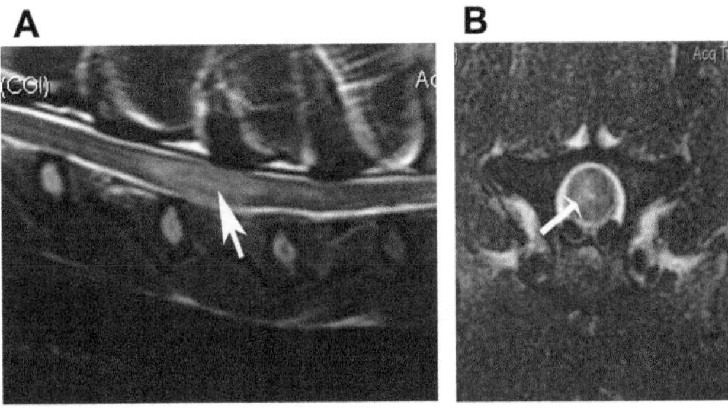

Fig. 2. (*A*) Mid-sagittal T2-weighted FSE image of a 9-year-old golden retriever with peracute onset of nonambulatory tetraparesis. An extensive hyperintense lesion (*arrow*) is seen within the spinal cord parenchyma over the vertebral body of C5. Histopathology confirmed a fibrocartilaginous embolus within the vasculature of the cord. (*B*) Transverse T2-weighted FSE image through the intramedullary hyperintensity depicted in *A*. The focal and relatively sharply demarcated lesion (*arrow*) involves the white and gray mater and is lateralized to the left.

The severity of neurologic dysfunction at initial examination has been associated with the longitudinal and transverse extent of the intramedullary ischemic lesions on MRI.[8] Repeated MRI studies have been used in humans to detect an ischemic lesion that was not apparent in the acute stage of the disease,[34,35] and may also be helpful in evaluating certain veterinary patients with suspected FCEM.

Diffusion-weighted (DW) MRI has been used in humans to increase the sensitivity and specificity for diagnosing spinal cord infarction in the early stage of the disorder.[35] DW MRI presents a technical challenge because of the relatively small size of the spinal cord (particularly in veterinary patients), low spatial resolution, and the magnetic susceptibility to artifacts caused by vascular and CSF pulsation.[8,34,35] Some of these technical problems may be overcome by using a multishot technique, which improves signal-to-noise ratio and is less sensitive to off-resonance effects.[36,37] DW MRI has shown increasing intramedullary hyperintensity from 1 to 24 hours postembolization in experimental dogs with spinal cord infarction induced by embolization of the spinal branches of T9-11 intercostal arteries bilaterally.[37]

CFS Analysis

CSF analysis may be normal or may reveal nonspecific abnormalities, including xanthochromia, mild to moderate pleocytosis (7–84 white blood cells per microliter) and elevated protein concentration. CSF abnormalities (mainly elevated protein concentration) have been reported in up to 46% of dogs with a histologic diagnosis of FCEM and in 44% to 75% of dogs with an antemortem diagnosis of FCEM.[2,8] Polymerase chain reaction for different infectious agents on CSF may help rule out specific causes of meningomyelitis.

Histologic Examination

Histologic examination of the affected spinal cord segments shows fibrocartilaginous material in spinal vessels (arteries or veins) within or near an area of focal myelomalacia (**Fig. 3**). The distribution of the lesion reflects the territory of the embolized vessels and therefore is frequently asymmetric. The gray matter is generally more severely affected than the white matter. The lesion margins tend to be well delineated from

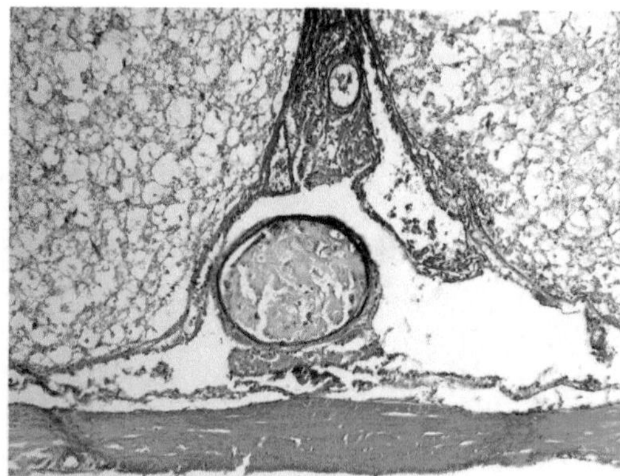

Fig. 3. Histopathologic transverse section of the midcervical spinal cord of a 13-year-old West Highland White Terrier with peracute nonambulatory tetraparesis. Intravascular fibrocartilaginous material is present within the ventral spinal artery and ischemic necrosis of dependent spinal cord parenchyma has occurred (Goldner stain, ×320). (*Courtesy of* Dr Carlo Cantile, University of Pisa, Italy.)

normal tissue. Infarcted areas are usually ischemic but sometimes may be accompanied by hemorrhage.

TREATMENT

Treatment of FCEM involves reducing secondary spinal cord injury (maintenance of spinal cord perfusion, neuroprotection) in the acute stage of the disease, nursing care, and physiotherapy. In patients with neurologic impairment of ventilation (eg, severe cervical spinal cord lesions, impaired phrenic nerve function) or with concurrent cardiovascular or respiratory disease, systemic blood pressure, ventilation, and oxygenation should be monitored and maintained within normal limits to ensure adequate spinal cord perfusion.

Neuroprotective agents such as methylprednisolone sodium succinate (MPSS) and polyethylene glycol could help minimize secondary spinal cord injury. However, the clinical benefits of these drugs require further investigation in dogs and cats with spinal cord injury and there are increasing concerns about the adverse effects of MPSS. Nursing care and physiotherapy play an essential role in the management of patients with FCEM (particularly those with severe neurologic impairment), because they promote recovery and help prevent complications. Nursing care includes providing adequate bedding, regular turning, skin care to prevent decubital ulcers and urine scalding, care of the respiratory system (prevention/treatment of hypoventilation, aspiration pneumonia, pulmonary atelectasis), bladder and bowel management, and adequate nutrition. Physiotherapy stimulates neuronal plasticity and therefore maximizes functional recovery mediated by unaffected neural tissue, and minimizes disuse and immobilization changes such as muscle atrophy and muscle and joint contractures.

PROGNOSIS

The prognosis for recovery in patients with FCEM depends on the severity and extent of the ischemic injury. Recovery rates have ranged from 58%[1] to 84%[8] in various studies, probably because of differences in inclusion criteria, severity and distribution of ischemic lesions, definition of outcome, and owner's commitment.[1,2,5,8] In a recent study, 42 of 50 (84%) dogs had either a complete clinical recovery or a partial recovery compatible with life as a functional pet (eg, urinary and fecally continent, being able to perform daily activities without extra care from the owner).[8]

Negative clinical prognostic factors reported include loss of nociception,[1,2,5] lower motor neuron signs,[1,2] symmetric neurologic deficits,[2,5] severity of neurologic signs at initial examination quantified by a neurologic score,[8] owner's reluctance to pursue nursing care and physiotherapy (particularly in large or giant breed dogs),[2] and lack of improvement within the first 14 days.[1]

Outcome has been associated with the extent of the ischemic intramedullary lesion on MRI, defined as the ratio between the length of the intramedullary hyperintensity on mid-sagittal T2-weighted images and the length of the vertebral body (referred to as *lesion length–vertebral length ratio*) of C6 (in dogs with cervical lesions) or L2 (in dogs with thoracolumbar lesions), and as the cross-sectional area of the largest intramedullary hyperintensity on transverse T2-weighted images expressed as a percentage of the cross-sectional area of the spinal cord at the same level (referred to as *percent cross-sectional area of the lesion*). Dogs with a lesion length–vertebral length ratio greater than 2.0 or a percent cross-sectional area of the lesion of 67% or greater were significantly more likely to have an unsuccessful outcome than those with lower values for these parameters.[8]

In one study, the presence of CSF abnormalities (increased protein concentration ± pleocytosis) was associated with a poorer outcome in dogs with FCEM.[5] However, a more recent study found no association between the presence of CSF abnormalities and outcome, or the extent of the ischemic intramedullary lesion on MRI.[8]

Intervals between onset of neurologic signs and recovery of voluntary motor activity, unassisted ambulation, and maximal recovery have been reported to be 6 days (range, 2.5–15 days), 11 days (range, 4–136 days), and 3.75 months (range, 1–12 months), respectively.[8] No statistically significant association has been identified between clinical or MRI variables and recovery times.[5,8]

Although reported cases are limited, prognosis for cats undergoing adequate nursing care for at least 2 weeks after onset of FCEM is likely to be as good as for dogs.[11]

SUMMARY

Prognosis for dogs and cats with FCEM is generally favorable. Severity of neurologic signs at initial examination and extent of the lesions seen on MRI can help predict outcome in dogs with FCEM.

ACKNOWLEDGMENTS

The authors would like to thank Allison Wright MS, CMI, for the illustrations and A. de Lahunta DVM, PhD, for his careful review of their anatomic detail.

REFERENCES

1. Gilmore DR, de Lahunta A. Necrotizing myelopathy secondary to presumed or confirmed fibrocartilaginous embolism in 24 dogs. J Am Anim Hosp Assoc 1986;23:373–6.
2. Cauzinille L, Kornegay JN. Fibrocartilaginous embolism of the spinal cord in dogs: review of 36 histologically confirmed cases and retrospective study of 26 suspected cases. J Vet Intern Med 1996;10:241–5.

3. Cauzinille L. Fibrocartilaginous embolism in dogs. Vet Clin North Am Small Anim Pract 2000;30:155–67.
4. Hawthorne JC, Wallace LJ, Fenner WR, et al. Fibrocartilaginous embolic myelopathy in miniature schnauzers. J Am Anim Hosp Assoc 2001;37:374–83.
5. Gandini G, Cizinauskas S, Lang J, et al. Fibrocartilaginous embolism in 75 dogs: clinical findings and factors influencing the recovery rate. J Small Anim Pract 2003;44:76–80.
6. Grunenfelder FI, Weishaupt D, Green R, et al. Magnetic resonance imaging findings in spinal cord infarction in three small breed dogs. Vet Radiol Ultrasound 2005;46:91–6.
7. Abramson CJ, Garosi L, Platt SR, et al. Magnetic resonance imaging appearance of suspected ischemic myelopathy in dogs. Vet Radiol Ultrasound 2005;46: 225–9.
8. De Risio L, Adams V, Dennis R, et al. Magnetic resonance imaging findings and clinical associations in 52 dogs with suspected ischemic myelopathy. J Vet Intern Med 2007;21:1290–8.
9. De Risio L, Adams V, Dennis R, et al. Association of clinical and magnetic resonance imaging findings with outcome in dogs suspected to have ischemic myelopathy: 50 cases (2000–2006). J Am Vet Med Assoc 2008;233:129–35.
10. Han JJ, Massagli TL, Jaffe KM. Fibrocartilaginous embolism—an uncommon cause of spinal cord infarction: a case report and review of the literature. Arch Phys Med Rehabil 2004;85:153–7.
11. MacKay AD, Rusbridge C, Sparkes AH, et al. MRI characteristics of suspected acute spinal cord infarction in two cats, and a review of the literature. J Feline Med Surg 2005;7:101–7.
12. Mikszewski JS, Van Winkle TJ, Troxel MT. Fibrocartilaginous embolic myelopathy in five cats. J Am Anim Hosp Assoc 2006;42:226–33.
13. Taylor HW, Vandevelde M, Firth EC. Ischemic myelopathy by fibrocartilaginous emboli in a horse. Vet Pathol 1977;14:479–81.
14. Tessaro SV, Doige CE, Rhodes CS. Posterior paralysis due to fibrocartilaginous embolism in two weaner pigs. Can J Comp Med 1983;47:124–6.
15. Stedman NL, Brown TP, Rowland GN. Intravascular cartilaginous emboli in the spinal cord of turkeys. Avian Dis 1998;42:423–8.
16. Jeffery M, Wells GA. Multifocal ischemic encephalomyelopathy associated with fibrocartilaginous emboli in the lamb. Neuropathol Appl Neurobiol 1986;12: 231–44.
17. Landolfi JA, Saunders GK, Swecker WS. Fibrocartilaginous embolic myelopathy in a calf. J Vet Diagn Invest 2004;16:360–2.
18. Adaska JM, Lynch S. Fibrocartilaginous embolic myelopathy in a Sumatran tiger (*Panthera tigris sumatrae*). J Zoo Wildl Med 2004;35(2):242–4.
19. Renner MS, Bryant W, Kennedy G. Fibrocartilaginous emboli in a tayra (*Eira Barbara*): a case report. J Zoo Wildl Med 1998;29:470–3.
20. Huneke RB, La Regina MC. Acute paralysis caused by fibrocartilaginous embolism in a pigtail macaque. Contemp Top Lab Anim Sci 1999;38(1):87–8.
21. Evans HE. The heart and arteries. Miller's anatomy of the dog. 3rd edition. Philadelphia: WB Saunders; 1993. p. 626–9, 647–8, 659.
22. Sharp NJH, Wheeler SJ. Functional anatomy. In: Sharp NJH, Wheeler SJ, editors. Small animal spinal disorders, diagnosis and surgery. 2nd edition. London: Elsevier Mosby; 2005. p. 14–7.
23. Caulkins SE, Purinton PT, Oliver JE. Arterial supply to the spinal cord of dogs and cats. Am J Vet Res 1989;50(3):425–30.

24. Evans HE. The veins. Miller's anatomy of the dog. 3rd edition. Philadelphia: WB Saunders; 1993. p. 713–5.
25. Zaki FA, Prata RG. Necrotizing myelopathy secondary to embolization of herniated intervertebral disk material in the dog. J Am Vet Med Assoc 1976;169:222–8.
26. Hayes MA, Creighton R, Boysen BG, et al. Acute necrotizing myelopathy from nucleus pulposus embolism in dogs with intervertebral disk degeneration. J Am Vet Med Assoc 1978;173:289–95.
27. Olby N, Jeffery N. Pathogenesis of diseases of the central nervous system. In: Slatter D, editor. Textbook of small animal surgery. 3rd edition. Philadelphia: WB Saunders; 2003. p. 1132–47.
28. Ueno H, Shimizu J, Uzuka Y, et al. Fibrocartilaginous embolism in a chondrodystrophoid breed dog. Aust Vet J 2005;83:142–4.
29. Junker K, van den Ingh T, Bossard MM, et al. Fibrocartilaginous embolism of the spinal cord (FCE) in juvenile Irish wolfhounds. Vet Q 2000;22:154–6.
30. Smith PM, Jeffery ND. Spinal Shock-Comparative aspects and clinical relevance. J Vet Intern Med 2005;19:788–93.
31. De Risio L, Adams V, Dennis R, et al. Association of clinical and magnetic resonance imaging findings with outcome in dogs with presumptive acute noncompressive nucleus pulposus extrusion: 42 cases (2000–2007). J Am Vet Med Assoc 2009;234:495–504.
32. Chang Y, Dennis R, Platt S, et al. Magnetic resonance imaging features of traumatic intervertebral disc extrusion in dogs. Vet Rec 2007;160:795–9.
33. Stein VM, Wagner F, Bull C, et al. Findings of magnetic resonance imaging in suspected canine fibro-cartilaginous embolization [abstract]. In: Proceedings of the XIX Symposium of the European Society of Veterinary Neurology. Barcelona, Spain, September 29–30, 2006. p. 157.
34. Luo CB, Chang FC, Teng MM, et al. Magnetic resonance imaging as a guide in the diagnosis and follow-up of spinal cord infarction. J Chin Med Assoc 2003;66: 89–95.
35. Kuker W, Weller M, Klose U, et al. Diffusion-weighted MRI of spinal cord infarction-high resolution imaging and time course of diffusion abnormality. J Neurol 2004;251:818–24.
36. Zhang J, Huan Y, Qian Y, et al. Multishot diffusion weighted imaging features in spinal cord infarction. J Spinal Disord Tech 2005;18:277–82.
37. Zhang J, Huan Y, Sun LJ, et al. Temporal evolution of spinal cord infarction in an in vivo experimental study of canine models characterized by diffusion-weighted imaging. J Magn Reson Imaging 2007;26:848–54.

Inflammatory Diseases of the Spine in Small Animals

Andrea Tipold, DVM*, Veronika M. Stein, DVM, PhD

KEYWORDS

• Meningitis • Myelitis • Discospondylitis • Dog • Cat

Inflammatory diseases of the central nervous system (CNS) or of the surrounding structures are an important disease category and have to be considered as differential diagnoses in small animals with clinical signs indicating a spinal cord lesion or spinal pain (cervical or thoracolumbar). Inflammatory lesions are commonly widespread and the whole CNS may be affected. Clinical signs may reflect a multifocal lesion. Pure myelitis cases are a rare finding in contrast to patients with meningitis. Of this last group, steroid responsive meningitis-arteritis (SRMA) is the most frequently occurring inflammatory lesion of the nervous system in our referral-teaching hospital. In most cases other than neurological abnormalities, additional clinical findings such as fever occur. This article focuses on the most important inflammatory diseases of the spine.

DISCOSPONDYLITIS

Discospondylitis is defined as an inflammation or infection of the intervertebral disk and osteomyelitis in adjacent vertebral end plates and bodies.

The most common cause is a bacterial infection with coagulase positive Staphylococci (*S aureus or S intermedius*) being the most frequent isolate.[1,2] Other frequently identified bacteria include *Streptococcus*, *Escherichia coli*, and *Brucella canis*. Less common causal agents are *Pasteurella* spp, *Proteus* spp, *Corynebacterium* spp, *Actinomyces*, *Nocardia* spp, *Bacteroides* spp, *Mycobacterium* spp, *Pseudomonas aeruginosa*, *Enterococcus faecalis*, and *Staphylococcus epidermidis*.[3–8] Fungal infections have also been reported, with *Aspergillus*, *Paecilomyces*, *Penicillium*, and *Fusarium* species, and *Coccidioides immitis* being cultured.[9–15]

Discospondylitis most commonly arises from hematogenous spread of organisms to the disk space, subsequently extending into the adjacent vertebrae. Primary sources can be the urogenital tract, skin or dental disease, and valvular endocarditis.[16–20] However, the initiating site of the infection usually cannot be identified. Additionally,

Department of Small Animal Medicine and Surgery, University for Veterinary Medicine Hannover, Buenteweg 9, D-30559 Hannover, Germany
* Corresponding author.
E-mail address: Andrea.Tipold@tiho-hannover.de

Vet Clin Small Anim 40 (2010) 871–879
doi:10.1016/j.cvsm.2010.05.008 **vetsmall.theclinics.com**
0195-5616/10/$ – see front matter

migrating foreign bodies (mostly plant material such as grass awns), extending body organ abscesses, iatrogenic trauma (such as spinal surgery or fenestration), and epidural injections can also cause discospondylitis.[8,16,21–23] Immunosuppressed animals or patients that underwent prior surgery might have a higher risk to develop discospondylitis.[20]

Discospondylitis typically affects young to middle-aged dogs. Purebred dogs are more commonly affected than mixed-breeds, and large-breed and male dogs are more often affected (ratio of male to female is 2:1).[18,24] Discospondylitis is very rare in cats.[25–27]

Clinical signs are variable. They range from systemic infection with depression, anorexia, fever, and weight loss to stiffness and reluctance to walk and jump. Spinal or paraspinal hyperesthesia is the most characteristic sign. With proliferation of inflammatory tissue, neurologic signs consistent with extradural compression can develop. Extension of inflammation through the meninges can also lead to meningitis and meningomyelitis. Clinical signs will be dependant on the site and severity of the lesions and include ataxia, paresis, and paralysis. The course of the disease is usually slowly progressive but vertebral pathological fractures or intervertebral disk protrusions can lead to acute deterioration of the clinical signs. The sites most commonly affected are L7-S1, caudal cervical, midthoracic, and thoracolumbar spine.[12,18,23,24,28]

The diagnosis is suggestive from patient history and physical and neurological examinations. A definitive diagnosis is made on the basis of characteristic findings in spinal radiographs such as concentric lysis of adjacent vertebral endplates with vertebral body osteolysis, shortening of vertebral bodies and proliferative sclerosis, and osseous bridging and narrowing of disk spaces in later stages. It has to be noted that unremarkable findings cannot rule out the existence of discospondylitis as it can take 2 to 6 weeks for radiographic changes to develop.[18,29]

MRI scans can reveal increased signal intensity on T2-weighted images and decreased signal on T1-weighted images in the affected intervertebral disk, vertebral end plates and bodies, and surrounding soft tissues before radiographic changes occur.[30] Post–gadolinium-diethylenetriamine pentetic acid (GdDTPA), T1-weighted images show enhancement between the disk and endplate (**Fig. 1**). CT scanning offers the possibility to guide fine-needle aspiration and tissue core biopsy.[29]

The large variety of potential causative agents underscores that it is essential to attempt bacterial isolation and sensitivity testing. Therefore, blood and urine cultures should be obtained before starting antibiotic therapy, but positive results are obtained in only 40% to 75% of affected dogs.[18,20] Percutaneous fluoroscopy-guided

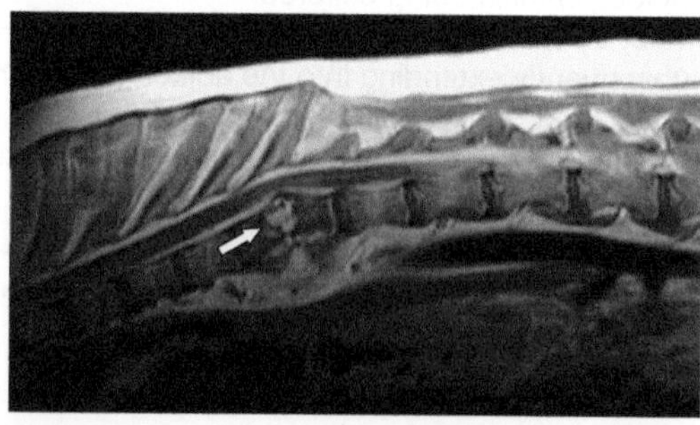

Fig. 1. Discospondylitis in a 3-year-old male Bernese Mountain dog. Sagittal T1-weighted image postintravenous injection of GdDTPA. The image reveals an irregular margin and enhancement between the end plates of T9 and T10 (*arrow*).

aspiration of the infected disk space can provide specimens for bacterial cultures.[31,32] This is particularly indicated in patients not responding to initial antibiotic therapy, cases where neoplasia has to be ruled out, or when the diagnosis is not clear.

Prognosis is usually favorable if neurological signs are mild, unless multiple lesions, vertebral fracture, instability, or dislocation occurs.[1,33] However, an aggressive long-term antibiotic therapy for at least 2 to 4 months is mandatory. Analgesics may be necessary. Prognosis may be guarded in dogs with fungal infections or infections with *B canis*.[5,6,18] Infections with *B canis* also bear the risk of a percutaneous fluoroscopy-guided aspiration zoonotic infection. Dogs with brucellosis should be neutered and antibiotic regimen switched to a combination of tetracyclines and aminoglycosides.

MENINGITIS

Dogs suffering from meningitis are mostly only painful and reluctant to move. Only if the adjacent spinal cord is affected might additional neurological deficits such as paresis or proprioceptive deficits be observed.

Bacterial Meningitis

Bacterial meningitis (BM) can be found occasionally in dogs. Bacteria commonly associated with BM in dogs and cats include *Staphylococcus* spp, *Escherichia coli, Pasteurella multocida, Actinomyces* spp, *Nocardia* spp, rarely *Streptococcus* spp, and various anaerobes.[34,35]

Bacterial invasion may occur via direct implantation (trauma, dog biting, surgery, cerebrospinal fluid (CSF) tap, local spread (discospondylitis), or hematogenous pathway (bacteremia)).

CSF examination, radiographs, and MRI are useful to establish the diagnosis and rule out other differential diagnosis. In the majority of the cases, CSF examination reveals neutrophilic pleocytosis and increased protein content. Bacterial culture of CSF samples is negative in most cases. More promising techniques may be universal bacterial polymerase chain reaction assays (PCR).[35] The search for a diagnosis of the cause is important for successful treatment. The focus of the infection has to be determined and treated surgically or medically. Changes in complete blood count and urinalysis may also be observed (leucocytosis, neutrophilia).

Treatment consists of a combination of antibiotics, such as ampicillin, amoxicillin, or cephalosporins for its high efficacy against gram-positive organisms, and metronidazole for its high potency against anaerobes. Based on sensitivity results, treatment has to be initiated as early as possible. Prognosis is variable depending on the sensitivity of the infectious agents causing the meningitis and the extent of the lesions. Because the disease occurs infrequently, studies on treatment outcome and on the effect of the application of glucocorticosteroids in dogs and cats are not currently available.

SRMA

SRMA occurs much more frequently than bacterial meningitis and is observed worldwide in young-adult dogs. A breed predisposition was described for Bernese mountain dogs, boxers, and beagles.[36,37] In recent years the Nova Scotia duck tolling retriever was found to be frequently affected and a familial predisposition has been reported.[38] Other medium- to large-breed dogs may also be affected.

SRMA is a systemic immune-mediated disorder with the main inflammatory lesions in the leptomeninges and associated vessels.[37,39] The etiopathogenesis is unknown; however, the epidemiology of the disease suggests an infectious origin. A large portion of the T cells are activated, suggesting the presence of a superantigen.[40] Several findings suggest an immunopathologic event: markedly increased IgA levels in CSF and serum, increased B-cell/T-cell ratio in the blood and CSF, a suggested Th2-mediated immune response, and autoantibodies in CSF and serum that are not specific for the disease and thought to be an epiphenomenon.[41–43] Elevated IL-8 levels and increased chemotactic activity in the CSF can explain the invasion of neutrophils in the leptomeninges in SRMA.[44] In addition, the pleocytosis in the CSF may be facilitated through upregulation of CD11a and matrixmetalloproteinases.[45,46]

Histopathology reveals changes in the meninges of the spinal cord and, to a much lesser degree, in the brain. Necrotizing arteritis of medium- and small-sized arteries and associated purulent leptomeningitis are the most important findings. In chronic lesions, proliferative changes of the vascular intima with stenosis and adventitial fibrosis occur. In rare cases vessels may be thrombosed.

Clinical signs are episodic and recurrent. Cervical pain of acute onset, reluctance to move, stiff gait, resistance to neck manipulation, paraspinal hyperesthesia, and fever are observed. In the chronic, protracted form, dogs develop neurologic deficits consistent with a multifocal or spinal cord lesion.[37] In rare cases, tetra- or paraplegia might occur due to spontaneous bleeding in the subarachnoidal space.

The diagnosis is supported by hematologic findings such as a neutrophilic leucocytosis. The examination of the CSF is the most important diagnostic tool in this disease. CSF samples may appear to be turbid from pleocytosis or xanthochromic from hemorrhage occurring in the subarachnoidal space. A marked neutrophilic CSF pleocytosis (up to several thousand cells/μl) (**Fig. 2**), erythrophagocytosis, and elevated immunoglobulin levels are prominent findings.

A combined elevation of high IgA levels in serum and CSF supports the diagnosis with a high sensitivity, but low specificity.[47] In addition, acute phase proteins (APPs), including C-reactive protein (CRP), have been shown to be elevated in the serum and CSF of dogs with SRMA.[39,48] MRI scans show enhancement in post-GdDTPA T1-weighted images in the meninges and enlarged vessels in severe cases.[37]

Response to antibiotics is thought to be incidental because spontaneous remission is observed and clinical signs are characterized by their waxing and waning nature. In dogs with only one episode of pain and a mild pleocytosis in the CSF, nonsteroidal antiinflammatory drugs are administered accompanied by careful patient monitoring.[37] If the clinical signs relapse or worsen, or if a severe pleocytosis is observed,

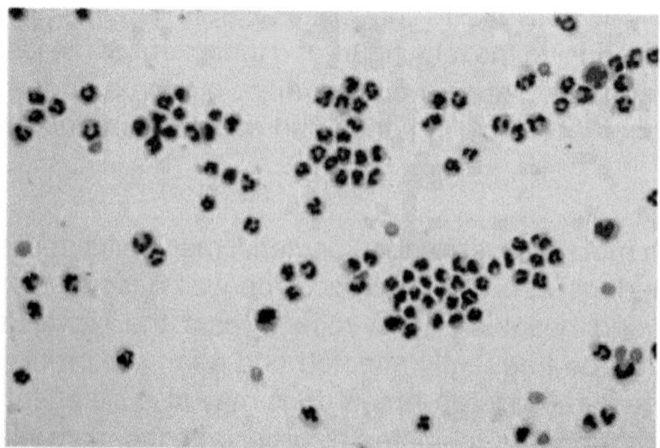

Fig. 2. Cerebrospinal fluid of a 6-month-old female Boxer with steroid-responsive meningitis-arteritis showing neutrophilic pleocytosis.

long-term treatment with glucocorticosteroids (approximately 6 months) is indicated. Prednisolone is given starting with 4 mg/kg of body weight for 1 to 2 days. The dose is reduced to 2 mg/kg daily for 1 to 2 weeks, than slowly reduced until a dose of 0.5 mg/kg every other day is reached. Response to treatment and follow-up examinations every 4 to 6 weeks with CSF analysis, hematology, and serum CRP levels determine the treatment protocol.[39,48] In refractory cases or in patients having side effects such as polydipsia or polyuria and polyphagia, immunosuppressive drugs and glucocorticoids are given on alternate days (eg, azathioprine 1.5–2 mg/kg every 48 hours). This treatment schedule does not influence the underlying immunopathologic condition, the disease seems to be self-limiting within a certain period. The application of glucocortocosteroids may prevent damage to the CNS that is related to hemorrhage or severe inflammation. Long-term treatment studies show a good prognosis in 60% to 80% of treated dogs.[49] Similar results were also found in a recent study.[48]

MYELITIS AND MENINGOMYELITIS

Pure myelitis or meningomyelitis is a rare disease in small animals. The inflammation of the spinal cord parenchyma (myelitis) and the surrounding meninges (meningomyelitis) mostly occurs in a combination with inflammatory brain disease (encephalitis).[34] Clinical signs associated with meningomyelitis depend on the affected region of the spinal cord and include paresis or paralysis, pain, and proprioceptive deficits. Spinal reflexes may or may not be reduced. In a survey of 28 cases,[50] the breeds more affected were hounds or toy breeds. Meningomyelitis of unknown cause and granulomatous meningomyelitis were the most common presumptive diagnoses. Diagnosis of meningomyelitis is supported by CSF and advanced imaging findings[50,51] such as MRI (**Fig. 3**). In rare cases the cause of the myelitis can be detected and includes organisms such as *Mycobacterium avium* or nematode larvae.[52,53] Specific treatment depends on the cause.

FELINE POLIOMYELITIS

The diagnosis of feline poliomyelitis is more of a description of a disease condition characterized by a subacute to chronic nonsuppurative myelitis with a predominance of pathological changes in the gray matter. Cats of any age and either sex can be affected, and no breed predisposition was found. The disease is sporadic and prevalent in different continents of the world, especially in northern Europe.[54–57]

The cause of the disease is unknown, although the histopathological findings reflect the typical conditions for a neurotropic viral infection. However, as in other idiopathic diseases, attempts for viral isolation were not successful and viral inclusions have not

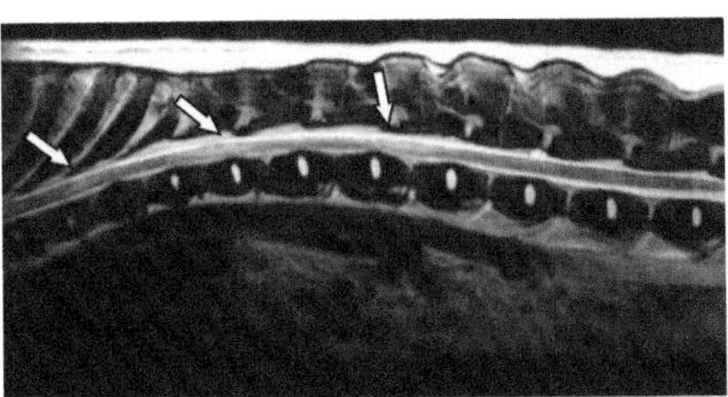

Fig. 3. Myelitis of unknown cause in a 5-year-old male mix breed dog. Sagittal T2-weighted images. Multiple hyperintense diffuse lesions (*arrows*) are seen.

been detected in histopathological exams. Although not proven, different viruses have been implicated as possible causative agents in feline poliomyelitis: Aujeszky disease virus, togavirus, Newcastle disease virus, feline parvovirus, and feline immunodeficiency virus have been considered but either ruled out by distinct pathological findings or could not be demonstrated.[56–59] Moreover, Bornavirus has been implicated in countries where the virus is endemic in certain areas, such as Austria, Switzerland, Germany, and Sweden. The disease condition caused by Bornavirus in cats is called "staggering disease". This Borna disease however, shows morphological and clinical differences to feline poliomyelitis. Moreover, poliomyelitis is also seen in countries where Borna disease has not been seen.[59–63]

Typical histopathological findings are disseminated inflammatory lesions in the brain and spinal cord with a predilection for gray matter. The lesions consist of perivascular mononuclear cuffing, gliosis, and neuronal degeneration predominantly in the spinal cord ventral horns.[55,56] In chronic cases only very slight inflammation can be seen but neuronal loss and astrogliosis are prominent. A marked Wallerian degeneration of lateral and ventral columns occurs which resembles a primary degenerative disorder.[57,58]

The course of the disease is subacute to chronic, and the neurological signs usually tend to progress over weeks to months but may also stabilize. Inflammatory lesions can be found histopathologically in the spinal cord and brain, which are most severe in the spinal cord and medulla. Therefore, clinical findings comprise predominantly paresis, ataxia, and proprioceptive deficits in pelvic and thoracic limbs, eventually accompanied by thoracic and lumbar spinal hyperesthesia. When the inflammation is spread to the nerve roots, signs of lower motor neuron involvement such as decreased tendon reflexes and muscle atrophy become visible. In some cases epileptic seizures, tremors, circling, opisthotonus, pupillary abnormalities, nystagmus, and impaired vision can be observed.[55,56,58] Some cats have fever and may be leukopenic or show a nonregenerative anemia.[56]

The diagnosis is based on suggestive clinical signs and possibly CSF changes such as a mild-to-moderate mononuclear pleocytosis with or without a moderate increase in protein levels.[59]

A curative treatment for feline poliomyelitis does not exist. Supportive therapy consists of anticonvulsants to control seizures, and possibly corticosteroids to reduce the CNS inflammation. The prognosis is guarded; some cats that mounted a sufficient immune response are known to have recovered from the disease.[56,58]

SUMMARY

Inflammatory diseases of the spine include diseases of unknown causes such as SRMA, but also a range of infectious agents are responsible for such destructive lesions. Advanced imaging techniques improved considerably the diagnostic workup. To improve treatment strategies, further studies on the pathogenesis and identification of possible causative agents should be encouraged.

REFERENCES

1. Gilmore DR. Lumbosacral diskospondylitis in 21 dogs. J Am Anim Hosp Assoc 1987;23:57–61.
2. Kornegay JN. Diskospondylitis. In: Kirk RW, editor. Current veterinary therapy IX. Philadelphia: WB Saunders; 1986. p. 810.
3. Hurov L, Troy G, Turnwald G. Diskospondylitis in the dog: 27 cases. J Am Vet Med Assoc 1978;173:275.

4. Jones JC, Sorjonen DC, Simpson ST, et al. Comparison between computed tomographic and surgical findings in large-breed dogs with lumbosacral stenosis. Vet Radiol Ultrasound 1996;37:247–56.
5. Kerwin SC, Lewis DD, Hribernik TN, et al. Diskospondylitis associated with *Brucella canis* infection in dogs: 14 cases (1980–1991). J Am Vet Med Assoc 1992;201:1253–7.
6. Kornegay JN, Barber DL. Diskospondylitis in dogs. J Am Vet Med Assoc 1980; 177:337–41.
7. Adamo PF, Cherubini GB. Discospondylitis associated with three unreported bacteria in the dog. J Small Anim Pract 2001;42:352–5.
8. Schwartz M, Boettcher IC, Kramer S, et al. Two dogs with iatrogenic discospondylitis caused by meticillin-resistant *Staphylococcus aureus*. J Small Anim Pract 2009;50:201–5.
9. Patnaik AK, Liu S-K, Wilkins RJ, et al. Paecilomycosis in a dog. J Am Vet Med Assoc 1972;161:806–13.
10. Wood GL, Hirsh DC, Selcer RR, et al. Disseminated aspergillosis in a dog. J Am Vet Med Assoc 1978;172:704–7.
11. Johnson RG, Prata RG. Intradiskal osteomyelitis: a conservative approach. J Am Anim Hosp Assoc 1983;19:743–50.
12. Butterworth SJ, Barr FJ, Pearson GR, et al. Multiple discospondylitis associated with Aspergillus species infection in a dog. Vet Rec 1995;136:38–41.
13. Booth MJ, van der Lugt JJ, van Heerden A, et al. Temporary remission of disseminated paecilomycosis in a German shepherd dog treated with ketoconazole. J S Afr Vet Assoc 2001;72:99–104.
14. Watt PR, Robins GM, Galloway AM, et al. Disseminated opportunistic fungal disease in dogs: 10 cases (1982–1990). J Am Vet Med Assoc 1995;207:67–70.
15. Moore MP. Discospondylitis. Vet Clin North Am Small Anim Pract 1992;22: 1027–34.
16. Siems JS, Jakovljevic S, Adams LG, et al. Discospondylitis in association with an intra-abdominal abscess in a dog. J Small Anim Pract 1999;40:123–6.
17. Dallman MJ, Dew TL, Tobias L, et al. Disseminated aspergillosis in a dog with diskospondylitis and neurologic deficits. J Am Vet Med Assoc 1992;200:511–3.
18. Thomas WB. Diskospondylitis and other vertebral infections. Vet Clin North Am Small Anim Pract 2000;30:169–82.
19. Betbeze C, McLaughlin R. Canine diskospondylitis: its etiology, diagnosis, and treatment. Vet Med 2002;97:673–81.
20. Greene CE, Budsberg SC. Musculoskeletal infections. In: Greene CD, editor. Infectious diseases of the dog and cat. St. Louis (MO): WB Saunders; 2006. p. 823–41, Chapter 86.
21. Johnson DE, Summers BA. Osteomyelitis of the lumbar vertebrae in dogs caused by grass-seed foreign bodies. Aust Vet J 1971;47:289–94.
22. Jacob F, Bagley RS, Moore MP, et al. Cervical intervertebral disk protrusion, discospondylitis, and porcupine quill foreign body in a dog. Prog Vet Neurol 1996;7:53–5.
23. Remedios AM, Wagner R, Caulkett NA, et al. Epidural abscess and discospondylitis in a dog after administration of a lumbosacral epidural analgesic. Can Vet J 1996;37:106–7.
24. Burkert BA, Kerwin SC, Hosgood GL, et al. Signalment and clinical features of diskospondylitis in dogs: 513 cases (1980–2001). J Am Vet Med Assoc 2005; 227(2):268–75.
25. Malik R, Latter M, Love DN. Bacterial discospondylitis in a cat. J Small Anim Pract 1990;31:404–6.

26. Watson E, Roberts RE. Discospondylitis in a cat. Vet Radiol Ultrasound 1993;34:397–8.
27. Aroch I, Shamir M, Harmelin A. Lumbar diskospondylitis and meningomyelitis caused by *Escherichia coli* in a cat. Feline Pract 1999;27:20–2.
28. Auger J, Dupuis J, Quesnel A, et al. Surgical treatment of lumbosacral instability caused by discospondylitis in four dogs. Vet Surg 2000;29:70–80.
29. Gonzalo-Orden JM, Altonaga JR, Orden MA, et al. Magnetic resonance, computed tomographic and radiologic findings in a dog with discospondylitis. Vet Radiol Ultrasound 2000;41:142–4.
30. Kraft SL, Mussman JM, Smith T, et al. Magnetic resonance imaging of presumptive lumbosacral discospondylitis in a dog. Vet Radiol Ultrasound 1998;39:9–13.
31. Fischer A, Mahaffey MB, Oliver JE. Fluoroscopically guided percutaneous disk aspiration in 10 dogs with diskospondylitis. J Vet Intern Med 1997;11:284–7.
32. Kinzel S, Koch J, Buecker A, et al. Treatment of 10 dogs with discospondylitis by fluoroscopy-guided percutaneous discectomy. Vet Rec 2005;156(3):78–81.
33. van Bree H, de Rick A, Verschooten F, et al. Successful conservative treatment of cervical discospondylitis in a dog. J Small Anim Pract 1981;22:59–65.
34. Tipold A. Diagnosis of inflammatory and infectious diseases of the central nervous system in dogs: a retrospective study. J Vet Intern Med 1995;9:304–14.
35. Messner JH, Wagner SO, Baumwart RD, et al. A case of canine streptococcal meningoencephalitis diagnosed using universal bacterial polymerase chain reaction assays. J Am Anim Hosp Assoc 2008;44:205–9.
36. Tipold A, Jaggy A. Steroid responsive meningitis-arteritis in dogs: long-term study of 32 cases. J Small Anim Pract 1994;35:311–6.
37. Tipold A, Schatzberg SJ. An update on steroid responsive meningitis-arteritis. J Small Anim Pract 2010;51(3):150–4.
38. Anfinsen KP, Berendt M, Liste FJ, et al. A retrospective epidemiological study of clinical signs and familial predisposition associated with aseptic meningitis in the Norwegian population of Nova Scotia duck tolling retrievers born 1994–2003. Can J Vet Res 2008;72:350–5.
39. Bathen-Noethen A, Carlson R, Menzel D, et al. Concentrations of acute-phase proteins in dogs with steroid responsive meningitis-arteritis. J Vet Intern Med 2008;22:1149–56.
40. Tipold A, Somberg R, Felsburg P. Involvement of a superantigen in sterile purulent meningitis and arteritis of dogs. Tieraerztliche Praxis 1996;24:514–8.
41. Schwartz M, Moore PF, Tipold A. Disproportionally strong increase of B cells in inflammatory cerebrospinal fluid of dogs with Steroid-responsive Meningitis-Arteritis. Vet Immunol Immunopathol 2008;125:274–83.
42. Schwartz M. Puff C. Stein VM. Pathogenetic factors for excessive IgA production: Th2-dominated immune response in canine steroid-responsive Meningitis-Arteritis. Vet J 2010. [Epub ahead of print]. DOI: 10.1016/j.tvjl.2009.12.001.
43. Schulte K, Carlson R, Tipold A. [Autoantibodies against structures of the central nervous system in steroid responsive meningitis-arteritis in dogs]. Berl Munch Tierarztl Wochenschr 2006;119:55–61 [in German].
44. Burgener I, Van Ham L, Jaggy A, et al. Chemotactic activity and IL-8 levels in the cerebrospinal fluid in canine steroid responsive meningitis-arteritis. J Neuroimmunol 1998;89:182–90.
45. Schwartz M, Carlson R, Tipold A. Selective CD11a upregulation on neutrophils in the acute phase of steroid-responsive meningitis-arteritis in dogs. Vet Immunol Immunopathol 2008;126:248–55.

46. Schwartz M, Puff C, Stein VM, et al. Marked MMP-2 transcriptional up-regulation in mononuclear leukocytes invading the subarachnoidal space in aseptic suppurative steroid-responsive meningitis-arteritis in dogs. Vet Immunol Immunopathol 2010;133:198–206.
47. Maiolini A, Carlson R, Schwartz M, et al. Determination of IgA levels in serum and cerebrospinal fluid: assessment of its diagnostic value for canine steroid-responsive meningitis-arteritis in a large number of cases. Proceedings of the 22nd Symposium ECVN, Bologna (Italy), 2009. p. 85.
48. Lowrie M, Penderis J, Eckersall PD, et al. The role of acute phase proteins in diagnosis and management of steroid-responsive meningitis arteritis in dogs. Vet J 2009;182:125–30.
49. Cizinauskas S, Jaggy A, Tipold A. Long-term treatment of dogs with steroid-responsive meningitis-arteritis: clinical, laboratory and therapeutic results. J Small Anim Pract 2000;41:295–301.
50. Griffin JF, Levine JM, Levine GJ, et al. Meningomyelitis in dogs: a retrospective review of 28 cases. J Small Anim Pract 2008;49:509–17.
51. Parry AT, Penning VA, Smith KC, et al. Imaging diagnosis—necrotizing meningomyelitis and polyarthritis. Vet Radiol Ultrasound 2009;50:412–5.
52. Kim DY, Cho DY, Newton JC, et al. Granulomatous myelitis due to *Mycobacterium avium* in a dog. Vet Pathol 1994;31:491–3.
53. Snook ER, Baker DG, Bauer RW. Verminous myelitis in a pitt bull puppy. J Vet Diagn Invest 2009;21:400–2.
54. Kronevi T, Nordström M, Moreno W, et al. Feline ataxia due to nonsuppurative meningoencephalomyelitis of unknown aetiology. Nord Vet Med 1974;26:720–5.
55. Hoff EJ, Vandevelde M. Non-suppurative encephalomyelitis in cats suggestive of a viral origin. Vet Pathol 1981;18:170–80.
56. Vandevelde M, Braund KG. Polioencephalomyelitis in cats. Vet Pathol 1979;16: 420–7.
57. Tipold A, Vandevelde M. Neurologic diseases of suspected infectious origin and prion disease. In: Greene CD, editor. Infectious diseases of the dog and cat. St Louis (MO): WB Saunders; 2006. p. 800–2.
58. Palmer AC, Cavanagh JB. Encephalomyelopathy in young cats. J Soc Adm Pharm 1995;36:57–64.
59. Lundgren AL. Feline non-suppurative meningoencephalomyelitis. A clinical and pathological study. J Comp Pathol 1992;107:411–25.
60. Lundgren AL, Ludwig H. Clinically diseased cats with non-suppurative meningoencephalomyelitis have Borna disease virus-specific antibodies. Acta Vet Scand 1993;34:101–3.
61. Lundgren AL, Czech G, Bode L, et al. Natural Borna disease in domestic animals others than horses and sheep. Zentralbl Veterinarmed B 1993;40:298–303.
62. Berg AL, Berg M. A variant form of feline Borna disease. J Comp Pathol 1998; 119:323–31.
63. Nakamura Y, Watanabe M, Kamitani W, et al. High prevalence of Borna disease virus in domestic cats with neurological disorders in Japan. Vet Microbiol 1999; 70:153–69.

Cervical Spondylomyelopathy (Wobbler Syndrome) in Dogs

Ronaldo C. da Costa, DMV, MSc, PhD

KEYWORDS

- Wobbler syndrome • Cervical • Spine • Dog • Canine
- Spinal cord • Myelopathy • Instability

Cervical spondylomyelopathy (CSM) is a common disease of the cervical spine of large and giant breed dogs. CSM is characterized by dynamic and static compressions of the cervical spinal cord, nerve roots, or both, leading to variable degrees of neurologic deficits and neck pain. CSM is a controversial disease. There are few diseases in veterinary medicine that have been referred to by 14 different names. Wobbler syndrome, caudal cervical spondylomyelopathy, cervical spondylopathy, cervical spondylopathy disc associated compression, cervical vertebral instability, cervical malformation/malarticulation syndrome, cervical spondylolisthesis, cervical stenotic myelopathy, disc-associated wobbler syndrome, cervical spinal stenosis, cervical subluxation, cervical vertebral instability-malformation syndrome, and cervical spondylotic myelopathy are all terms that have been used to describe the disease.[1–13] The pathogenesis, diagnosis, and treatment of CSM are also controversial. No fewer than 21 surgical techniques have been proposed to treat CSM. This diversity of treatment approaches reflects the lack of understanding of the basic mechanisms of CSM. Fortunately, recent studies have aimed at understanding the mechanisms leading to CSM. Only with a thorough knowledge of the disease will the treatment of CSM evolve.

Palmer and Wallace,[1] in 1967, were the first to describe CSM in young Basset hounds. Later in the 1970s, Great Danes appeared as the most commonly affected breed.[2,14] Since the early 1980s, Dobermans have accounted for the majority of the reported cases.[4,9,15–17] Although no prevalence study has been performed, it is likely that CSM is the most common disease of the cervical spine of large and giant breed dogs. Canine CSM bears similarities with the cervical spondylotic myelopathy of humans and the Doberman breed has been proposed as a natural model to study this disease in humans.[18] Not surprisingly, much more is known about cervical

Department of Veterinary Clinical Sciences, College of Veterinary Medicine, The Ohio State University, Columbus, 601 Vernon Tharp Street, OH 43210-1089, USA
E-mail address: dacosta.6@osu.edu

Vet Clin Small Anim 40 (2010) 881–913
doi:10.1016/j.cvsm.2010.06.003
vetsmall.theclinics.com
0195-5616/10/$ – see front matter

spondylotic myelopathy than its canine counterpart. Therefore, when applicable, parallels between the 2 diseases are emphasized herein.

ETIOLOGY

The etiology of CSM is still unknown. Proposed etiologies include genetic, congenital, body conformation, and nutritional.

Genetic

Many investigators have proposed a genetic origin.[1,19–21] The first description of the syndrome in Basset hounds suggested that the disease was inherited, but only 6 dogs (all males younger than 6 months of age) were studied and the specific mode of inheritance could not be established.[1] A Swiss study in Borzois suggested that CSM was inherited with an autosomal recessive pattern, but no explanation was given why only females were affected.[22] Other studies proposed a hereditary or familial basis,[14] but the methodology to support such conclusions was not reported. Two large studies with more than 370 Dobermans failed to demonstrate an inheritable trait.[16,23] However, no well-designed prospective study has yet specifically evaluated the genetic aspects of CSM in Dobermans or Great Danes.

Congenital

A study of neonatal Dobermans investigated the computed tomography (CT) features of the cervical spine in 27 dogs, comparing it to the cervical spine of neonatal dogs of other breeds.[24] Stenosis of the cranial aspect of the vertebral canal and asymmetry of the vertebral body were identified in the fifth, sixth, and seventh cervical vertebrae of Dobermans. The most severely affected vertebra was the seventh. The findings of the study indicate that Dobermans are born with congenital vertebral canal stenosis.[24]

Body Conformation

Body conformation has been proposed as a predisposing factor since the early study by Wright and colleagues[3] in 1973. The abnormal forces exerted by a large head in a long neck and the association with a rapid growth rate were proposed to lead to abnormal stresses in the vertebral bodies, causing vertebral changes and spinal cord compression. However, a study found no correlation between body conformation (head size, neck length, body length, and height at withers) and radiographic evidence of CSM in 138 Dobermans aged 1 to 13 years.[16] It seems unlikely that body conformation has a significant role in the development of CSM.

Nutritional

Dietary factors, including overfeeding and excessive dietary calcium, were implicated as contributory factors in Great Danes,[25,26] but these factors do not seem to have the same importance in Dobermans.[27] Even in Great Danes, their importance is questionable because the practices of overfeeding and calcium supplementation have been abandoned for many years, and the disease is still commonly seen.

PATHOPHYSIOLOGY

As stated in the definition of CSM, the disease involves both static and dynamic factors. Traditionally, spinal cord compression was thought to be a key factor leading to the signs of CSM. Of note, 2 recent magnetic resonance imaging (MRI) studies found that 25% to 30% of clinically normal Dobermans have clinically silent spinal cord compression.[28,29] Similarly, other spinal changes previously thought to be associated with CSM have been found in a high percentage of clinically normal Dobermans. Such abnormalities are intervertebral disc degeneration (75% of dogs), intervertebral disc protrusion (100% of dogs), and intervertebral foraminal stenosis (68% of dogs).[28] These findings in normal dogs called into question the traditional assumptions of CSM and prompted consideration of other mechanisms potentially involved in the pathogenesis of the disease.[28,30]

A key mechanistic difference between normal and CSM-affected Dobermans that explains why disc-associated spinal cord compression does not necessarily lead to neurologic signs is the vertebral canal stenosis.[28] Vertebral canal stenosis was consistently present throughout the entire cervical spine of CSM-affected Dobermans, even at C2 and C7-T1 regions.[28] Clinically normal Dobermans have a larger vertebral canal. A narrow canal lowers the threshold at which the cumulative effects of various structures encroaching on the spinal cord cause signs of myelopathy.[31] In humans a smaller vertebral canal is considered the most important static factor for the development of cervical spondylotic myelopathy.[32–34]

All dogs with CSM have some degree of vertebral canal stenosis. It may be an absolute vertebral canal stenosis (which then causes direct spinal cord compression and neurologic signs) or a relative vertebral stenosis, which by itself does not lead to myelopathic signs, but predisposes the patient to develop myelopathy.[28] Despite some degree of overlap, the pathophysiology of the spinal cord compressions can be basically divided into osseous- or disc-associated compression.[4]

Disc-Associated Compressions

Disc-associated compression is typically seen in middle-aged large breed dogs. This form of CSM is commonly seen in Doberman Pinschers and most studies have focused on this breed. Disc-associated CSM is primarily associated with ventral spinal cord compression. This compression may be symmetric or asymmetric (**Fig. 1**). It can also be complicated by dorsal compressions caused by either vertebral canal stenosis or hypertrophy of the ligamentum flavum. Affected dogs are apparently born with a congenital relative vertebral canal stenosis.[24] This relative vertebral canal stenosis *per se* does not lead to clinical signs, but predisposes to the development of signs. The vast majority of the disc-associated spinal cord compressions are located in the caudal cervical spine, affecting the discs C5-6 and C6-7.[16] The biomechanical features of the caudal cervical spine explain the high incidence of caudal cervical disc lesions. The caudal cervical spine was recently shown to experience 3 times more torsion than the cranial cervical spine,[35] confirming the findings of a morphometric study.[36] Torsion is the main biomechanical force leading to intervertebral disc degeneration in nonchondrodystrophic dogs, more so than axial compression.[37] In addition, a recent study found that Dobermans with CSM have larger intervertebral discs than clinically normal Dobermans.[28] This difference would cause a larger volume of disc protrusion into the vertebral canal. Therefore, 3 factors act in combination to explain the pathophysiology of disc-associated CSM: relative vertebral canal stenosis, more pronounced torsion in the caudal cervical spine leading to intervertebral disc degeneration, and protrusion of larger volume of disc material in the caudal cervical spine.[30]

Osseous-Associated Compressions

The pathophysiology of osseous or bony-associated CSM is different. Osseous-associated CSM is seen predominantly in young adult giant breed dogs. Because the disease is seen at an earlier age, a congenital cause seems likely. Affected dogs have severe, absolute vertebral canal stenosis secondary to proliferation of the vertebral arch (dorsally), articular facets (dorsolaterally), or articular facets and pedicles (laterally) (**Fig. 2**).[11,14,38,39] The cause of the compression appears to be

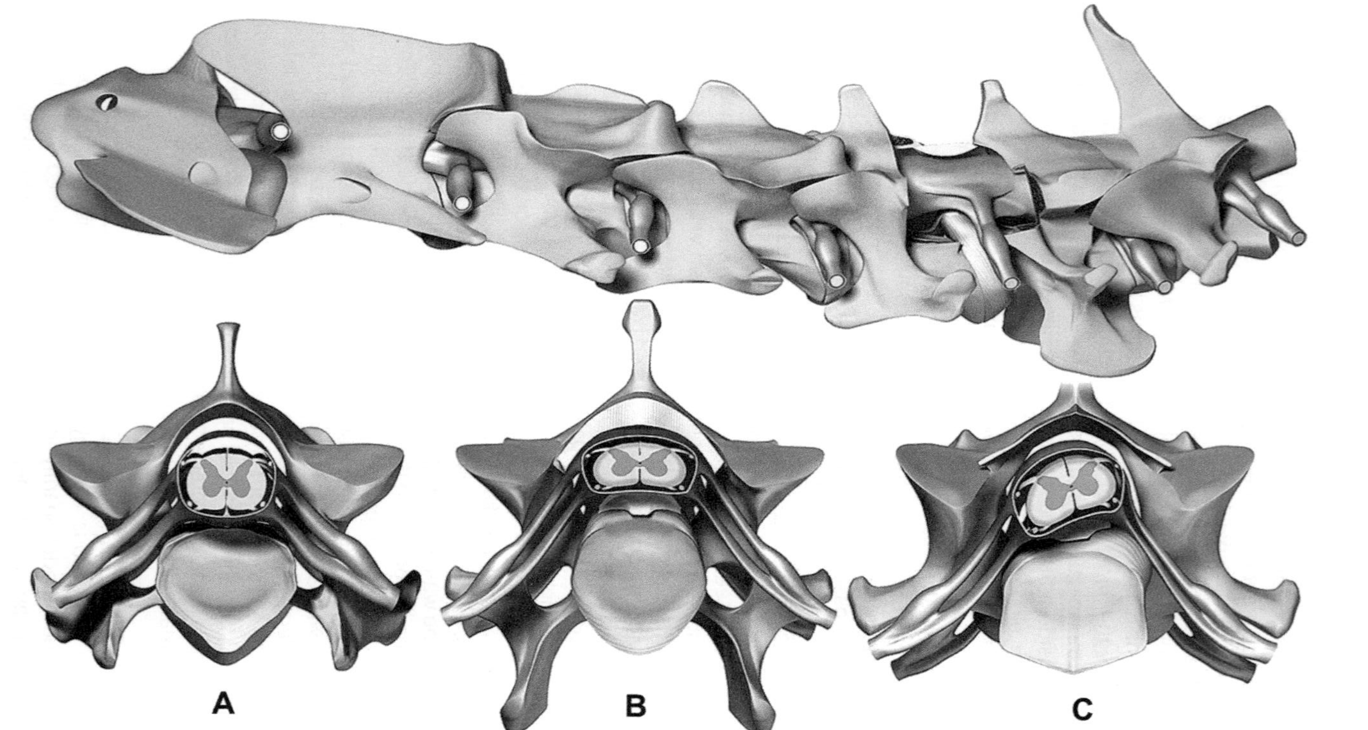

Fig. 1. Disc-associated CSM. (*Top*) Ventral spinal cord compression and nerve root compression at C5-6 caused by intervertebral disc protrusion. Dorsally, hypertrophy of the ligamentum flavum causes mild spinal cord compression. (*Bottom*) (*A*) Transverse section at the level of the C4-5 disc region showing normal spinal cord and vertebral canal. (*B*) Ventral compression at C5-6 region caused by intervertebral disc protrusion and hypertrophy of the dorsal longitudinal ligament (*yellow*) and ligamentum flavum (causing mild dorsal compression). (*C*) Asymmetric intervertebral disc protrusion at C6-7 causing spinal cord and nerve root compressions. (*Courtesy of* The Ohio State University; with permission.)

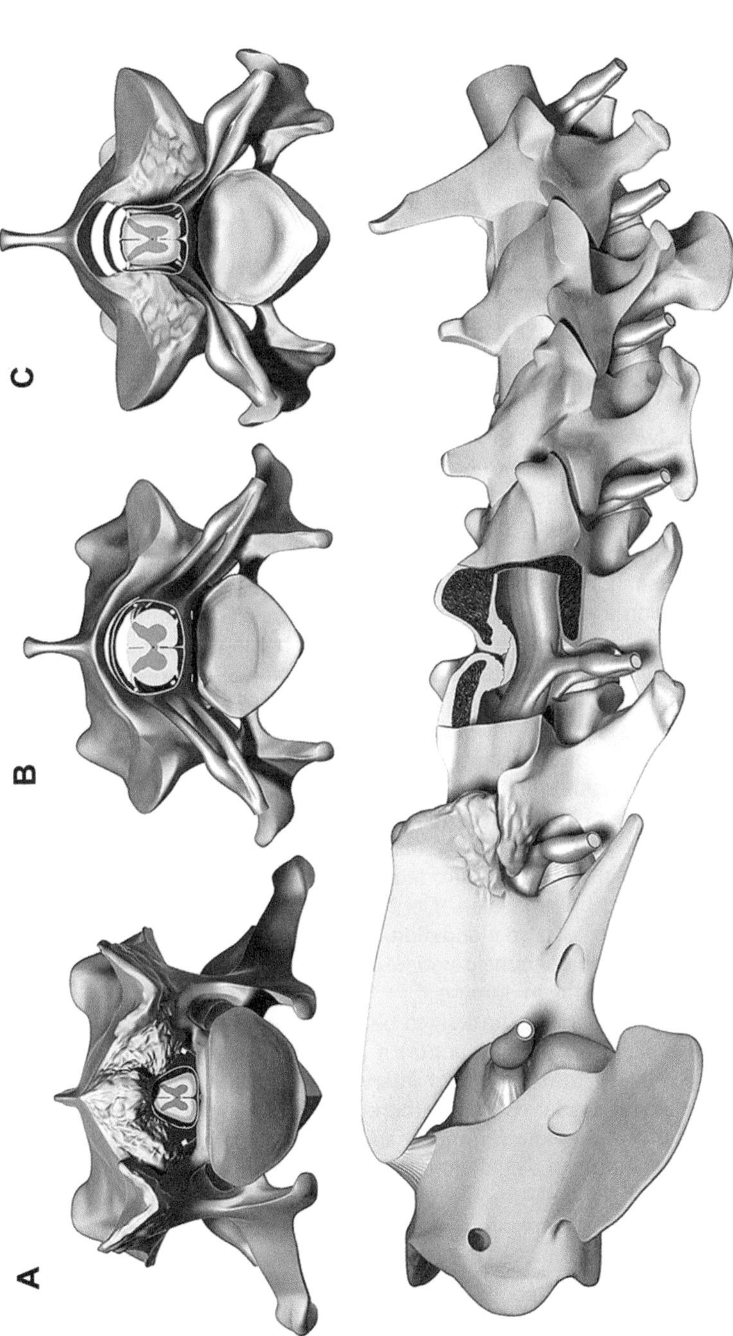

Fig. 2. Osseous-associated CSM. (*Top*) (*A*) Severe dorsolateral spinal cord compression at C2-3 caused by osseous malformation and osteoarthritic changes. (*B*) Normal C3-4 disc region. (*C*) Bilateral compression at C4-5 caused by osteoarthritic changes and medial proliferation of the facets causing absolute vertebral canal stenosis and foraminal stenosis, leading to spinal cord and nerve root compressions, respectively. (*Bottom*) Dorsal spinal cord compression at C3-4 caused by lamina malformation and hypertrophy of the ligamentum flavum. Osteoarthritic changes are also shown at C2-3. (*Courtesy of* The Ohio State University; with permission.)

a combination of vertebral malformations and osteoarthritic changes of the articular facets. Even though most giant breed dogs have osseous compressions, occasionally these compressions are complicated by disc protrusion in older dogs. Extradural synovial cysts may also be present secondary to degenerative arthritic facet changes, leading to uni- or bilateral axial compression.[40,41] Large breed dogs also have purely osseous compressions, but not as commonly as disc-associated compressions.

Ligamentous compression (ligamentum flavum) may be part of the disease in giant and large breed dogs, but pure ligamentous compression as the single source of compression does not appear often.

Dynamic Compressions

An important mechanism to explain the development of clinical signs in dogs with either disc- or osseous-associated CSM is the concept of dynamic lesions.[30,42–44] Confusion appears in the literature regarding the concepts of instability and dynamic lesions. These 2 concepts are completely distinct. Instability in cervical myelopathies is defined as "the loss of ability of the cervical spine under physiologic loads to maintain relationships between vertebrae in such a way that there is neither initial nor subsequent damage to the spinal cord or nerve roots, and in addition, there is neither development of incapacitating deformity nor severe pain."[45] A dynamic lesion is one that worsens or improves with different positions of the cervical spine.[46] The fact that the spinal cord appears to be compressed on neck flexion or extension on a myelogram does not necessarily mean that there is instability. Variations on the degree of spinal cord compression are expected because it is a physiologic pattern of motion in dogs and humans.[47–52] Cervical extension in healthy humans causes an 11% to 16% reduction of the area of the vertebral canal due to infolding of the ligament flavum, annulus fibrosus, and posterior dura.[47,48] At the same time, extension increases the spinal cord area by 9% to 17%.[48] This fact explains why cervical extension or dorsiflexion causes worsening of cord compression and clinical signs in dogs.[4] Neck flexion generates the opposite effect in the spinal cord, stretching the cord between C2 and T1 for up to 17.6% of its length in humans, with the maximal stretch occurring in the caudal cervical region.[47,53] With spinal cord stretch, a ventrally positioned space-occupying lesion, such as a protruded intervertebral disc, will cause more severe ventral spinal cord compression. Continuous flexion and extension of the cervical spine can lead to spinal cord elongation, causing axial strain and stress within the spinal cord, both of which are considered key mechanisms of spinal cord injury in cervical spondylotic myelopathy in humans.[30,42–44]

Instability as previously defined is unlikely to be present in dogs with CSM, and the evidence currently available does not support it as a factor in the pathogenesis of CSM.[30] A study compared the amount of intervertebral disc distraction between normal and CSM-affected Dobermans and found no difference between groups.[28] In addition, it appears that restricted, rather than excessive, intervertebral motion is more likely to occur at the sites of disc degeneration.[54–56] When subjectively evaluated in dogs with CSM, instability was thought to be either absent or rarely present.[21,57] Nonetheless, specific investigations are needed to define the specific role of dynamic lesions in dogs with CSM, and assess the presence or absence of instability.

In summary, the pathogenesis of CSM involves an association of static and dynamic factors independent of the cause and direction of the compressive spinal cord lesion.

Distribution and location of compressive lesions

Two recent studies of 118 dogs with CSM indicated that approximately 50% of large breed dogs with CSM have a single site of spinal cord compression, whereas the other

50% have 2 or mores sites of compression.[38,39] Other studies have found lower prevalence of multiple compressive lesions (approximately 25%).[15] The prevalence of single compressive lesion in large breed dogs contrasts with that seen giant breed dogs, in which a single site of compression was seen in 20% of dogs, with multiple sites of spinal cord compression observed in 80%.[38,39] Others have reported an even higher incidence of multiple compressive sites in giant breeds.[11]

The most commonly affected intervertebral region in large breed dogs is C6-7, followed closely by the C5-6. The main lesion is located in 1 of these 2 sites in 90% of dogs.[38,39] In giant breed dogs, the C6-7 region is also the most commonly affected, followed by C5-6 and C4-5. The main spinal cord compression is located in 1 of these 3 regions in approximately 80% of cases. The remaining 20% have involvement of C2-3 and C3-4 regions.[38,39] A recent CT study of 58 dogs identified lesions affecting the T1-T2 and T2 regions in 14% of giant breed dogs, and the C7-T1 region in 22% of dogs.[38] Although these lesions were not considered the primary source of compression, their identification is important in the decision-making process of treatment planning. The cranial thoracic spine should therefore always be examined, and the need to investigate this area should be considered when selecting an imaging modality for diagnosis.

DIAGNOSIS

Signalment

CSM can affect dogs of all ages and breeds, even small dogs, albeit uncommonly.[17,58] The majority of Dobermans and large breed dogs (Weimaraners, Dalmatians) with CSM are presented after 3 years of age. The mean age for Dobermans with CSM is 6.8 years, whereas for all large breeds it is 7.9 years.[9,15,38,39] Earlier reports described Dobermans younger than 1 year old,[2,5] but this presentation is currently uncommon. Although most affected Dobermans tend to be middle-aged, Great Danes and giant breeds (Mastiffs, Rottweilers, Bernese, and Swiss Mountain dogs) are usually younger. The mean age of giant breed dogs with CSM is 3.8 years, and the disease may be seen in dogs just a few months old.[9,15,38,39]

The author has recently seen several middle-aged to old German shepherds with osseous-associated CSM. This illustrates that large and giant breeds may have either osseous- or disc-associated forms of the disease, with a great overlap of clinical presentations.

Both males and females are affected by CSM, and many studies report a similar incidence between males and females.[2,21,59,60] Studies having a higher proportion of giant breed dogs usually report a higher incidence in males.[11,38]

History and Clinical Signs

A chronic progressive history (several weeks to months) is typical. Acute presentations are usually associated with neck pain. Occasionally, acute decompensation of a chronic lesion is observed.

Neck pain or cervical hyperesthesia is a common historical finding, but typically is not the main reason for presentation. Neck pain is part of the clinical findings in approximately 65% to 70% of Dobermans, and in 40% to 50% of other breeds, but it is the chief complaint in only 5% to 10% of dogs with CSM.[17] Forceful manipulations of the cervical spine are unnecessary to document the presence of neck pain, and can lead to severe neurologic decompensation. Careful assessment of posture and evaluation of voluntary range of motion (side-to-side, ventrally, and dorsally) using a food treat is recommended to assess cervical pain. Deep palpation of the transverse processes can also assist in the identification of neck pain. Supraspinatus muscle atrophy is frequently observed in large and giant breed dogs with CSM, and reflects involvement of the suprascapularis nerve or cell bodies of the sixth spinal cord segment. Elbow abduction with internal rotation of the digits ("toe-in posture"), is seen in approximately one-third of Dobermans with CSM (**Fig. 3**).[61]

Gait evaluation is the most important component of the examination in dogs suspected of having CSM because it reliably identifies proprioceptive ataxia, even in the absence of conscious proprioceptive deficits.[62,63] Proprioceptive ataxia is seen in most dogs with CSM. Dogs with lesions in the cranial or midcervical spine tend to present with ataxia affecting all 4 limbs more equally. However, affected dogs typically have obvious pelvic limb ataxia with milder abnormalities in the thoracic limbs. In some cases, the thoracic limb ataxia or weakness may be very mild in comparison with the pelvic limbs signs, making the thoracic limb abnormalities go unnoticed. The thoracic limb gait can appear short-strided or spastic with a pseudo-hypermetric ("floating") appearance.[62] This pseudo-hypermetria is the result of upper motor neuron release causing stiffness/spasticity, and it differs from the true hypermetria whereby the limbs show the "high-stepping" secondary to hyperflexion of the thoracic limb joints. Occasionally, thoracic limb lameness can be seen, suggesting nerve root entrapment. The pelvic limb gait is often wide-based (abducted) and markedly uncoordinated. The stride length of the pelvic limbs is prolonged, causing the swaying movements of the hind end typical of the disease. Scuffing of the pelvic or

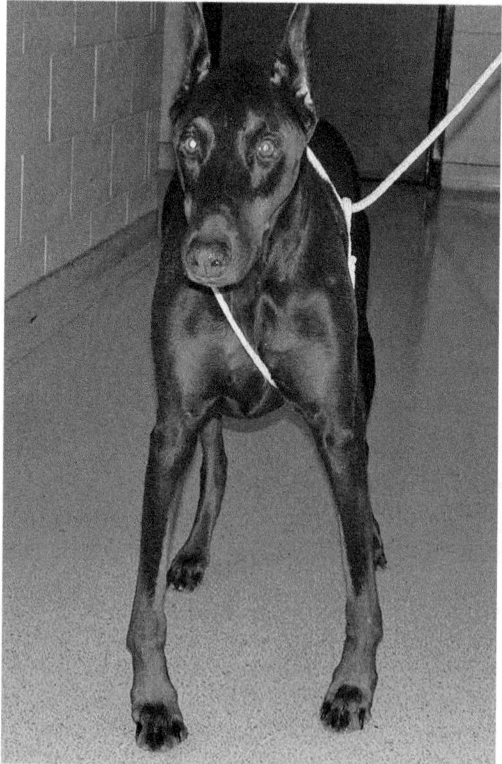

Fig. 3. Elbow abduction with internal rotation of digits ("toe-in posture") in a Doberman pinscher dog with CSM.

thoracic limb toes/nails can also be seen. A short-strided thoracic limb gait, with a wide-based, long-strided pelvic limb gait has been called a “2-engine” gait. In general, the faster the dog is walked, the less obvious the abnormalities are, so the dog should be walked at a slow pace. In severely affected dogs, weakness may be pronounced and they may collapse in their pelvic, thoracic, or all 4 limbs. Postural reaction deficits (proprioceptive positioning deficits) are seen in most dogs with CSM, but may not be evident in those with a chronic history despite the presence of proprioceptive ataxia. The reason for this discrepancy is that different tracts carry the pathways for conscious and unconscious proprioception.[62,63] Mildly asymmetric neurologic signs are seen in approximately 50% of dogs with CSM.[61] Approximately 10% of dogs with CSM present initially with nonambulatory tetraparesis.[17,61] Evaluation of the spinal reflexes in dogs with CSM will indicate a lesion located either at C1-5 spinal cord segments (normal to increased spinal reflexes in all 4 limbs, with neurologic signs as described above) or C6-8 spinal cord segments. A C6-8 myelopathy is typical because the osseous and disc lesions are concentrated in the C5-6 and C6-7 regions. In these cases, the gait is affected in all 4 limbs but more severely in the pelvic limbs. Evaluation of the spinal reflexes in the thoracic limbs will show a decreased flexor (withdrawal) reflex indicating involvement of the musculocutaneous nerve from C6-8 spinal cord segments, with normal to increased extensor tone suggesting an upper motor neuron lesion and release of the radial nerve from spinal cord segments C7, C8, T1, and mostly C8-T1. The pelvic limb reflexes will be normal to increased.

Radiography

Survey radiographs cannot confirm a diagnosis of CSM but often are used as a screening test to rule out other differential diagnoses for cervical myelopathies such as osseous neoplasia, trauma, vertebral osteomyelitis, and discospondylitis.[64] Radiographic findings seen in disc-associated CSM are primarily changes in the shape of the vertebral body (assuming a triangular shape in severe cases), narrowing of the intervertebral disc space, and vertebral canal stenosis.[64] Osteoarthritic, sclerotic changes of the articular facets are the radiographic hallmarks in giant breed dogs with osseous compressions, and can be seen on lateral and ventrodorsal projections (**Fig. 4**). Some of the radiographic findings seen in dogs with CSM (eg, vertebral

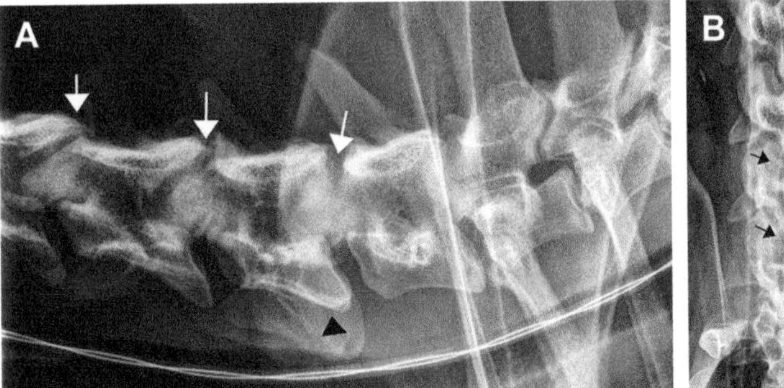

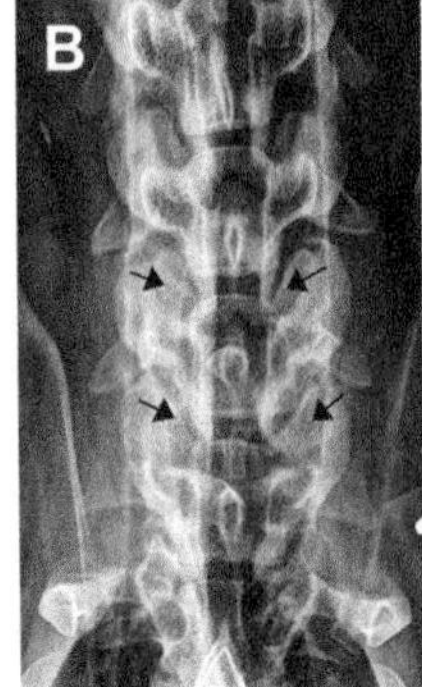

Fig. 4. Radiographs of a 1-year-old Mastiff with CSM. (*A*) Lateral radiograph. Observe severe osteoarthritic changes in the articular processes of C4-5, C5-6, and C6-7 regions (*white arrows*). The black arrowhead indicates C6 vertebra. (*B*) Ventrodorsal radiograph shows medial proliferation of the enlarged/arthritic facets (*arrows*).

tipping), also are seen in normal dogs. Studies in Dobermans indicate that approximately 20% to 25% of clinically normal dogs have radiographic changes comparable with those seen in dogs with CSM.[16,23,28] Cervical vertebral ratios are used routinely in the diagnosis and screening of humans and horses with cervical stenosis.[65–67] Two recent studies have revisited the use of vertebral ratios in dogs, more specifically in Dobermans.[68,69] Although the methodologies were different, the results of one of these studies indicate that cervical vertebral ratios may be useful as a screening test for dogs with CSM.[68]

Myelography

For many years, and up to recently, myelography has been considered the method of choice to diagnose CSM.[70] Myelography defines the site or sites and direction (ventral, dorsal, lateral) of the spinal cord compression, and allows stress myelographic studies.[4,64] Lateral and ventrodorsal views should be obtained, and oblique views may increase the diagnostic sensitivity of myelography. Stress myelography is defined as the radiographic examination of the cervical spine in various positions (ventral flexion, dorsal extension, and linear traction). Due to the risk of severe neurologic decompensation after myelography, only traction views are routinely used. For the last 30 years, traction myelographic views have been extensively used to distinguish dynamic from static lesions.[4] This differentiation has since been considered fundamental for surgery planning. Surprisingly, guidelines have not been established for performance or interpretation of traction myelography. Some clinicians indicate that a dynamic lesion is one that improves with traction, whereas others consider a lesion dynamic when it reduces completely.[71] The technique of traction also has never been standardized. The original description of grasping and holding the dog's head violates radiation safety and cannot be standardized.[4] A recent study proposed using a cervical harness and traction forces not greater than 25% of the dog's weight.[61] Comparative myelographic and MRI studies have shown how the concept of static and dynamic lesions is subjective.[61] A lesion that appears dynamic on myelography may appear static on MRI (**Fig. 5**). It appears that any compressive lesion will improve with traction (**Fig. 6**).[61] Others have also indicated that the concept of dynamic and static lesions is highly subjective and dependent on personal opinion.[71] As such, caution should be used when trying to apply this concept clinically. In dogs with multiple sites of spinal cord compression, it may be difficult to establish the clinically relevant site on myelography. Postmyelographic seizures and temporary deterioration of the patient's neurologic status are important adverse effects in large and giant breed dogs with CSM.[72–74]

Computed Tomography

CT is a rapid test that allows visualization of transverse sections of the cervical spine. CT is used mostly after myelography in dogs with CSM, and has been found to be complementary to standard myelography in the evaluation of Dobermans with CSM.[60] CT provides superior visualization of the direction and severity of the spinal cord compression (**Fig. 7**) and more precise identification of the most severely affected site when compared with myelography alone. An advantage of CT myelography is the visualization of spinal cord atrophy,[60] which has been identified in CT myelographic studies of 20%–30% of dogs with CSM.[38,60] Atrophy is identified on CT myelography as a widening of the subarachnoid space surrounding the spinal cord, with the cord assuming a triangular shape.[60] It is currently unknown whether spinal cord atrophy is associated with a poor prognosis in affected dogs. Disadvantages

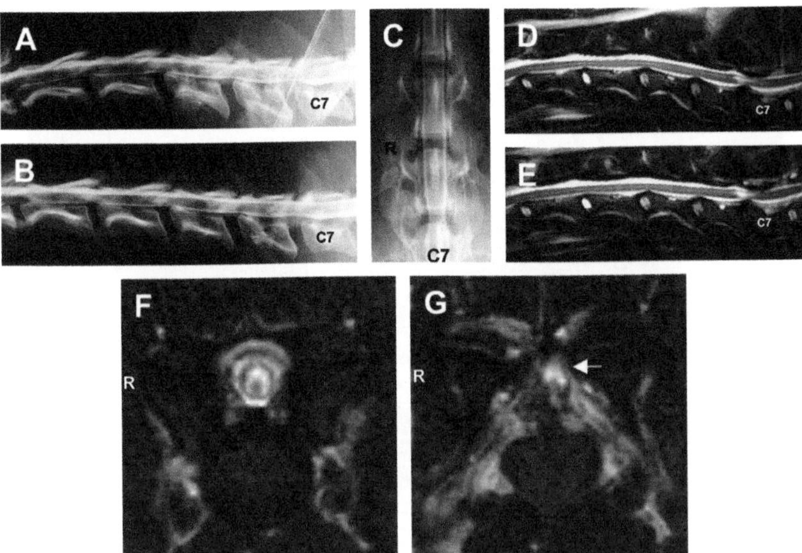

Fig. 5. (*A–G*) Cervical myelogram and T2-weighted (T2W) MR images of a 7-year-old Doberman with disc-associated CSM. (*A*) Pretraction cervical myelogram shows a ventral extradural compression at C6-7. (*B*) Posttraction cervical myelogram reveals improvement in the degree of ventral compression. This lesion could be considered dynamic. (*C*) Ventrodorsal myelogram shows bilateral extradural compression worse on the right. (*D*) Pretraction sagittal T2W image shows ventral and dorsal spinal cord compression with marked spinal cord hyperintensity at C6-7. Complete intervertebral disc degeneration is also seen at C6-7. (*E*) Posttraction sagittal T2W image reveals minimal improvement in the ventral spinal cord compression. On MRI the lesion appears static. (*F*) Transverse T2W image at the cranial region of the spinal cord compression shows bilateral spinal cord compression with cord hyperintensity. (*G*) Transverse T2W image at the central aspect of the cord compression. Marked circumferential compression reveals a small, atrophic spinal cord that is seen as an irregular area of hyperintensity (*arrow*). C7, seventh cervical vertebra. (*From* da Costa RC, Parent JP, Dobson H, et al. Comparison of magnetic resonance imaging and myelography in 18 Doberman pinscher dogs with cervical spondylomyelopathy. Vet Radiol Ultrasound 2006;47(6):527; with permission.)

of CT myelography are their invasiveness compared with MRI, and the risk of seizures and transient neurologic deterioration after the procedure.

Magnetic Resonance Imaging

MRI is the gold standard test for evaluation of dogs suspected of having CSM. The main advantage of MRI is that it detects signal changes in the spinal cord and thus allows assessment of the spinal cord parenchyma.[11,61] These signal changes are seen in approximately 50% of dogs with CSM, and allow precise identification of the site most severely affected.[39] A recent study compared myelography and MRI in the diagnosis of CSM and concluded that MRI was more accurate in predicting the site, severity, and nature of spinal cord compression (see **Figs. 5** and **6**).[61]

The presence of spinal cord signal changes, namely hyperintensity on T2-weighted images (T2WI), seems to be associated with severity of clinical signs, seen most commonly in dogs with moderate to severe neurologic deficits and a chronic history.[61] Although not yet documented in naturally occurring canine CSM, the correlation of spinal cord signal changes on MRI and histopathology has been well described in

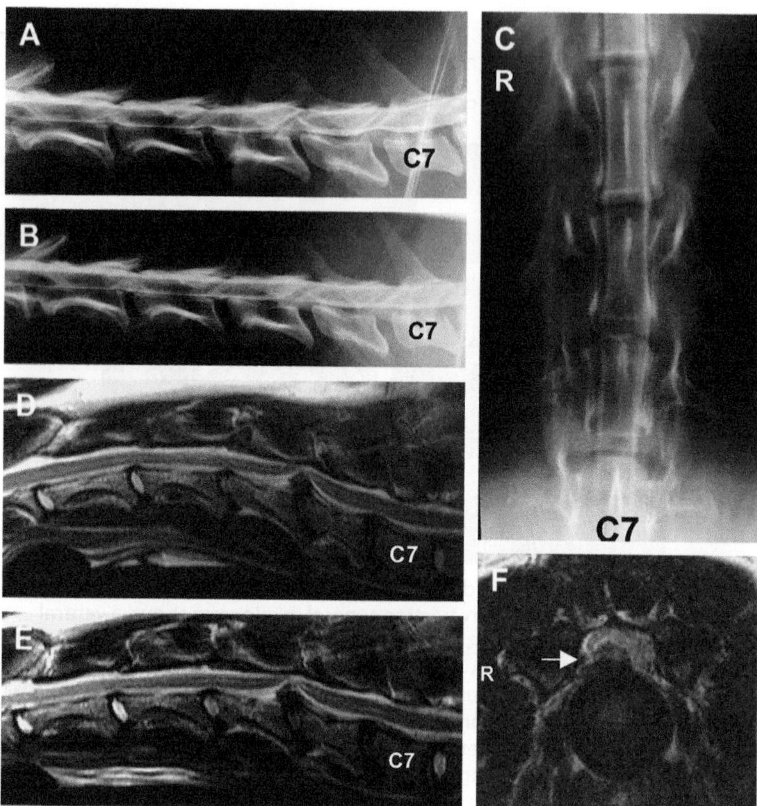

Fig. 6. (*A–F*) Cervical myelogram and T2W MR images of a 9-year-old Doberman with CSM. (*A*) Pretraction cervical myelogram shows ventral extradural compression at C6-7 and splitting of the ventral contrast column at C5-6. (*B*) Posttraction cervical myelogram shows improvement in the ventral compression and in the splitting of the contrast column. This lesion can be considered dynamic. (*C*) Ventrodorsal myelogram shows bilateral widening of the contrast columns at C5-6. No asymmetric compression is seen. (*D*) Pretraction sagittal T2W image shows marked spinal cord compression at C5-6, with minimal cord compression at C6-7. Intervertebral disc degeneration is observed at C4-5, C5-6, and C6-7. (*E*) Posttraction sagittal T2W image still shows the marked spinal cord compression at C5-6. On MRI the lesion appears static. (*F*) Transverse T2W image shows markedly asymmetric spinal cord compression, worse on the right side (*arrow*). C7, seventh cervical vertebra. (*From* da Costa RC, Parent JP, Dobson H, et al. Comparison of magnetic resonance imaging and myelography in 18 Doberman pinscher dogs with cervical spondylomyelopathy. Vet Radiol Ultrasound 2006;47(6):528; with permission.)

affected humans.[75] Hyperintensity in T2WI and isointensity in T1WI were characterized by slight loss of nerve cells, gliosis, and edema in the gray matter, as well as demyelination, edema, and Wallerian degeneration in the white matter. The combination of T2 hyperintensity and T1 hypointensity was characterized by severe lesions such as necrosis, myelomalacia, and spongiform changes in the gray matter, as well as white matter necrosis.[75] Hyperintensity on T2WI does not appear to correlate with prognosis in dogs, but preliminary evidence suggests that the combination of hyperintensity on T2WI and hypointensity on T1WI may be associated with a worse prognosis.[76] Current evidence in humans suggests that multilevel hyperintensity on T2WI and hypointensity on T1WI are associated with a poorer prognosis.[77–79]

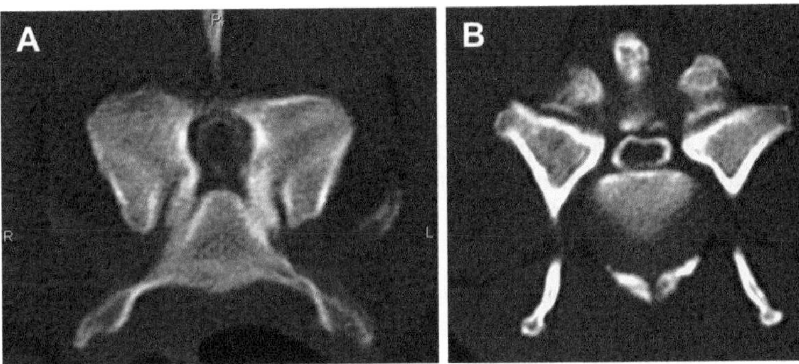

Fig. 7. Computed tomographic images of 2 Great Danes with CSM caused by osseous compressions. (*A*) Bilateral spinal cord and nerve root compressions at C6-7. (*B*) Dorsal spinal cord compression at C4-5.

The observed MRI changes are dependent on the cause of spinal cord compression. Osseous compressions are observed as hypointense proliferations associated with the articular processes, lamina, and pedicles in both T1- and T2-weighted images. Transverse and dorsal images are useful to assess the degree of vertebral canal stenosis in these cases. On disc-associated CSM, disc hypointensity or isointensity relative to the vertebral bodies on T2WI is seen along with variable degrees of protrusion. Even when not clearly visible on imaging, relative vertebral canal stenosis is present in dogs with disc-associated CSM.[28] The disc-associated compression leads to ventral spinal cord compression and displacement. Intervertebral foraminal stenosis can be an important cause of cervical spinal pain, and it is important to evaluate the foraminal diameter in all dogs with CSM. T2WI are more useful for assessment of foraminal size. Synovial spinal cysts may be seen in giant breed dogs as hyperintense regular areas associated with the articular processes on T2WI.

In some cases, the degree of spinal compression is minimal relative to the severity of clinical signs. Dynamic spinal cord compressions are assumed to be present in such cases.[30] Testing for dynamic compression using traction MRI can be performed, and guidelines for testing have been published.[61,80]

Cerebrospinal Fluid Analysis

Cerebrospinal fluid abnormalities are uncommon and nonspecific in dogs with CSM. Mild pleocytosis (≤12 cells/μL) was seen in approximately 20% of dogs with CSM, mainly in those with acute onset of signs. Mild increases in protein concentration (<40 mg/dL) also were observed in 27% of dogs with CSM, primarily in dogs with a chronic history.[81]

Electrodiagnostics

Electromyography (EMG) may be used to document neurogenic muscle atrophy in dogs with supraspinatus muscle or thoracic limb atrophy. However, the EMG may be normal in these dogs even when obvious muscle atrophy is present. Transcranial magnetic motor-evoked potentials (MEPs) are a sensitive way to assess spinal cord function.[82,83] All imaging modalities provide anatomic, but not functional information. MEPs of the cranial tibial muscle were shown to correlate with neurologic and MRI findings in dogs with CSM.[83] An advantage of the MEP is that is a rapid test that can be performed under mild sedation. Transcranial magnetic MEPs can provide an objective way to assess treatment outcome in dogs with CSM.[83]

Additional Diagnostic Tests

Many large breed dogs suffer from concurrent medical conditions that can potentially increase anesthetic or surgical risk, or affect long-term prognosis. The following tests should be considered in addition to the minimum database and previously mentioned tests:

Thyroid function: Hypothyroidism is very common in Doberman pinschers and has been identified in a high percentage of dogs in association with CSM.[61,84] Hypothyroidism can interfere with neurologic function and anesthetic recovery.

von Willebrand status: Deficiency of von Willebrand factor can lead to severe hemorrhage. A prevalence of 73% of von Willebrand disease has been found in Dobermans.[85] Buccal mucosal bleeding time is a rapid and efficient method to evaluate von Willebrand status.

Cardiac function: Electrocardiogram (5-minute ECG or Holter monitor) and echocardiogram are recommended before surgical treatment. General anesthesia can worsen cardiac function and lead to decompensation in dogs with occult dilated cardiomyopathy.[86]

Differential Diagnosis

Other differentials should be considered in large and giant breed dogs with neck pain, tetraparesis, and/or proprioceptive ataxia. Many neurologic diseases can cause at least one of these signs, and the primary differentials to consider are spinal neoplasia, intervertebral disc disease, trauma, discospondylitis, vertebral osteomyelitis, meningitis or meningomyelitis, synovial or subarachnoid spinal cysts, fibrocartilaginous embolic myelopathy, and polyneuropathies or polymyopathies. Orthopedic conditions frequently occur in older large and giant breed dogs and can coexist with neurologic disturbances, but no matter how severe a musculoskeletal disease may be, it will never cause proprioceptive ataxia.

TREATMENT

Conservative (Medical) Treatment

Traditionally, medical treatment for CSM has been considered a temporary measure to alleviate clinical signs. Without surgery, the disease was thought to be progressive, and euthanasia would have to be contemplated.[13,87] The only evidence to support these statements came from a study of primarily Great Danes that essentially received no treatment, more than 30 years ago.[14] Medical management for CSM was recently revisited in 2 studies.[17,88] A study compared the outcome of dogs treated medically and surgically and found that 54% of dogs treated medically improved and 27% were unchanged in a long-term follow-up.[17] Therefore, the clinical signs of CSM are either improved or stable in 81% of dogs managed medically.[17] Of note, the overall percentage of improvement and the owner's perception of the dog's quality of life were similar between dogs treated medically and those treated surgically.[17] Although many surgical techniques offer a higher success rate (approximately 80%), the index of improvement or stabilization of clinical status seen with medical management is quite acceptable, and may be preferred by some owners because of financial constraints or concerns about anesthetic and surgical risks, predominantly in Dobermans due to the high incidence of dilated cardiomyopathy in the breed.

A key component of medical management is exercise restriction to minimize high-impact activities that would exacerbate the dynamic component of spinal cord compression. Dogs can be leash walked but free, unsupervised activity is strongly discouraged. A body harness should be worn instead of a neck collar.

Corticosteroids appear to benefit dogs with CSM, and anti-inflammatory dosages of prednisone often are used (0.5–1.0 mg/kg every 12–24 h), progressively tapering the dosage over the course of 2 to 3 weeks, even though no scientific evidence is available to support their use.[17] In some patients, dexamethasone appears to elicit a better response, and so can be used for more severely affected patients or as a rescue therapy for dogs with sudden deterioration. Only low doses of dexamethasone should be used, never more than 0.25 mg/kg every 24 hours. No therapeutic benefit is gained by the higher dosage, and the risk of adverse effects is higher.[89] The severe complications reported with dexamethasone use were seen mainly when much higher dosages were used (1–2 mg/kg/d).[90] When using dexamethasone, the author uses a dosage of 0.2 to 0.25 mg/kg every 24 hour (avoiding doses higher than 8 mg/dog) initially for 1 to 3 days, depending on the severity of clinical signs, and then continues with 0.1 mg/kg every 24 hours. Corticosteroids, particularly dexamethasone, improve neurologic function in chronic spinal cord compression predominantly by decreasing vasogenic edema.[91] Other proposed mechanisms include protection from glutamate toxicity and reduction of neuronal and oligodendroglial apoptosis.[92–94] Despite the potential benefits associated with corticosteroid therapy, the use of corticosteroids, particularly for long periods, can be associated with important adverse effects. Gastrointestinal ulceration, colonic perforation, iatrogenic hypoadrenocorticism, pulmonary thromboembolism, risk of infections, overt diabetes mellitus, and behavioral changes all have been associated with corticosteroid treatment.[95] Due to the possibility of gastrointestinal complications, omeprazole (0.7 mg/kg every 24 hours) or famotidine (0.5 mg/kg every 12–24 hours) often are used in conjunction with corticosteroid therapy. Nonsteroidal anti-inflammatory drugs (NSAIDs) can be used in place of corticosteroids if neck pain appears to be a main component of the syndrome or if the adverse effects of the corticosteroids cannot be tolerated. Although many NSAIDs can be effectively used, the author often uses meloxicam (0.2 mg/kg initially, followed by 0.1 mg/kg every 24 hours). Independent of the NSAID used, corticosteroids and NSAIDs should never be used in combination. The response to medical management (corticosteroids and exercise restriction) can be used to indirectly assess the degree of reversible spinal cord lesions.[70]

One reason for the success with medical management is the slow progression of spinal changes associated with the disease (**Figs. 8** and **9**).[76] Surviving demyelinated axons also may remyelinate with treatment. Remyelination has been shown in the spinal cords of horses and humans with cervical myelopathy treated medically.[96,97]

Physical therapy also has been reported in the treatment of dogs with severe cervical myelopathies, and can also be used in the treatment of dogs with CSM.[98] A study also described the use of electroacupuncture in the treatment of CSM.[99] Anecdotally, protein and calorie reduction have been used in the treatment of CSM in young dogs with osseous lesions. No controlled studies are currently available, but as nutrition seems to have a questionable role in CSM, the efficacy of this therapy is uncertain.

As previously mentioned, some dogs with CSM have concurrent hypothyroidism (8 out of 12 dogs in a recent study).[61] Hypothyroid dogs with CSM may show remarkable improvement in strength and energy when thyroid supplementation is started. In these cases, improvement usually is noticeable within a week.

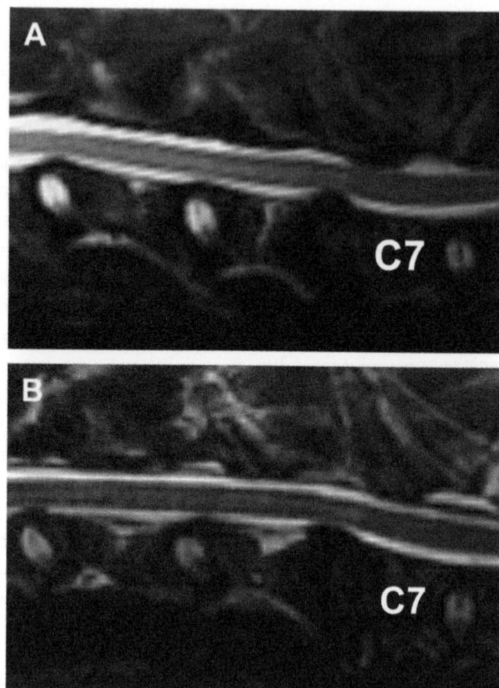

Fig. 8. MR images of the cervical spine of a 5-year-old male Doberman with CSM treated conservatively. (*A*) Midsagittal T2W image showing spinal cord compression and mild cord hyperintensity at C6-7. (*B*) Midsagittal T2W image obtained 15 months after the first MRI. The area of spinal cord hyperintensity is still present, and adjacent discs do not show degenerative changes. Clinically the dog had improved and was stable. The spinal cord compression appears less severe but the dog actually had spinal cord atrophy on the follow-up MR images. (*From* da Costa RC, Parent JM. One-year clinical and magnetic resonance imaging follow-up of Doberman Pinschers with cervical spondylomyelopathy treated medically or surgically. J Am Vet Med Assoc 2007;231(2):247; with permission.)

SURGICAL TREATMENT

The decision to recommend surgical treatment should be based on several factors such as severity of neurologic signs, degree of pain, type and severity of compressive lesion(s), response (or lack of response) to medical management, short- and long-term expectations of the owner, and presence of other concurrent neurologic or orthopedic problems or extraneurologic diseases such as dilated cardiomyopathy that would affect the long-term outcome. Once a decision has been made that surgery is the ideal method of treatment, the selection of the specific method of surgical treatment to be used can be complicated. Few diseases in veterinary medicine have had so many proposed surgical techniques as CSM. Direct decompressive techniques reported include dorsal laminectomy, dorsal laminoplasty, ventral slot, inverted cone slot, and hemilaminectomy.[58,100–105] Indirect decompressive techniques typically are grouped into the distraction-stabilization category, and have been reported using bone grafts of several types, pins (smooth, threaded) or screws and polymethyl methacrylate (PMMA), interbody screws, washers, metallic spacers, metallic plates, plastic

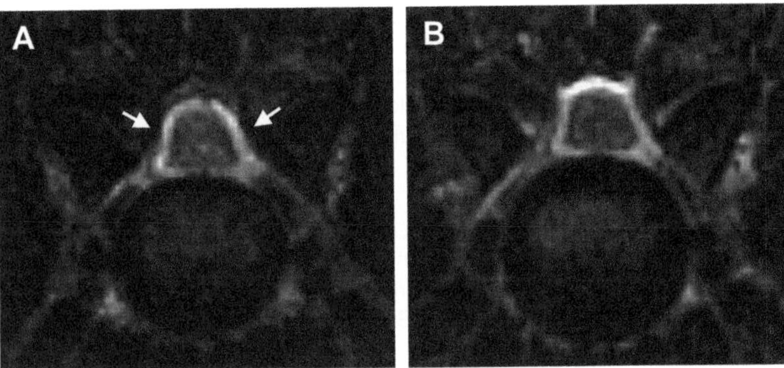

Fig. 9. Transverse T2W MR images of a 4-year-old male Doberman with CSM with mild ataxia and neck pain treated conservatively. (*A*) Bilateral spinal cord deformation caused by medial proliferation of the articular processes is observed (*arrows*). (*B*) MR image obtained 12 months after the first MRI. The spinal cord compression was unchanged. Clinically the dog still had mild ataxia but no neck pain. Identical cord area to the first MRI was confirmed by morphometry. (*From* da Costa RC, Parent JM. One-year clinical and magnetic resonance imaging follow-up of Doberman Pinschers with cervical spondylomyelopathy treated medically or surgically. J Am Vet Med Assoc 2007;231(2):246; with permission.)

plates, k-wire spacer, Harrington rods, interbody PMMA plug, and fusion cage. All of these techniques have been combined either with discectomy or with partial or complete ventral slots.[12,14,15,57,59,70,84,106–118] Intervertebral disc fenestration also has been used, and more recently, motion-preserving techniques, using disc arthroplasty or artificial disc replacement, have been proposed.[119–121] With so many choices, the decision on which technique to use may be difficult.

In general, as the source and direction of compression can be broadly divided into disc-associated or osseous-associated, treatment recommendations can be made as follows.

Disc-Associated CSM

Disc-associated CSM is the most common form of CSM and the one with the largest number of surgical techniques proposed to treat it. Many, if not most, of the surgical techniques have been based on the concept of static or dynamic lesions following stress or traction myelography which, as discussed in the diagnosis section, is highly subjective. Nevertheless, the outcome for most surgical techniques is quite similar and generally positive.[8] Ventral static compressions are usually treated with the traditional ventral slot or the inverted cone slot. Dynamic compressions can be treated with distraction-stabilization techniques, and the PMMA plug or pins/screws combined with PMMA, are commonly used. Multiple compressive sites can be treated with distraction-stabilization techniques, the most common being distraction with a PMMA plug.[70] Dorsal laminectomy is an alternative for multiple ventral compressions.[103]

Osseous Compressions

These compressions typically are thought to be primarily static and, as such, direct decompression of the affected sites is recommended[105]; this is typically achieved by dorsal laminectomy, but can also be achieved by cervical hemilaminectomy.[58,104]

Another way to treat osseous lesions is by distraction-stabilization of the affected segments ventrally.[70,113] Stabilization and fusion of the affected segments does not directly decompress the affected sites, but eliminates the dynamic component of the spinal cord compression. It also may allow regression of the osseous and ligamentous lesions over time.[70,122] The technique used in these cases was the PMMA plug.[70,122]

Pure Ligamentous Compressions

Ligamentous hypertrophy is usually combined with either disc- or osseous-associated compressions. Pure ligamentous compression (hypertrophy of the ligamentum flavum) is currently a rare presentation. Surgical treatment can be achieved either by decompressing the affected sites (dorsal laminectomy) or by using the PMMA plug technique.

Surgical Techniques

Direct decompressive techniques

Ventral slot Ventral slot is primarily indicated for single ventral static compressions. As the determination of a static or dynamic lesion is subjective, it can be considered for any ventral compression, as there are no data indicating that it is less successful or carries a worse outcome with dynamic lesions.[8,105] Two slots (preferably using the inverted cone technique) can be performed but the risk of complications is higher. Ideally, the slot should not exceed one-third of the length and width of the vertebral bodies (**Fig. 10**).[101,123] Care should be exercised to avoid injuring the internal vertebral venous plexus, which can cause very severe hemorrhage. All disc protrusion and ligament hypertrophy should be removed to effectively decompress the spinal cord. The ventral slot technique offers adequate spinal cord decompression, and fusion is expected to occur at the slot site 8 to 12 weeks postoperatively (**Fig. 11**).[101,123] Serious complications can occur after a ventral slot procedure, including respiratory compromise, cardiac dysrhythmias, vertebral subluxations, and hemorrhage. These complications were reported to occur in 14.9% of dogs in one study.[124] The reported long-term success rate of the ventral slot procedure is 72%.[71,100,106] An alternative to the traditional ventral slot procedure is the inverted cone technique (see **Fig. 10**C). This modification aims at minimizing bone removal, and therefore reducing the risk of vertebral subluxation, and hemorrhage.[102] The decompression window resembles an inverted cone in which the base of the cone lies adjacent to the ventral vertebral canal, allowing maximal surgical access cranially, caudally, and laterally.

Dorsal laminectomy Dorsal laminectomy is indicated for dorsal compressions associated with osteoarthritic changes of the articular facets, lamina malformation, or ligamentum flavum hypertrophy. It can be used to decompress one or multiple sites (**Fig. 12**).[11,58] Dorsal laminectomy also has been recommended to treat multiple ventral spinal cord compressive lesions.[103] No direct comparisons of dorsal laminectomy with other surgical techniques have been published. An important complication of dorsal laminectomy is worsening of neurologic status, which has been reported to occur in 70% of treated dogs postoperatively.[58] Dogs that became or remained nonambulatory after surgery took an average of 2.5 months to recover their ability to walk without assistance.[58]

Postlaminectomy membrane is a major problem after decompressive spinal surgery in humans, being responsible for 8% of all failures of spinal surgery.[125] Although reported in one dog after dorsal cervical laminectomy,[58] its true incidence is unknown. Typically a free fat graft is placed over the laminectomy defect to minimize the

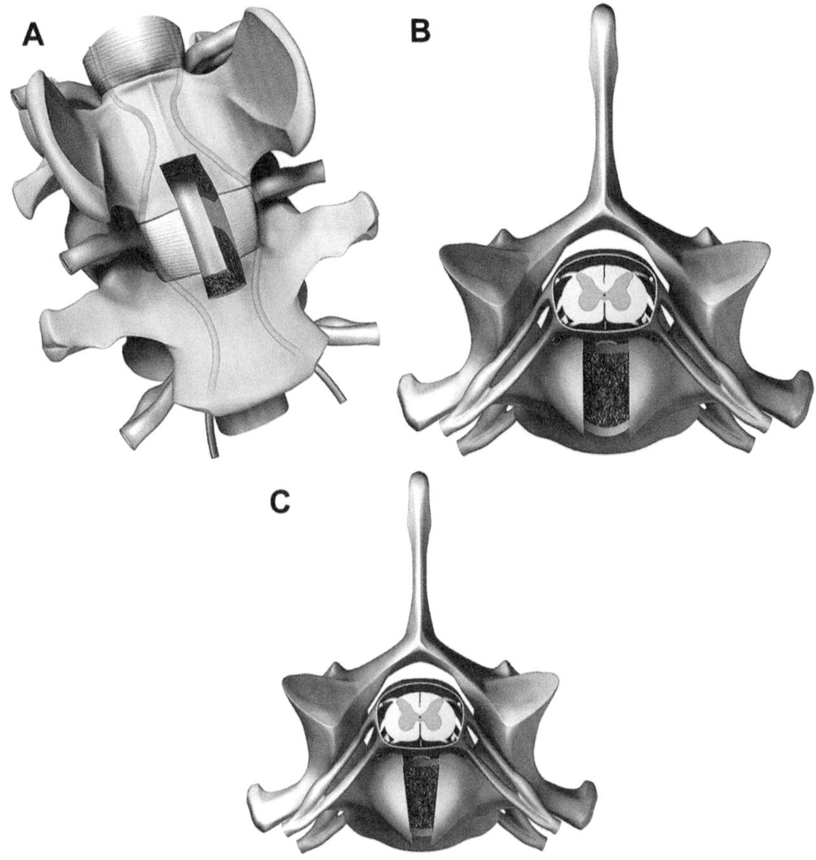

Fig. 10. Ventral slot at C6-7. (*A*) Ventral view. (*B*) Transverse view. The slot width and length should ideally be kept at about one-third of the vertebral bodies. The internal vertebral venous plexus are represented by the blue vessels running in the ventral aspect of the vertebral canal. (*C*) Inverted cone slot; this is a modification of the traditional ventral slot that minimizes the risk of hemorrhage and subluxation. (*Courtesy of* The Ohio State University; with permission.)

development of a postlaminectomy membrane. However, a study in dogs indicated a high incidence of graft failure and neurologic complications after the use of a free fat graft in the thoracolumbar spine.[126] Whether or not the same occurs in the cervical spine, explaining the common neurologic deterioration seen postoperatively, is unknown at this time. Considering the high incidence of graft failure and the neurologic complications documented in dogs, the use of free fat grafts after dorsal laminectomy is not recommended at this time.

The success rate for dorsal laminectomies ranges from 79% to 95%.[11,58,103] The mean time to reach optimal improvement is long (3.6 months), and in one report, 30% of dogs had recurrence of signs postoperatively.[58] Dorsal laminoplasty is an alternative to dorsal laminectomy that has not been sufficiently explored in dogs.[105]

Cervical hemilaminectomy A technique of lateral approach for cervical hemilaminectomy was used in the treatment of CSM in dogs with either disc- or

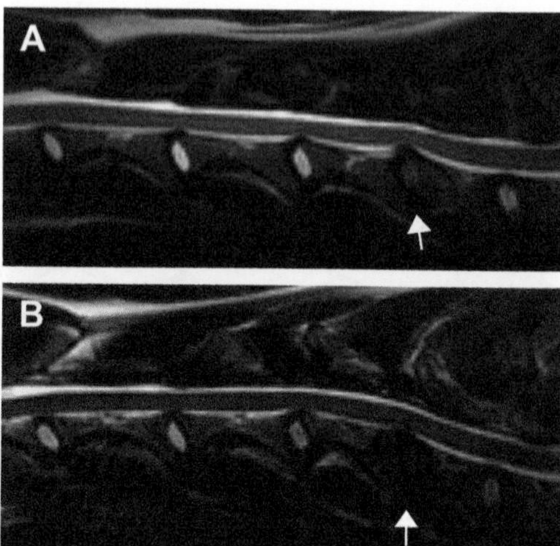

Fig. 11. Magnetic resonance (MR) images of the cervical spine of a 4-year-old female Doberman dog with CSM treated with ventral slot decompression at C5-6. (*A*) Initial MR images show ventral spinal cord compression at C5-6 (*arrow*). (*B*) Follow-up MR image 12 months after the ventral slot shows effective decompression with residual compression. Bone proliferation at the slot site suggests that fusion developed at that site (*arrow*). Clinically the dog had improved after surgery and was stable.

osseous-associated CSM.[104] The investigators reported no postoperative worsening of neurologic status, which is an attractive benefit for dogs with osseous lesions.[104]

Indirect decompression: vertebral distraction techniques

Pins and PMMA This technique is recommended primarily for single ventral dynamic compressive lesions.[107] It can be used for 2 affected segments, but the risk of failure

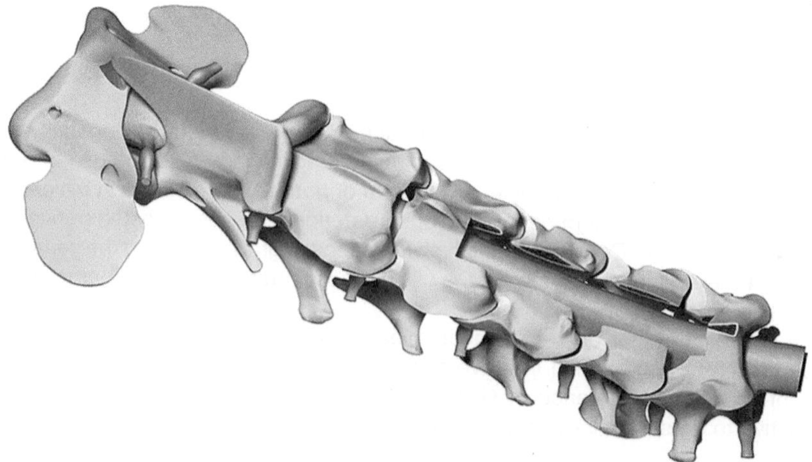

Fig. 12. Dorsal laminectomy from C4 to C7. (*Courtesy of* The Ohio State University; with permission.)

increases. Either a partial or complete ventral slot is created. The metal implant can be either 2 Steinmann pins, threaded pins, or bone screws (**Fig. 13**). A recent study suggested that positive profile pins provide more rigid fixation than smooth pins.[127] The original recommended angle of implant insertion was 30° to 35°.[107] A recent study indicated that these angles are relatively safe for the vertebrae C5 and C6, but that an angle of approximately 45° should be used for implants at C7, which is very challenging at this location.[128] The long-term success rate of this technique is 73%.[107] Vertebral or transverse foramina penetration is a major risk of this procedure, and has been reported to occur in 25% to 57% of cases studied experimentally.[127,128]

Several modifications of this procedure have been reported using different techniques and materials for distraction.[109,116] A recent study reported the use of screws inserted into the transverse processes, using a U-shaped Steinmann pin that was wired to the screws and covered with PMMA.[115] The advantage of this technique is that it avoids the risk of penetration into the vertebral canal or transverse foramina. A disadvantage of some of the distraction techniques is that the instrumentation used for vertebral body fixation can cause severe imaging artifacts, predominantly with MR imaging, making postoperative spinal cord visualization difficult or impossible.

Distraction using the PMMA plug Distraction using the PMMA plug is a popular technique and has been used for either single or multiple ventral and dorsal compressions,

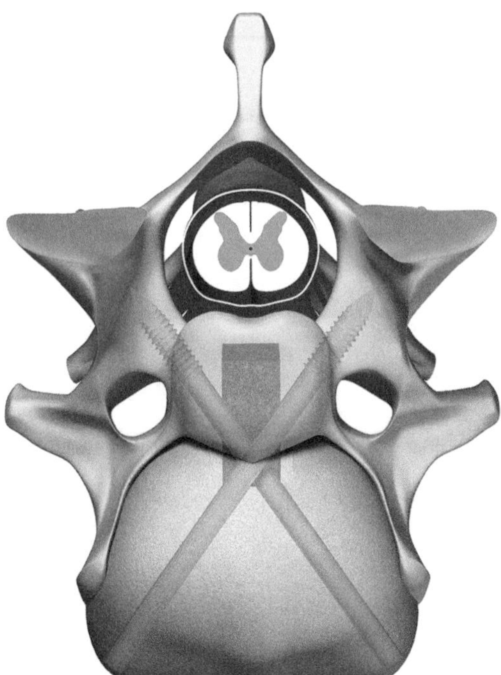

Fig. 13. The technique of pins and PMMA combined with a partial slot. Note the location of pin insertion avoiding the transverse foramina and vertebral canal. (*Courtesy of* The Ohio State University; with permission.)

static and dynamic. The original report focused on ventral disc-associated dynamic lesions, and the investigators did not recommend the technique for dorsal or ventral static lesions.[84] However, others have indicated that it can be used for up to 3 ventral sites and can also be indicated to treat sites with dorsal osseous compressions.[70,122] A discectomy is performed, traction is applied, and multiple holes (including an anchor hole) are drilled into the cranial and caudal end plates before application of PMMA (**Fig. 14**). Modifications of this technique have included a retention screw or pin ventral to the plug, and its application combined with a complete ventral slot.[70,112] The reported long-term success with the PMMA plug technique is 82%.[84]

Locking plate Locking plates have been used with either partial ventral slots or discectomies. Screws of the locking plates are less likely to loosen than are conventional screws, and can be inserted monocortically with sustained stability, thus decreasing the risk of vertebral canal penetration and spinal cord injury.[114] A variety of bone grafts was used in the reported cases including cancellous autograft, cortical allograft with cancellous autograft, and cancellous bone block graft.[12,113,114] The success rate based on the follow-up information of 3 cases series is 73%.[12,113,114] An important disadvantage of this system is the cost of the plate and screws.

Motion-preserving techniques

Cervical disc arthroplasty Disc arthroplasty is an area of intensive investigation in humans with cervical spondylotic myelopathy. Fusion or distraction may increase the risk of adjacent segment disease or "domino" lesion by altering the biomechanics of the adjacent segments.[129,130] Disc arthroplasty allows reestablishment of the normal disc space with motion preservation of the affected intervertebral segment.

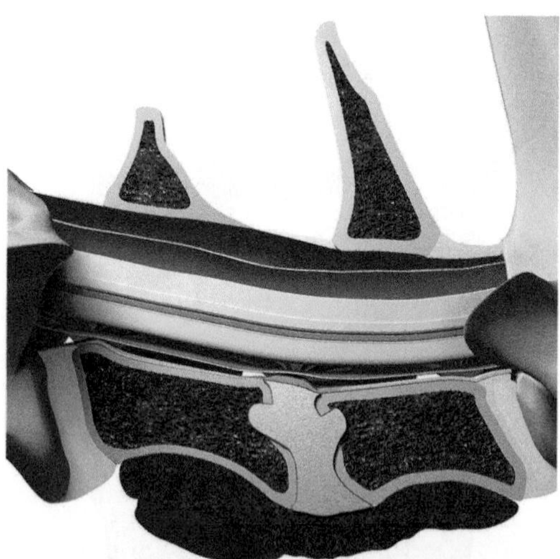

Fig. 14. The PMMA plug distraction technique. The PMMA plug is in place (*gray*). Two anchor holes in the cranial and caudal endplates prevent plug displacement. The dorsal annulus is left intact. Multiple small holes should be drilled in the ventral aspect of the vertebral bodies to promote incorporation of the cancellous bone graft (*dark red*) and fusion. (*Courtesy of* The Ohio State University; with permission.)

An artificial disc was recently introduced for treatment of CSM in dogs.[120,121] The technique was combined with complete ventral slot allowing direct spinal cord decompression. Long-term results of large patient series are not yet available.

Complications

Several complications, including death, can occur with surgical treatment of CSM. The mean mortality rate associated with decompressive surgery on the cervical spine of 771 reported cases was 3% (range 0%–6.3%).[124,131–135] Common complications are postoperative worsening of the neurologic status (which is challenging in large and giant breed dogs), penetration of the vertebral canal or transverse foramina with implants, and implant failure, ranging from 7.5% to 30%.[12,14,15,57,59,70,71,84,106–118]

Adjacent segment disease or "domino" effect

"Domino" effect or adjacent segment disease is a late postoperative complication after surgical treatment of CSM that occurs in approximately 20% of dogs after surgery, mainly with distraction-stabilization techniques.[8,112,136] Ventral slot techniques reportedly decrease the risk of "domino" lesion.[8,71] The domino effect may occur secondary to bone fusion.[70,106] Evidence in humans, however, suggests there is no difference in the incidence of adjacent segment syndrome in sites with or without fusion.[137] The domino effect typically affects only one disc region, either cranial or caudal to the operated area.[15,64,106,136] However, a recent study documented involvement of 3 sites after lack of fusion after ventral slot (**Fig. 15**).[76] Experimentally, ventral slots always developed bone proliferation and fusion 2 to 3 months after surgery.[101,123] Apparently this does not always occur in clinical patients, which then can lead to postoperative instability.[76] Motion-preserving techniques potentially could decrease the incidence of domino lesions by preserving the local biomechanics, but this still needs to be proved. Questions have been raised about whether these domino lesions are simply part of the natural history of CSM.[8] A recent study suggests that they are in fact a surgically induced phenomenon. A 1-year follow-up MRI study found no evidence of adjacent lesions in 9 dogs treated medically, whereas 2 of 3 dogs treated with ventral slots developed spinal cord lesions in the sites adjacent to surgery.[76] Long-term MRI follow-up investigations of other surgical techniques have not yet been reported.

Outcome and Prognosis

The outcome of surgical treatment of disc-associated CSM is usually successful, with approximately 80% (70%–90%) of dogs improving after surgery.[8,17] No surgical technique stands out as being clearly superior, even for dogs with disc-associated CSM. Intervertebral disc fenestration is not recommended because the reported success rate was only 33%.[119] In contrast to older studies, new reports on medical management indicate an improvement rate of approximately 50% (45%–54%).[17,88] Several factors were recently investigated to assess if they would be associated with a successful or unsuccessful outcome after surgical or medical treatment in 104 dogs with CSM. Age, duration of clinical signs, presence or absence of neck pain, severity of ataxia, nonambulatory status, and location of the lesion all were deemed nonsignificant.[17]

Considering the success rate of surgical and medical treatments for CSM, surgery more consistently leads to clinical improvement, and should always be considered in the treatment of dogs with CSM. Surgery, however, does not alter the long-term survival of dogs with CSM. The survival time of 76 dogs with CSM (33 dogs treated

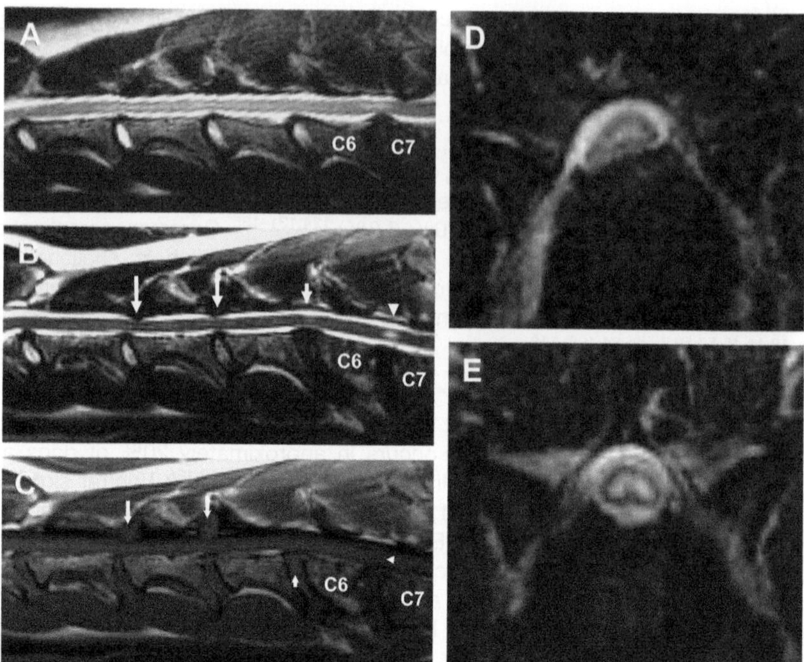

Fig. 15. Magnetic resonance (MR) images of the cervical spine of a 7-year-old Doberman pinscher with CSM treated with ventral slot decompression at C6-7. (*A*) Midsagittal T2W image shows spinal cord compression and cord hyperintensity at C6-7. (*B*) Midsagittal T2W image obtained 14 months after the first MRI. Spinal cord compression is no longer visible at C6-7, but cord hyperintensity is more evident (*arrowhead*). There are new areas of spinal cord compression at C5-6 and at C3-4 and C4-5 dorsally (*long arrows*). Mild cord hyperintensity can be seen associated with the compression at C5-6 (*short arrow*). (*C*) Follow-up midsagittal T1W image. Observe an area of hypointensity within the spinal cord at C6-7 (*arrowhead*), minimal bone proliferation between the vertebral bodies of C6-7, and the intermediate signal of the structures compressing the spinal cord dorsally (*long arrows*) and ventrally (*short arrow*). Apparently bone fusion did not occur at this site. Contrast the images of this dog with the dog in **Fig. 11**. (*D*) Transverse T2W image at the level of C6-7 before surgery. (*E*) Follow-up transverse T2W image. Adequate cord decompression is seen with marked cord hyperintensity and atrophy. C6, C7, sixth and seventh cervical vertebrae. (*From* da Costa RC, Parent JM. One-year clinical and magnetic resonance imaging follow-up of Doberman Pinschers with cervical spondylomyelopathy treated medically or surgically. J Am Vet Med Assoc 2007;231(2):245; with permission.)

surgically and 43 dogs treated medically) was reported recently. The median survival time of dogs with CSM was identical (36 months), regardless of whether the dog was treated medically or surgically.[17] This finding indicates that CSM continues to progress independent of the method of treatment, and that the clinical deterioration seen months to years after treatment may not be due solely to failure of the surgery or development of adjacent segment disease, but also may occur secondary to other mechanisms, such as ischemia, apoptosis, or other molecular changes within the spinal cord.[30]

SUMMARY

Many advances have been made in the diagnosis and treatment of cervical spondylomyelopathy in recent years. However, much is still unknown on the mechanisms causing the disease. Molecular investigations aiming to unveil the causes of the CSM are needed to enable us to prevent rather than only treat the disease. Newer surgical techniques are proposed continuously, but the criteria for patient evaluation and outcome assessment often do not allow meaningful comparisons among different surgical techniques. Objective inclusion criteria and valid methods of outcome assessment are needed to facilitate assessment of treatments for CSM. Routine MRI investigation of dogs that deteriorate postoperatively is also important to address the mechanisms leading to late-onset postoperative deterioration. This could lead to refinement of treatment strategies and improvement in survival times beyond those currently available.

ACKNOWLEDGMENTS

The author acknowledges Tim Vojt from The Ohio State University for preparation of figures 1, 2, 10, 12, 13, 14, and Dr. Stephen DiBartola for reviewing this manuscript.

REFERENCES

1. Palmer AC, Wallace ME. Deformation of cervical vertebrae in Basset hounds. Vet Rec 1967;80(14):430–3.
2. Trotter EJ, de Lahunta A, Geary JC, et al. Caudal cervical vertebral malformation-malarticulation in Great Danes and Doberman Pinschers. J Am Vet Med Assoc 1976;168(10):917–30.
3. Wright F, Rest JR, Palmer AC. Ataxia of the Great Dane caused by stenosis of the cervical vertebral canal: comparison with similar conditions in the Basset Hound, Doberman Pinscher, Ridgeback and the thoroughbred horse. Vet Rec 1973;92(1):1–6.
4. Seim HB, Withrow SJ. Pathophysiology and diagnosis of caudal cervical spondylo-myelopathy with emphasis on the Doberman Pinscher. J Am Anim Hosp Assoc 1982;18:241–51.
5. Parker AJ, Park RD, Cusick PK, et al. Cervical vertebral instability in the dog. J Am Vet Med Assoc 1973;163(1):71–4.
6. Raffe MR, Knecht CD. Cervical vertebral malformation—a review of 36 cases. J Am Anim Hosp Assoc 1980;16:881–3.
7. Shores A. Canine vertebral malformation/malarticulation syndrome. Compend Contin Educ Pract Vet 1984;6:326–34.
8. Jeffery ND, McKee WM. Surgery for disc-associated wobbler syndrome in the dog—an examination of the controversy. J Small Anim Pract 2001;42(12):574–81.
9. Lewis DG. Cervical spondylomyelopathy ('wobbler' syndrome) in the dog: a study based on 224 cases. J Small Anim Pract 1989;30(12):657–65.
10. de Lahunta A. Cervical spinal cord contusion from spondylolisthesis (a wobbler syndrome in dogs). In: Kirk RW, editor. Current veterinary therapy IV—Small animal practice. 4th edition. Philadelphia: Saunders; 1971. p. 503–4.
11. Lipsitz D, Levitski RE, Chauvet AE, et al. Magnetic resonance imaging features of cervical stenotic myelopathy in 21 dogs. Vet Radiol Ultrasound 2001;42(1):20–7.
12. Trotter EJ. Cervical spine locking plate fixation for treatment of cervical spondylotic myelopathy in large breed dogs. Vet Surg 2009;38(6):705–18.

13. Seim HB. Diagnosis and treatment of cervical vertebral instability-malformation syndromes. In: Bonagura JD, editor. Current veterinary therapy: small animal practice. 13th edition. Philadelphia: Saunders; 2000. p. 992–1000.
14. Denny HR, Gibbs C, Gaskell CJ. Cervical spondylopathy in the dog—a review of thirty-five cases. J Small Anim Pract 1977;18(2):117–32.
15. McKee WM, Butterworth SJ, Scott HW. Management of cervical spondylopathy-associated intervertebral disc protrusions using metal washers in 78 dogs. J Small Anim Pract 1999;40(10):465–72.
16. Burbidge HM, Pfeiffer DU, Blair HT. Canine wobbler syndrome: a study of the Doberman pinscher in New Zealand. N Z Vet J 1994;42(6):221–8.
17. da Costa RC, Parent JM, Holmberg DL, et al. Outcome of medical and surgical treatment in dogs with cervical spondylomyelopathy: 104 cases. J Am Vet Med Assoc 2008;233(8):1284–90.
18. Sharp NJ, Cofone M, Robertson ID, et al. Cervical spondylomyelopathy in the Doberman dog: a potential model for cervical spondylotic myelopathy in humans. J Invest Surg 1989;2:333.
19. Selcer RR, Oliver JE Jr. Cervical spondylopathy—wobbler syndrome in dogs. J Am Anim Hosp Assoc 1975;11(2):175–9.
20. Mason TA. Cervical vertebral instability (wobbler syndrome) in the Doberman. Aust Vet J 1977;53(9):440–5.
21. Olsson SE, Stavenborn M, Hoppe F. Dynamic compression of the cervical spinal cord. Acta Vet Scand 1982;23(1):65–78.
22. Jaggy A, Gaillard C, Lang J, et al. Hereditary cervical spondylopathy (wobbler syndrome) in the Borzoi dog. J Am Anim Hosp Assoc 1988;4:453–60.
23. Lewis DG. Radiological assessment of the cervical spine of the Doberman with reference to cervical spondylomyelopathy. J Small Anim Pract 1991;32(2): 75–82.
24. Burbidge HM. Caudal cervical malformation in the Doberman pinscher [PhD thesis]. New Zealand: Massey University; 1999. p. 121–35.
25. Hedhammar A, Wu FM, Krook L, et al. Overnutrition and skeletal disease. An experimental study in growing Great Dane dogs. Cornell Vet 1974;64(2) (Suppl 5):5–160.
26. Hazewinkel HA, Goedegebuure SA, Poulos PW, et al. Influences of chronic calcium excess on the skeletal development of growing Great Danes. J Am Anim Hosp Assoc 1985;21(3):377–91.
27. Burbidge HM, Pfeiffer DU, Guilford WG. Presence of cervical vertebral malformation in Doberman puppies and the effects of diet and growth rate. Aust Vet J 1999;77(12):814–8.
28. da Costa RC, Parent JM, Partlow G, et al. Morphologic and morphometric magnetic resonance imaging features of Doberman pinscher dogs with and without clinical signs of cervical spondylomyelopathy. Am J Vet Res 2006; 67(10):1601–12.
29. De Decker S, Gielen IM, Duchateau L, et al. Low-field magnetic resonance imaging findings of the caudal portion of the cervical region in clinically normal Doberman Pinschers and Foxhounds. Am J Vet Res 2010;71(4):428–34.
30. da Costa RC. Pathogenesis of cervical spondylomyelopathy: lessons from recent years. ACVIM Forum Proceedings. Lakewood (CO): American College of Veterinary Internal Medicine; 2007. p. 318–20.
31. Bernhardt M, Hynes RA, Blume HW, et al. Cervical spondylotic myelopathy. J Bone Joint Surg Am 1993;75(1):119–28.

32. Okada Y, Ikata T, Katoh S, et al. Morphologic analysis of the cervical spinal cord, dural tube, and spinal canal by magnetic resonance imaging in normal adults and patients with cervical spondylotic myelopathy. Spine 1994;19(20):2331–5.
33. Yu YL, du Boulay GH, Stevens JM, et al. Computed tomography in cervical spondylotic myelopathy and radiculopathy: visualisation of structures, myelographic comparison, cord measurements and clinical utility. Neuroradiology 1986;28(3):221–36.
34. Okada Y, Ikata T, Yamada H, et al. Magnetic resonance imaging study on the results of surgery for cervical compression myelopathy. Spine 1993;18(14):2024–9.
35. Johnson JA, da Costa RC, Allen MJ, et al. Kinematics of the cranial and caudal cervical spine in large breed dogs. ACVIM Forum Proceedings. Lakewood (CO): American College of Veterinary Internal Medicine; 2010. p. 338.
36. Breit S, Kunzel W. Shape and orientation of articular facets of cervical vertebrae (C3-C7) in dogs denoting axial rotational ability: an osteological study. Eur J Morphol 2002;40(1):43–51.
37. Farfan HF, Cossette JW, Robertson GH, et al. The effects of torsion on the lumbar intervertebral joints: the role of torsion in the production of disc degeneration. J Bone Joint Surg Am 1970;52(3):468–97.
38. da Costa RC, Echandi RL, Beauchamp D. Computed tomographic findings in large and giant breed dogs with cervical spondylomyelopathy: 58 cases. J Vet Intern Med 2009;23(3):709.
39. da Costa RC, Parent JM. Magnetic resonance imaging findings in 60 dogs with cervical spondylomyelopathy. J Vet Intern Med 2009;23(3):740.
40. Levitski RE, Chauvet AE, Lipsitz D. Cervical myelopathy associated with extradural synovial cysts in 4 dogs. J Vet Intern Med 1999;13(3):181–6.
41. Gray MJ, Kirberger RM, Spotswood TC. Cervical spondylomyelopathy (wobbler syndrome) in the Boerboel. J S Afr Vet Assoc 2003;74(4):104–10.
42. Levine DN. Pathogenesis of cervical spondylotic myelopathy. J Neurol Neurosurg Psychiatry 1997;62(4):334–40.
43. Henderson FC, Geddes JF, Vaccaro AR, et al. Stretch-associated injury in cervical spondylotic myelopathy: new concept and review. Neurosurgery 2005;56(5):1101–13 [discussion: 1101–13].
44. Ichihara K, Taguchi T, Sakuramoto I, et al. Mechanism of the spinal cord injury and the cervical spondylotic myelopathy: new approach based on the mechanical features of the spinal cord white and gray matter. J Neurosurg 2003; 99(Suppl 3):278–85.
45. Panjabi MM, Yue JJ, Dvorak J, et al. Cervical spine kinematics and clinical instability. In: The Cervical Spine Research Society, editor. The cervical spine. 4th edition. Philadelphia: Lippincott Williams & Wilkins; 2005. p. 55–78.
46. White AA 3rd, Panjabi MM. Biomechanical considerations in the surgical management of cervical spondylotic myelopathy. Spine 1988;13(7):856–60.
47. Reid JD. Effects of flexion-extension movements of the head and spine upon the spinal cord and nerve roots. J Neurol Neurosurg Psychiatry 1960;23: 214–21.
48. Waltz TA. Physical factors in the production of the myelopathy of cervical spondylosis. Brain 1967;90(2):395–404.
49. Wright F, Palmer AC. Morphological changes caused by pressure on the spinal cord. Pathol Vet 1969;6(4):355–68.
50. Wright JA. A study of the radiographic anatomy of the cervical spine in the dog. J Small Anim Pract 1977;18:341–57.

51. Morgan JP, Miyabayashi T, Choy S. Cervical spine motion: radiographic study. Am J Vet Res 1986;47(10):2165–9.
52. Penning L, Badoux DM. Radiological study of the movements of the cervical spine in the dog compared with those in man. Anat Histol Embryol 1987; 16(1):1–20.
53. Muhle C, Resnick D, Ahn JM, et al. In vivo changes in the neuroforaminal size at flexion-extension and axial rotation of the cervical spine in healthy persons examined using kinematic magnetic resonance imaging. Spine 2001;26(13): E287–93.
54. Dai L. Disc degeneration and cervical instability. Correlation of magnetic resonance imaging with radiography. Spine 1998;23(16):1734–8.
55. Kumaresan S, Yoganandan N, Pintar FA, et al. Contribution of disc degeneration to osteophyte formation in the cervical spine: a biomechanical investigation. J Orthop Res 2001;19(5):977–84.
56. Kaigle AM, Wessberg P, Hansson TH. Muscular and kinematic behavior of the lumbar spine during flexion-extension. J Spinal Disord 1998;11(2):163–74.
57. Read RA, Robins GM, Carlisle CM. Caudal cervical spondylo-myelopathy (wobbler syndrome) in the dog—a review of thirty cases. J Small Anim Pract 1983;24(10):605–21.
58. De Risio L, Munana K, Murray M, et al. Dorsal laminectomy for caudal cervical spondylomyelopathy: postoperative recovery and long-term follow-up in 20 dogs. Vet Surg 2002;31(5):418–27.
59. Mason TA. Cervical vertebral instability (wobbler syndrome) in the dog. Vet Rec 1979;104(7):142–5.
60. Sharp NJ, Cofone M, Robertson ID, et al. Computed tomography in the evaluation of caudal cervical spondylomyelopathy of the Doberman Pinscher. Vet Radiol Ultrasound 1995;36(2):100–8.
61. da Costa RC, Parent JP, Dobson H, et al. Comparison of magnetic resonance imaging and myelography in 18 Doberman pinscher dogs with cervical spondylomyelopathy. Vet Radiol Ultrasound 2006;47(6):523–31.
62. de Lahunta A, Glass EN. General sensory systems: general proprioception and general somatic afferent. In: de Lahunta A, Glass EN, editors. Veterinary neuroanatomy and clinical neurology. 3rd edition. St Louis (MO): Saunders; 2009. p. 221–42.
63. da Costa RC. Ataxia, paresis and paralysis. In: Ettinger SJ, Feldman EC, editors. Textbook of veterinary internal medicine. 7th edition. St Louis (MO): Elsevier; 2010. p. 222–5.
64. Sharp NJ, Wheeler SJ, Cofone M. Radiological evaluation of 'wobbler' syndrome—caudal cervical spondylomyelopathy. J Small Anim Pract 1992; 33(10):491–9.
65. Moore BR, Reed SM, Biller DS, et al. Assessment of vertebral canal diameter and bony malformations of the cervical part of the spine in horses with cervical stenotic myelopathy. Am J Vet Res 1994;55(1):5–13.
66. Hahn CN, Handel I, Green SL, et al. Assessment of the utility of using intra- and intervertebral minimum sagittal diameter ratios in the diagnosis of cervical vertebral malformation in horses. Vet Radiol Ultrasound 2008;49(1): 1–6.
67. Yue WM, Tan SB, Tan MH, et al. The Torg-Pavlov ratio in cervical spondylotic myelopathy: a comparative study between patients with cervical spondylotic myelopathy and a nonspondylotic, nonmyelopathic population. Spine 2001; 26(16):1760–4.

68. da Costa RC, Johnson JA, Parent JM. Are cervical vertebral ratios useful in the diagnosis of cervical spondylomyelopathy in Dobermans? ACVIM Forum Proceedings. Lakewood (CO): American College of Veterinary Internal Medicine; 2010. p. 332.
69. De Decker S, Saunders J, Duchateau P, et al. Radiographic vertebral canal and body ratios in Doberman pinschers with and without clinical signs of disk associated wobbler syndrome. J Vet Intern Med 2010;24(3):737.
70. Sharp NJ, Wheeler SJ. Cervical spondylomyelopathy. In: Sharp NJH, Wheeler SJ, editors. Small animal spinal disorders diagnosis and surgery. 2nd edition. Philadelphia: Elsevier Mosby; 2005. p. 211–46.
71. Rusbridge C, Wheeler SJ, Torrington AM, et al. Comparison of two surgical techniques for the management of cervical spondylomyelopathy in Dobermans. J Small Anim Pract 1998;39(9):425–31.
72. Barone G, Ziemer LS, Shofer FS, et al. Risk factors associated with development of seizures after use of iohexol for myelography in dogs: 182 cases (1998). J Am Vet Med Assoc 2002;220(10):1499–502.
73. Lewis DD, Hosgood G. Complications associated with the use of iohexol for myelography of the cervical vertebral column in dogs: 66 cases (1988-1990). J Am Vet Med Assoc 1992;200(9):1381–4.
74. da Costa RC, Parent JM, Dobson H. Incidence and risk factors of postmyelographic seizures in dogs: 503 cases. J Vet Intern Med 2009;23(3):707–8.
75. Ohshio I, Hatayama A, Kaneda K, et al. Correlation between histopathologic features and magnetic resonance images of spinal cord lesions. Spine 1993;18(9):1140–9.
76. da Costa RC, Parent JM. One-year clinical and magnetic resonance imaging follow-up of Doberman Pinschers with cervical spondylomyelopathy treated medically or surgically. J Am Vet Med Assoc 2007;231(2):243–50.
77. Chatley A, Kumar R, Jain VK, et al. Effect of spinal cord signal intensity changes on clinical outcome after surgery for cervical spondylotic myelopathy. J Neurosurg Spine 2009;11(5):562–7.
78. Mastronardi L, Elsawaf A, Roperto R, et al. Prognostic relevance of the postoperative evolution of intramedullary spinal cord changes in signal intensity on magnetic resonance imaging after anterior decompression for cervical spondylotic myelopathy. J Neurosurg Spine 2007;7(6):615–22.
79. Yagi M, Ninomiya K, Kihara M, et al. Long-term surgical outcome and risk factors in patients with cervical myelopathy and a change in signal intensity of intramedullary spinal cord on magnetic resonance imaging. J Neurosurg Spine 2010;12(1):59–65.
80. Penderis J, Dennis R. Use of traction during magnetic resonance imaging of caudal cervical spondylomyelopathy ("wobbler syndrome") in the dog. Vet Radiol Ultrasound 2004;45(3):216–9.
81. da Costa RC. Cervical spondylomyelopathy in Doberman pinscher dogs: anatomic, functional, diagnostic and follow-up investigations [PhD thesis]. Ontario Veterinary College, University of Guelph; 2006. p. 189–220.
82. Poma R, Parent JM, Holmberg DL, et al. Correlation between severity of clinical signs and motor evoked potentials after transcranial magnetic stimulation in large-breed dogs with cervical spinal cord disease. J Am Vet Med Assoc 2002;221(1):60–4.
83. da Costa RC, Poma R, Parent JM, et al. Correlation of motor evoked potentials with magnetic resonance imaging and neurological findings in Doberman pinscher dogs with and without signs of cervical spondylomyelopathy. Am J Vet Res 2006;67(10):1613–20.

84. Dixon BC, Tomlinson JL, Kraus KH. Modified distraction-stabilization technique using an interbody polymethyl methacrylate plug in dogs with caudal cervical spondylomyelopathy. J Am Vet Med Assoc 1996;208(1):61–8.
85. Brooks M, Dodds WJ, Raymond SL. Epidemiologic features of von Willebrand's disease in Doberman pinschers, Scottish terriers, and Shetland sheepdogs: 260 cases (1984-1988). J Am Vet Med Assoc 1992;200(8):1123–7.
86. Calvert CA, Jacobs GJ, Pickus CW. Unfavorable influence of anesthesia and surgery on Doberman pinschers with occult cardiomyopathy. J Am Anim Hosp Assoc 1996;32(1):57–62.
87. VanGundy TE. Disc-associated wobbler syndrome in the Doberman pinscher. Vet Clin North Am Small Anim Pract 1988;18(3):667–96.
88. De Decker S, Bhatti SF, Duchateau L, et al. Clinical evaluation of 51 dogs treated conservatively for disc-associated wobbler syndrome. J Small Anim Pract 2009; 50(3):136–42.
89. Delattre JY, Arbit E, Rosenblum MK, et al. High dose versus low dose dexamethasone in experimental epidural spinal cord compression. Neurosurgery 1988; 22(6 Pt 1):1005–7.
90. Toombs JP, Collins LG, Graves GM, et al. Colonic perforation in corticosteroid-treated dogs. J Am Vet Med Assoc 1986;188(2):145–50.
91. Delattre JY, Arbit E, Thaler HT, et al. A dose-response study of dexamethasone in a model of spinal cord compression caused by epidural tumor. J Neurosurg 1989;70(6):920–5.
92. Ogata T, Nakamura Y, Tsuji K, et al. Steroid hormones protect spinal cord neurons from glutamate toxicity. Neuroscience 1993;55(2):445–9.
93. Melcangi RC, Cavarretta I, Magnaghi V, et al. Corticosteroids protect oligodendrocytes from cytokine-induced cell death. Neuroreport 2000;11(18): 3969–72.
94. Zurita M, Vaquero J, Oya S, et al. Effects of dexamethasone on apoptosis-related cell death after spinal cord injury. J Neurosurg 2002;96(Suppl 1): 83–9.
95. Boothe DM, Mealey KA. Glucocorticoid therapy in the dog and cat. In: Boothe DM, editor. Small animal clinical pharmacology and therapeutics. 1st edition. Philadelphia: Saunders; 2001. p. 313–29.
96. Yovich JV, leCouteur RA, Gould DH. Chronic cervical compressive myelopathy in horses: clinical correlations with spinal cord alterations. Aust Vet J 1991; 68(10):326–34.
97. Ito T, Oyanagi K, Takahashi H, et al. Cervical spondylotic myelopathy. Clinicopathologic study on the progression pattern and thin myelinated fibers of the lesions of seven patients examined during complete autopsy. Spine 1996; 21(7):827–33.
98. Speciale J, Fingeroth JM. Use of physiatry as the sole treatment for three paretic or paralyzed dogs with chronic compressive conditions of the caudal portion of the cervical spinal cord. J Am Vet Med Assoc 2000;217(1):43–7 29.
99. Sumano H, Bermudez E, Obregon K. Treatment of wobbler syndrome in dogs with electroacupuncture. Dtsch Tierarztl Wochenschr 2000;107(6):231–5.
100. Chambers JN, Oliver JE, Bjorling DE. Update on ventral decompression for caudal cervical disk herniation in Doberman Pinschers. J Am Anim Hosp Assoc 1986;22(6):775–8.
101. Swaim SF. Ventral decompression of the cervical spinal cord in the dog. J Am Vet Med Assoc 1974;164(5):491–5.

102. Goring RL, Beale BS, Faulkner RF. The inverted cone decompression technique: a surgical treatment for cervical vertebral instability "wobbler syndrome" in Doberman Pinschers. J Am Anim Hosp Assoc 1991;27(4):403–9.
103. Lyman R. Continuous dorsal laminectomy for the treatment of caudal cervical instability and malformation. ACVIM Forum Proceedings. Lakewood (CO): American College of Veterinary Internal Medicine; 1989. p. 13–6.
104. Rossmeisl JH Jr, Lanz OI, Inzana KD, et al. A modified lateral approach to the canine cervical spine: procedural description and clinical application in 16 dogs with lateralized compressive myelopathy or radiculopathy. Vet Surg 2005;34(5):436–44.
105. Jeffery ND. The 'wobbler' syndrome. In: Jeffery ND, editor. Handbook of small animal spinal surgery. London: Saunders; 1995. p. 169–86.
106. Bruecker KA, Seim HB 3rd, Withrow SJ. Clinical evaluation of three surgical methods for treatment of caudal cervical spondylomyelopathy of dogs. Vet Surg 1989;18(3):197–203.
107. Bruecker KA, Seim HB, Blass CE. Caudal cervical spondylomyelopathy: decompression by linear traction and stabilization with Steinmann pins and polymethyl methacrylate. J Am Anim Hosp Assoc 1989;25(6):677–83.
108. Bruecker KA, Seim HB, Withrow SJ. Ventral decompression and lubra-plate stabilization for the treatment of caudal cervical spondylomyelopathy: results of 37 cases. Vet Surg 1987;16(1):84–5.
109. Ellison GW, Seim HB, Clemmons RM. Distracted cervical spinal fusion for management of caudal cervical spondylomyelopathy in large-breed dogs. J Am Vet Med Assoc 1988;193(4):447–53.
110. Queen JP, Coughlan AR, May C, et al. Management of disc-associated wobbler syndrome with a partial slot fenestration and position screw technique. J Small Anim Pract 1998;39(3):131–6.
111. McKee WM, Levelle RB, Mason TA. Vertebral stabilization for cervical spondylopathy using a screw and washer technique. J Small Anim Pract 1989;30(6): 337–42.
112. McKee WM, Sharp NJ. Cervical spondylopathy. In: Slatter DH, editor. Textbook of small animal surgery. 3rd edition. Philadelphia: Saunders; 2003. p. 1180–93.
113. Bergman RL, Levine JM, Coates JR, et al. Cervical spinal locking plate in combination with cortical ring allograft for a one level fusion in dogs with cervical spondylotic myelopathy. Vet Surg 2008;37(6):530–6.
114. Voss K, Steffen F, Montavon PM. Use of the ComPact UniLock System for ventral stabilization procedures of the cervical spine: a retrospective study. Vet Comp Orthop Traumatol 2006;19(1):21–8.
115. Hicks DG, Pitts MJ, Bagley RS, et al. In vitro biomechanical evaluations of screw-bar-polymethylmethacrylate and pin-polymethylmethacrylate internal fixation implants used to stabilize the vertebral motion unit of the fourth and fifth cervical vertebrae in vertebral column specimens from dogs. Am J Vet Res 2009;70(6):719–26.
116. Shamir MH, Chai O, Loeb E. A method for intervertebral space distraction before stabilization combined with complete ventral slot for treatment of disc-associated wobbler syndrome in dogs. Vet Surg 2008;37(2):186–92.
117. Walker TL. Use of Harrington rods in caudal cervical spondylomyelopathy. In: Bojrab MJ, editor. Current techniques in small animal surgery. 3rd edition. Philadelphia (PA): Lea & Febiger; 1990. p. 584–6.

118. Adrega Da Silva C, Bernard F, Bardet JF. Caudal cervical arthrodesis using a distractable fusion cage in a dog. Vet Comp Orthop Traumatol 2010;23(3): 209–13.
119. Lincoln JD, Petit GD. Evaluation of fenestration for treatment of degenerative disc disease in the caudal cervical region of large dogs. Vet Surg 1985;14(3): 240–6.
120. Adamo PF, Kobayashi H, Markel M, et al. In vitro biomechanical comparison of cervical disk arthroplasty, ventral slot procedure, and smooth pins with polymethylmethacrylate fixation at treated and adjacent canine cervical motion units. Vet Surg 2007;36(8):729–41.
121. Adamo PF, Burns G. Cervical arthroplasty in dogs with disc-associated caudal cervical spondylomyelopathy and cervical disc herniation: preliminary study of two cases. J Vet Intern Med 2009;23(3):710.
122. Galano H, Olby NJ, Sharp NJ, et al. Long-term effect of cervical fusion on neurological status and vertebral canal diameter in giant breed dogs with cervical stenotic myelopathy. J Vet Intern Med 2005;19(3):419.
123. Gilpin GN. Evaluation of three techniques of ventral decompression of the cervical spinal cord in the dog. J Am Vet Med Assoc 1976;168(4):325–8.
124. Smith BA, Hosgood G, Kerwin SC. Ventral slot decompression for cervical intervertebral disc disease in 112 dogs. Aust Vet Practit 1997;27(2):58–64.
125. Burton CV. Causes of failure of surgery on the lumbar spine: ten-year follow-up. Mt Sinai J Med 1991;58(2):183–7.
126. da Costa RC, Pippi NL, Graca DL, et al. The effects of free fat graft or cellulose membrane implants on laminectomy membrane formation in dogs. Vet J 2006; 171(3):491–9.
127. Koehler CL, Stover SM, LeCouteur RA, et al. Effect of a ventral slot procedure and of smooth or positive-profile threaded pins with polymethylmethacrylate fixation on intervertebral biomechanics at treated and adjacent canine cervical vertebral motion units. Am J Vet Res 2005;66(4):678–87.
128. Corlazzoli D. Bicortical implant insertion in caudal cervical spondylomyelopathy: a computed tomography simulation in affected Doberman Pinschers. Vet Surg 2008;37(2):178–85.
129. Rihn JA, Lawrence J, Gates C, et al. Adjacent segment disease after cervical spine fusion. Instr Course Lect 2009;58:747–56.
130. Hilibrand AS, Carlson GD, Palumbo MA, et al. Radiculopathy and myelopathy at segments adjacent to the site of a previous anterior cervical arthrodesis. J Bone Joint Surg Am 1999;81(4):519–28.
131. Clark DM. An analysis of intraoperative and early postoperative mortality associated with cervical spinal decompressive surgery in the dog. J Am Anim Hosp Assoc 1986;22(6):739–44.
132. Stauffer JL, Gleed RD, Short CE, et al. Cardiac dysrhythmias during anesthesia for cervical decompression in the dog. Am J Vet Res 1988;49(7):1143–6.
133. Beal MW, Paglia DT, Griffin GM, et al. Ventilatory failure, ventilator management, and outcome in dogs with cervical spinal disorders: 14 cases (1991–1999). J Am Vet Med Assoc 2001;218(10):1598–602.
134. Fry T, Johnson AL, Hungerford L, et al. Surgical treatment of cervical disc herniations in ambulatory dogs: ventral decompression vs. fenestration, 111 cases (1980-1988). Prog Vet Neurol 1991;2(3):165–73.
135. Cherrone KL, Dewey CW, Coates JR, et al. A retrospective comparison of cervical intervertebral disk disease in nonchondrodystrophic large dogs versus small dogs. J Am Anim Hosp Assoc 2004;40(4):316–20.

136. Wilson ER, Aron DN, Roberts RE. Observation of a secondary compressive lesion after treatment of caudal cervical spondylomyelopathy in a dog. J Am Vet Med Assoc 1994;205(9):1297–9.
137. Hilibrand AS, Robbins M. Adjacent segment degeneration and adjacent segment disease: the consequences of spinal fusion? Spine J 2004;4(Suppl 6):190S–4S.

Spinal Neoplasms in Small Animals

Rodney S. Bagley, DVM

KEYWORDS

• Dog • Cat • Spine • Neoplasm • Tumor • Spinal cord

Spinal cord disease can result from a variety of disease processes.[1–3] Neoplastic disease can similarly involve the spinal cord, dura, exiting peripheral nerves, or perispinal tissues (eg, the vertebrae and ligaments) and result in clinical signs of spinal cord dysfunction. Because of the fact that many of these neoplastic processes are locally aggressive, early recognition of such diseases is important. This recognition often requires some type of advanced imaging of the spinal cord unless the abnormality obviously involves the vertebra. Surgical treatments are often employed for definitive diagnosis of the tumor and for decompression of the spinal cord. Other treatments, such as radiation therapy and chemotherapy, are used in some instances. Outcomes of animals affected with spinal tumors are dependent upon the growth characteristics and biologic behavior of the tumor itself and the degree of associated spinal cord damage.

CLASSIFICATION

Spinal neoplasms are often categorized initially based upon the anatomic area, in relation to the dura and spinal cord, of spinal involvement.[4–17] Tumors are grouped into those primarily arising from an extradural location (extradural), within the dura but outside the spinal cord proper (intradural/extramedullary), or arising within the spinal cord parenchyma proper (intramedullary). Obviously, depending upon growth characteristics and tumor aggressiveness, tumors can expand and extend from one of these strict anatomic areas to involve another. This expansion is most often seen with peripheral nerve sheath tumors that may begin in an extradural location but may traverse the dura into the intradural/extramedullary space, and eventually, into the spinal cord gray matter.

Spinal tumors may also be classified into primary tumors (those tumors that arise from cells native to the spinal, dural, and perispinal tissues) or secondary tumors (those tumors that have metastasize from another location within the body).[18–27] This system lends information as to whether the disease is localized or systemic and influences treatment and prognosis.

Neurology and Neurosurgery, Department of Clinical Sciences, Iowa State University, College of Veterinary Medicine, 1600 South 16th street, Ames, IA 50011-1250, USA
E-mail address: rsbagley@iastate.edu

Vet Clin Small Anim 40 (2010) 915–927
doi:10.1016/j.cvsm.2010.05.010 **vetsmall.theclinics.com**
0195-5616/10/$ – see front matter

Understanding the initial anatomic location of the cell of origin of the tumor aids in predicting the type of tumor present. Extradural tumors are the most common of all spinal tumors in dogs and cats (**Fig. 1**). These tumors include primary and secondary bone tumors (osteosarcoma, fibrosarcoma, chondrosarcoma), hemangiosarcoma, multiple myeloma and other plasma cell tumors, liposarcoma, and lymphosarcoma. Carcinomas are often found to metastasize to the extradural spinal location.[20] Lymphosarcoma is the most commonly recognized spinal tumor in cats.[28–30]

Less commonly, benign neoplasms of bone, such as osteomas, fibromas, chondromas, and lipomas, may be present.[31,32] Vascular expansile lesions have been seen in cats.[33] In some instances, proliferations of bone and connective tissues mimic tumors but are not neoplastic. One example is multiple cartilaginous exostoses.[34–37] These abnormalities are proliferations of bone and cartilage that are thought to result from aberrant growth displaced chondrocytes from the metaphyseal growth plates of bone. Subsequently, this disease is most often seen in younger animals (<18 months of age). Dogs, cats, and other species, including humans, have been reported with this disease. The boney and cartilaginous proliferations are often multiple and can affect the long bones, ribs, or vertebrae. The bony protuberances may be palpable. If these proliferations of cartilage affect the vertebrae, varying degrees of spinal pain, paresis, or paralysis may result. Radiographs of the affected bones often show proliferations of bone that are smooth, contoured, irregular, and multilobulated. These bony proliferations, however, may eventually become malignant as the animal ages.[38,39]

Intradural but extramedullary tumors include meningiomas and nerve sheath tumors.[10,15,40–45] Meningiomas are most often found in the cervical area followed by the lumbar area. These tumors are infrequently found in the thoracic area. In the lumbar area, these tumors often proliferate around, entwine, and become adherent to exiting peripheral nerves.

Primary neoplasia may involve numerous peripheral nerves within or around the spinal cord (**Figs. 2** and **3**). Clinical signs are related to dysfunction of the involved

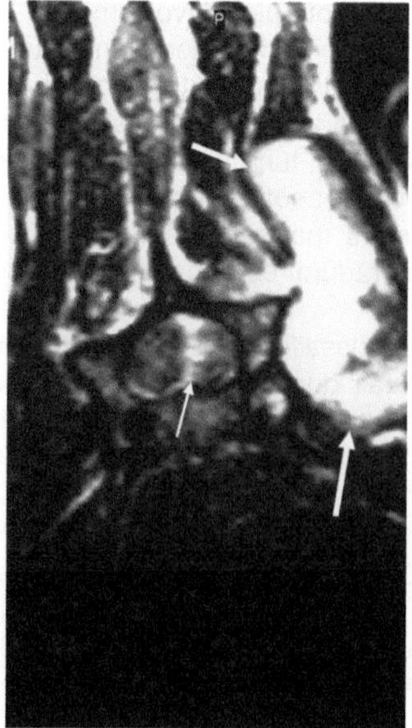

Fig. 1. Transverse, T2-weighted MRI of the cervical spine of a dog with an extradural tumor. There is tumor both extradural (*small arrow*) and lateral to the vertebrae (*larger arrows*).

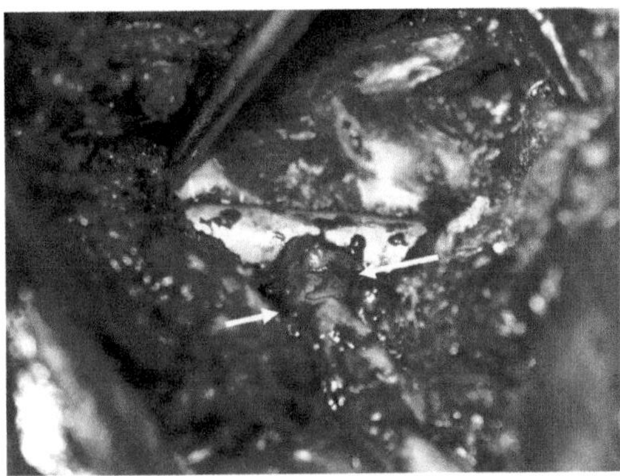

Fig. 2. Intraoperative view following laminectomy of a dog with a nerve sheath tumor abutting the dura (*arrows*).

peripheral nerves. General clinical signs reflect lower motor neuron dysfunction. These signs include hyporeflexia to areflexia, hypotonia to atonia, neurogenic atrophy, and abnormal proprioception. Primary neoplasia involving the peripheral nervous system usually results in clinical dysfunction localized to one body area or nerve segment.

Nerve sheath tumors are one of the most common types of primary neoplasia of the peripheral nervous system. These tumor types include schwannomas, neurofibromas, and neurofibrosarcomas. Histologic differentiation is sometimes difficult and the biologic behavior is similar allowing for the use of the generic grouping within the nerve sheath tumor category. These tumor types can arise from the Schwann (myelinated) cell of the peripheral nervous system, from connective tissue elements associated with the peripheral nerve, or from the axon and cell body. Tumors often involve nerves of the thoracic limbs but any peripheral nerve, including cranial nerves, may be involved. Nerve sheath tumor, for example, may involve the sciatic nerve and result in pelvic limb lameness. Importantly, nerve sheath tumors may involve the nerve at any site along its length. Distally located tumors may be focally painful if palpated, and may sometimes result in firm enlargements that may be tubular or spherical in shape. These tumors tend to feel firm upon palpation.

Additionally, there is an unusual intradural but extramedullary tumor that has been referred to by various terms, including neuroepithelioma and spinal cord

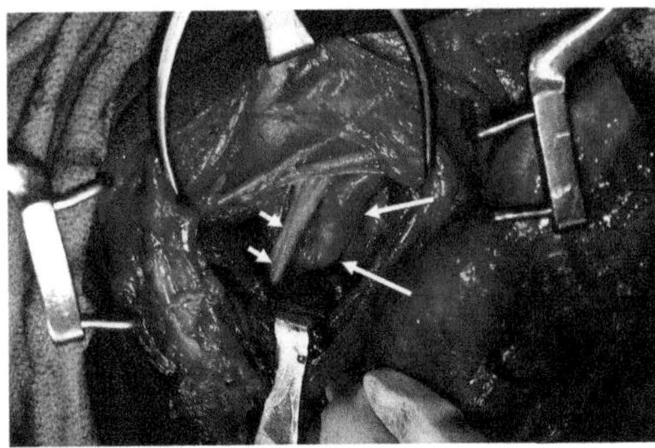

Fig. 3. Intraoperative view following brachial plexus exploration from a dog with a peripheral nerve sheath tumor. Note the enlarged, discolored nerve (*Larger arrows*) compared with an adjacent normal nerve (*smaller arrows*).

blastoma.[4,46–49] This tumor tends to occur in young animals and often occurs in the T11 to L2 area of the spinal cord. German shepherds may be overrepresented with this tumor type.[4] In some instances a histologically similar tumor may be present in other locations rather than limited to the T11 to L2 region, and in other breeds of dogs besides German Shepherds.

Intramedullary tumors include astrocytomas, oligodendrogliomas, and ependymomas. These tumors arise from cells within the spinal cord parenchyma.[4,6,10,15,50] They are often poorly encapsulated and sometimes difficult to differentiate from normal spinal cord tissue (**Fig. 4**). In some instances, however, the tumors are well encapsulated and firm, making differentiation easier.

Metastatic disease can also affect the spinal cord.[18–20,25,26,51] Both extradural and intramedullary metastasis is possible. Carcinomas are one of the most common types of tumors associated with extradural metastasis. In some instances, clinical signs of the metastasis may be apparent before clinical signs of the primary tumor. Hemangiosarcoma has resulted in intramedullary spinal cord metastasis.[26]

CLINICAL FEATURES

Clinical signs of spinal tumor are never pathognomonic because these signs are prototypical of spinal cord dysfunction and pain.[3,10,33,36,40,41,52] The location that the spinal cord is involved will determine the presence of associated upper-motor or lower-motor neuron (LMN) signs.

If the tumor begins in a peripheral nerve, clinical signs usually involve a nonlocalizable lameness, monoparesis, localized appendicular muscle atrophy, or pain.[53] Dogs with nerve sheath tumor may initially present for lameness and may be initially diagnosed as having some orthopedic and musculoskeletal causes for the dysfunction. Complicating the ultimate diagnosis, many animals will concurrently have minor

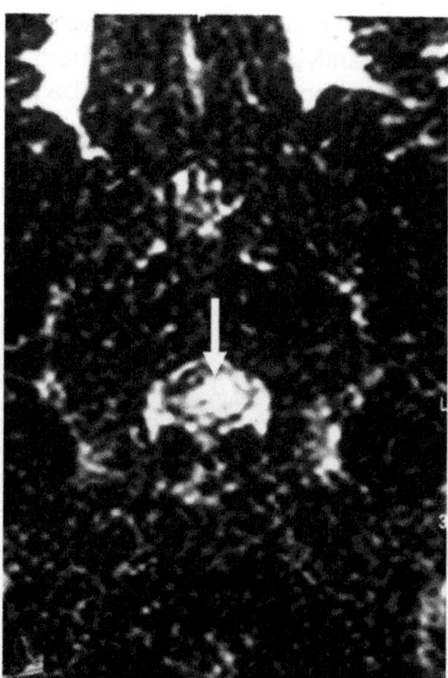

Fig. 4. Transverse, T2-weighted MRI of the spinal cord of a dog with an intramedullary lesion. There is a hyperintense lesion presence within the spinal parenchyma. Histologic diagnosis was a glioma (*arrow*).

orthopedic or musculoskeletal abnormalities. Progression of signs reflective of an LMN dysfunction ultimately suggests a nervous-system origin of the problem. Pain upon direct palpation may be present, with some dogs requiring sedation or anesthesia for adequate palpation of this area. Some animals, even at seemingly adequate depths of anesthesia, will awaken quickly during palpation indicative of a painful reaction. Occasionally an obvious mass or tissue enlargement is palpated. These masses may be linear, tubular, or spherical as they course along the affected nerve.

Nerve sheath tumors may also result in a chronically painful condition. In some animals this manifests only in signs of depression and behavioral change and obvious localized pain may not be found on physical examination. Associated behavior abnormalities include aggression toward owners, unwillingness to play, and a general lethargy. These clinical signs could reflect a variety of clinical diseases and may prompt pursuit of diagnostic evaluations for systemic disease.

If the nerve roots involved are not associated with the cervical or lumbar intumescence, the animal may only have spinal pain. The limb may be positioned in a more flexed posture (nerve root signature). Clinical signs usually progress to proprioceptive impairment. Occasionally an animal will present with acute paraplegia or tetraplegia caused by spinal cord compression. This compression may result from the effects of the mass itself or from associated spinal cord pathophysiologic alterations, including edema, ischemia, infarction, or hemorrhage as a consequence of the mass. These latter abnormalities often account for the acuity of onset of clinical signs that often accompany spinal tumors. Importantly, a spinal tumor should not be overlooked as a cause of acute spinal cord dysfunction.

Clinical signs of all tumor types depend upon the level of spinal cord involvement. Tumors of the C6 to T2 segments or brachial plexus nerves may be associated with ipsilateral Horner's syndrome or ipsilateral loss of cutaneous trunci contraction. Generally, extradural and intradural extramedullary tumors result in some form of pain, whereas the intramedullary tumors may be nonpainful. If, however, the tumor causes expansion of the spinal cord resulting in stretching of nerve roots or compression of the dura, hyperesthesia may be present. The progression of clinical signs is often more chronic with the extradural tumors and more acute with the intramedullary tumors.

SPINAL TUMORS IN CATS

Cats have some different features with regards to spinal tumors.[26–30,37,45,51,52,54] Lymphosarcoma appears to be the most common tumor affecting the spinal cord followed by osteosarcoma.[29] Cats with lymphosarcoma were typically younger at initial examination, had a shorter duration of clinical signs, and had lesions in more regions of the central nervous system than did cats with other types of tumors. In 22 of 26 (84.6%) cats with lymphosarcoma, the tumor was also found in extraneural sites. Feline leukemia virus status was inconsistent. Osteosarcoma in the vertebrae of cats may act less aggressively compared with similar tumors in dogs.

DIAGNOSIS

Diagnosis of a spinal tumor is often presumptively made using survey spinal radiographs, myelography, or advanced imaging (CT and MRI).[10,55,56] Tumors of bone may be evident on survey radiographs as osteolytic/osteoproliferative processes. These bony changes need to be differentiated from diskospondylitis and vertebral bony osteomyelitis. Classically, vertebral tumors do not cross the joint space (intervertebral disk). Rarely, however, vertebral tumors invade adjacent vertebral bodies and therefore appear to "jump" the joint. Extradural compression of the spinal cord overlying the vertebral body rather than the intervertebral disk space is suspicious for neoplasia.

Soft tissue tumors are usually not apparent on survey radiographs. Nerve sheath tumors, however, may involve exiting peripheral nerves within the intervertebral foramina.[10] The foramen where the abnormal nerve is exiting may be enlarged and visible on survey radiographs.

Myelography has historically been used to outline the subarachnoid space and determine if spinal cord compression or expansion is present. However, myelography is now increasingly less used with the advent of advanced imaging, such as MRI. MRI is superior to myelography in almost all instances of spinal imaging. The principle location description of tumor categories still remains from the myelography era. In extradural tumors, one or both of the contrast columns may be shifted axial (toward the center of the spinal canal). Clues to the presence of an extradural tumor include compression of the spinal cord primarily overlying a vertebral body rather than the intervertebral disk space and annular compressive lesions of the dura. These same imaging features may also be seen with intervertebral disk disease and other spinal cord compressive diseases and therefore should not be considered pathognomonic for extradural spinal tumor.

With intradural but extramedullary tumors, spinal imaging will often result in a characteristic pattern of expansion of the subarachnoid space and outlining of the tumor in negative shadow, referred to as a *golf tee* (**Fig. 5**).[10,33,57] Nerve sheath tumors may also expand to either side of where the nerve traverses the dura, giving these tumors a dumbbell-shaped appearance. Conversely, expansion of the dural tube in 90° opposed radiographic views is indicative of an intramedullary lesion.

Advanced imaging studies, such as CT or MRI, have greatly improved the ability to determine the extent of any spinal tumor.[58] The major advantage of both CT and MRI techniques is the ability to noninvasively image structures below to the surface of the body. Advantages of CT imaging include the ability to image in planes giving a spatial orientation to abnormalities seen. Disadvantages include its use of ionizing radiation (radiation exposure) and the poor imaging of the spinal cord. Spatial resolution, especially for small animals like as cats, may not be adequate to determine small (<5 mm) lesions.

With CT, a myelogram is often necessary as part of the CT evaluation process to more accurately outline the subarachnoid space. Unfortunately, by having to perform myelography, the inherent risks to the animal from myelography are introduced into the cost/benefit of the procedure. In some instances, a series of scans are performed before and after intravenous injection of an iodinated contrast material. Abnormalities disrupting the blood-spinal cord or blood-nerve barrier may become more apparent

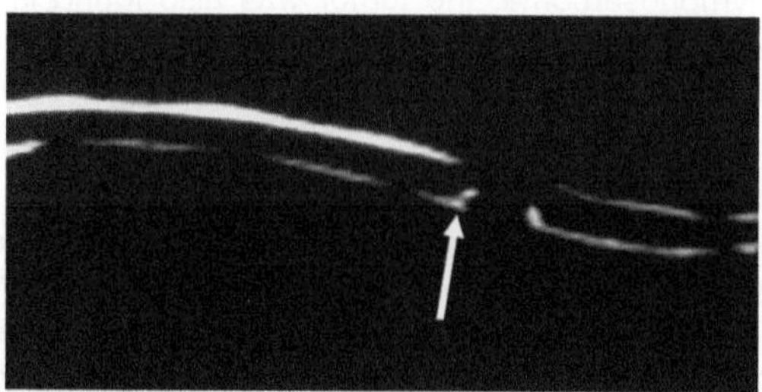

Fig. 5. Lateral, MRI myelographic view of a dog with an intradural but extramedullary lesion showing a golf-tee sign (*arrow*).

with this technique. Loss of integrity of these barriers or increased vascularity may result in an area of increased uptake (whiteness) after intravenous contrast enhancement. Contrast enhancement is most often seen with tumors, vascular abnormalities, and inflammatory foci; however, it may also be seen with intervertebral disk disease.

MRI is the imaging modality of choice for a variety of spinal lesions.[58] MRI affords superior anatomic evaluation of soft tissue structures. Similar to myelography, MRI is helpful in determining the presence of a spinal cord compressive or expansile lesion. MRI, however, is superior to all other spinal studies in delineating soft tissue components of spinal lesions.[36,59]

Most epidural tumors invade the surrounding vertebral body before impinging on the spinal cord. Thus, bony destruction of the vertebrae may be a clue to an underlying neoplastic process. In general, on T1-weighted images, vertebral bone marrow signal should be roughly equivalent to disk material. In instances of diffuse marrow involvement, the disk spaces will show greater signal intensity than the vertebral marrow.

Tumors are typically vascular and invasive, breaking the normal integrity of the blood brain barrier thus intravenous injection of a contrast agent generally results in some degree of either diffuse or focal enhancement in the area affected by tumor. Contrast enhancement does not precisely define the tumor borders; neoplastic cells are generally found outside the enhanced portion of the mass. Gadolinium administration may not be as helpful in identifying tumors that involve the vertebral bodies, because gadolinium-enhanced osseous lesions may have an appearance similar to that of normal marrow. Particular enhancing characteristics have been inconsistent various tumors.

Intradural, extramedullary tumors may result in a similar golf-tee appearance to the subarachnoid space, which is most evident on T2-weighted images. These tumors are occasionally less obvious because they may have little contrast with respect to the adjacent spinal cord. These tumors may also not be as obvious on sagittal images if they are primarily lateral to the spinal cord. Intravenous gadolinium-DTPA (Magnevist, Berlex Laboratories, Cedar Knolls, NJ, USA), enhances these tumors increasing their signal intensity on T1-weighted images. Dorsal and transverse contrast-enhanced images are helpful images to detect this category of tumors.

Intramedullary tumors generally cause the spinal cord to be expanded. On T1-weighted images, most intramedullary neoplasms have diminished signal intensity with respect to the cord. On T2-weighted images, they usually have a brighter signal than cord, which often reflects associated spinal cord edema or hemorrhage. Most tumors have a nonhomogenous signal intensity and indistinct margins between tumor and surrounding normal cord.

TREATMENT

Treatment options for spinal tumors include surgical removal and possibly radiation therapy.[36,40–42,47,60–64] Surgical removal is most often reserved for extradural tumors, however, both intradural/extramedullary and intramedullary tumors have also been successfully resected. The ultimate prognosis depends upon degree of local resection, degree of spinal infiltration, associated spinal damage before and during surgery, surgeon experiences with spinal neoplastic conditions, and tumor type.

SURGERY

Extradural tumors are removed by laminectomy, either dorsal or hemilaminectomy. Ventral slotting is inadequate for removal of most cervical tumors. Abnormal tissue is identified and removed via blunt or sharp dissection. Advanced imaging studies before surgery help in determining the extent of the tumor and involved vital structures but even with MRI the extent of the neoplastic process may be underappreciated. The surgical keys are obviously adequate lesion exposure and subsequent removal. Most surgical problems and failures result from inadequate surgical exposure. In some instances, increased bone removal necessary for tumor resection will result in a need for surgical stabilization through internal fixation. If the surgeon is not experienced in surgical spinal stabilization (if that becomes necessary) this can result in surgical failure.

For spinal tumor removal, especially with intradural or intramedullary lesions, the vertebral structure needs to be removed. Caution is used during drilling with lesions that involve the vertebrae because the consistency and strength of this bone may be compromised, which may lead to unwarranted entry of the spinal canal with the drill. Also, if the tumor involves large vascular structures, such as the vertebral artery or sinus, bleeding during resection can be significant and life threatening.

One of the most important aspects of surgical tumor removal is the surgeon's experience either visually or through touch in determining the border between tumor and normal or normal, but damaged tissue. General surgical oncologic principles are often not applicable for neurosurgical oncology. Wide surgical margins are a main tenet of surgical oncology, however, they are often an unrealistic goal when dealing with neoplasia in the vertebrae or spinal cord because of the obvious vital nature of the surrounding nervous system. With vertebral neoplasia a significant portion, if not all of a vertebral body, lamina, or pedicles, may be involved requiring extensive surgical resection.[65] Although total vertebrectomy is possible, tumor margins often extend to the edge and beyond reasonable limits of vertebral resection. If the amount of bone removal is excessive, surgical stabilization of the involved spinal segments is necessary. This stabilization can be accomplished with spinal fractures using a combination of bone screws, Steinmann pins, K-wires, and polymethylmethacrylate or other techniques.

If the tumor is located within the proximal brachial plexus or associated peripheral nerve, an approach to this area may be necessary concurrently with an approach that will afford lateral access to the cervical spinal cord.[53,66–68] In this situation, the animal is positioned in lateral recumbency with the side of the exploration facing upward. Some prefer, if a hemilaminectomy is also to be performed, to tilt the dorsal aspect of patients in a dorsolateral direction to varying degrees (20°–45°). A hemilaminectomy can also be performed with the animal in lateral recumbency. Nerve sheath tumors tend to expand intradurally and form bulbous enlargements into the spinal cord. The enlargements tract inward with the nerve rootlets and often hide underneath the spinal cord ventrally. Magnification and microdissectors and scissors are used for tumor removal.

Hemorrhage from venous sinuses is controlled by adequate removal of compressive material, absorbable gelatin sponge (Gelfoam) or similar material (autogenous muscle), or some combination of the two. Once the spinal cord is decompressed it should be visible lying flat along the floor of the vertebral canal. Gelatin sponge is placed in the bony defect. The muscles, subcutaneous tissues, and skin are routinely apposed.

RADIATION THERAPY

Conventional radiation therapy is being used with increasing frequency in dogs with spinal tumor.[60,69] Overall, however, small numbers of animals with spinal tumors have been treated. Radiation therapy is more apt to control tumor progression; however, in some instances it may eradicate the tumor completely. Significant and rapid reduction in spinal lymphoma, for example, may occur following radiation therapy. The main goal of the treatment is to administer to the tumor the highest possible dose while minimizing the dose to the surrounding normal tissue. Radiation protocols vary.[69] Fractional dosing schemes have been used to decrease the acute toxicity of the radiation. The majority of dogs treated for spinal tumors receive 38 to 48 Gy total dose administered in smaller (3–4 Gy) fractions each. These doses appeared to be generally well tolerated for the periods studied. Some of the reports indicated neurologic and pathologic change compatible with acute radiation induced necrosis. A fraction size of 3 Gy may reduce the incidence of late-responding tissue response. It is recommended, therefore, that daily fractions of 3 Gy be given with the total normal tissue dose below 50 to 55 Gy.

Side effects include radiation damage to normal structures surrounding the abnormality. Both acute, early delayed, and late delayed affects can be seen. The acute affects may be the result of edema caused by tumor kill and may be reversed with antiedema medications. The later effects may not be reversible and may be as detrimental to the animals as the underlying disease.

CHEMOTHERAPY

Chemotherapies are infrequently used for primary spinal tumors.[70] In some instances, similar chemotherapeutic agents used for appendicular osteosarcoma (cisplatin, carboplatin) are used for vertebral osteosarcoma. Spinal or perispinal lymphoma may be responsive to similar chemotherapeutic agents as for systemic lymphoma. Because of the good cerebrospinal fluid penetration of cytosine arabinoside, this drug is often added to spinal lymphoma treatment regimes.

PROGNOSIS OF ANIMALS WITH SPINAL TUMOR

There are too few large series assessing prognoses of animals with spinal tumors to make accurate treatment recommendations for affected animals. Individual animals with tumors in each of the 3 locations (extradural, intradural/extramedullary, and intramedullary) have been successfully treated with combinations of surgery or radiation therapy, but overall efficacy of specific treatments in statistically significant numbers of affected animals is not determined. Advances in microsurgical techniques have afforded the ability to successful operate tumors involving the spinal cord; however, reports of larger numbers of similarly affected animals will be required to make objective outcome conclusions. In one report of 37 dogs with a variety of spinal tumors, median survival of all dogs that survived 20 days following diagnosis was 240 days.[9] A total of 40% of these dogs, however, were euthanized or died within the first 20 days following diagnosis. These dogs were not figured into the overall survival statistics. Tumors primary involving the vertebral body may be associated with shorter survival times.

Reviews of spinal tumors and peripheral nerve sheath tumors have been reported.[9,40,41,71] Median survival in dogs with spinal tumors that had surgery varied depending upon whether the tumor was benign or malignant.[40] For nerve sheath tumors, prognosis was influenced by whether the tumor was more peripheral in location versus involving the nerve plexus or root (median survival plexus group 360 days, median survival root group 150 days).

Intramedullary tumors have historically been diagnosed at necropsy with infrequent reports of treatment. Surgical removal is occasionally successful and, with refinements in microsurgical experiences, should be used more frequently in the future following advancements in all types of primary spinal cord surgeries.

SUMMARY

Diagnosis and treatment of spinal neoplastic disease is increasingly occurring in the modern veterinary era. Most of the recent advancements in this field have resulted from (1) increased use of imaging modalities, such as MRI, which provide important anatomic information, such as tumor extent and involvement, and (2) increased surgical experiences with tumor removal in or surrounding the spinal cord. Surgery of the spine is more successful in the modern era as veterinarians better understand the limitations of the spinal cord to surgical manipulation during tumor removal. Increasing use of additional treatment modalities, such as radiation therapy, chemotherapies, and the like, will hopefully result in increased survival and quality of life for animals with spinal neoplastic disease.

REFERENCES

1. Bagley RS. Fundamentals of veterinary clinical neurology. Ames (IA): Wiley Blackwell; 1996.
2. de Lahunta A. Veterinary neuroanatomy and clinical neurology. 2nd edition. Philadelphia: WB Saunders; 1983.
3. Gilmore DR. Neoplasia of the cervical spinal cord and vertebrae in the dog. J Am Anim Hosp Assoc 1983;19:1009–14.
4. Gilmore DR. Intraspinal tumors in the dog. Comp Cont Educ Pract 1983;5:55–64.
5. Gruber A, Kneissl S, Vidoni B, et al. Cervical spinal chordoma with chondromatous component in a dog. Vet Pathol 2008;45(5):650–3.
6. Huisinga M, Henrich M, Frese K, et al. Extraventricular neurocytoma of the spinal cord in a dog. Vet Pathol 2008;45(1):63–6.
7. Levy MS, Kapatkin AS, Patnaik AK, et al. Spinal tumors in 37 dogs: clinical outcome and long-term survival (1987–1994). J Am Anim Hosp Assoc 1997;33:307–12.
8. Luttgen PJ, Braund KG, Brawner WR Jr, et al. A retrospective study of twenty-nine spinal tumours in the dogs and cat. J Soc Adm Pharm 1980;21:213–26.
9. Petersen SA, Sturges BK, Dickinson PJ, et al. Canine intraspinal meningiomas: imaging features, histopathologic classification, and long-term outcome in 34 dogs. J Vet Intern Med 2008;22(4):946–53.
10. Rizzo SA, Newman SJ, Hecht S, et al. Malignant mediastinal extra-adrenal paraganglioma with spinal cord invasion in a dog. J Vet Diagn Invest 2008;20(3):372–5.
11. Ródenas S, Pumarola M, Añor S. Imaging diagnosis–cervical spine chondroma in a dog. Vet Radiol Ultrasound 2008;49(5):464–6.
12. Summers BA, Cummings JF, de Lahunta A. Veterinary neuropathology. St. Louis (MO): Mosby; 1995.
13. Wright JA. The pathological features associated with spinal tumours in 29 dogs. J Comp Pathol 1985;95:549–57.
14. Wells MY, Weisbrode SE. Vascular malformations in the thoracic vertebrae of three cats. Vet Pathol 1987;24:360–1.
15. Zaki FA, Prata RG, Hurvitz AI, et al. Primary tumors of the spinal cord and meninges in six dogs. J Am Vet Med Assoc 1975;166:511–7.
16. Bentley JF, Simpson ST, Hathcock JT, et al. Metastatic thyroid solid-follicular carcinoma of the cervical portion of the spine of a dog. J Am Vet Med Assoc 1990;197:1498–500.
17. Byrne TN. Spinal cord compression from epidural metastasis. N Engl J Med 1992;327:614.
18. Cooley DM, Waters DJ. Skeletal metastasis as the initial clinical manifestation of metastatic carcinoma in 19 dogs. J Vet Intern Med 1998;12:288–93.

19. Jeffery ND, Phillips SM. Surgical treatment of intramedullary spinal cord neoplasia in two dogs. J Soc Adm Pharm 1995;36:553–7.
20. Macpherson GC, Chadwick BJ, Robbins PD. Intramedullary spinal cord metastasis of a primary lung tumour in a dog. J Soc Adm Pharm 1993;34:242–6.
21. Platt SR, Sheppard BJ, Graham J, et al. Pheochromocytoma in the vertebral canal of two dogs. J Am Anim Hosp Assoc 1998;34:365–71.
22. Uchida K, Morozumi M, Yamaguchi R, et al. Diffuse leptomeningeal malignant histiocytosis in the brain and spinal cord of a Tibetan Terrier. Vet Pathol 2001; 38:219–22.
23. Van Ham L, van Bree H, Maenhout T, et al. Metastatic pilomatrixoma presenting as paraplegia in a dog. J Soc Adm Pharm 1991;32:27–30.
24. Waters DJ, Hayden DW. Intramedullary spinal cord metastasis in the dog. J Vet Intern Med 1990;4:207–15.
25. Woo GH, Bak EJ, Lee YW, et al. Cervical chondroid chordoma in a Shetland sheep dog. J Comp Pathol 2008;138(4):218–23.
26. Lane SB, Kornegay JN. Spinal lymphosarcoma. In: August JR, editor. Consultations in feline internal medicine. Philadelphia: WB Saunders; 1991. p. 487.
27. Marioni-Henry K, Van Winkle TJ, Smith SH, et al. Tumors affecting the spinal cord of cats: 85 cases (1980–2005). J Am Vet Med Assoc 2008;232(2):237.
28. Suess RP Jr, Martin RA, Shell LG, et al. Vertebral lymphosarcoma in a cat. J Am Vet Med Assoc 1990;197:101.
29. Aloisio F, Levine JM, Edwards JF. Immunohistochemical features of a feline spinal cord gemistocytic astrocytoma. J Vet Diagn Invest 2008;20(6):836–8.
30. Appel SL, Moens NM, Abrams-Ogg AC, et al. Multiple myeloma with central nervous system involvement in a cat. J Am Vet Med Assoc 2008;233(5):743–7.
31. Marks SL, Bellah JR, Wells M. Resolution of quadriparesis caused by cervical tumoral calcinosis in a dog. J Am Anim Hosp Assoc 1991;27:72–6.
32. Reif U, Lowrie CT, Fitzgerald SD. Extradural spinal angiolipoma associated with bone lysis in a dog. J Am Anim Hosp Assoc 1998;34:373–6.
33. Wright JA, Bell DA, Clayton-Jones DG. The clinical and radiological features associated with spinal tumours in thirty dogs. J Soc Adm Pharm 1979;20:461–72.
34. Banks WC, Bridges CH. Multiple cartilaginous exostoses in a dog. J Am Vet Med Assoc 1956;110:156.
35. Chester DK. Multiple cartilaginous exostoses in two generations of dogs. J Am Vet Med Assoc 1971;159:895.
36. Gavin PG, Bagley RS. Practical small animal MRI. Ames (IA): Wiley Blackwell; 2009.
37. Pool RR, Carrig CB. Multiple cartilaginous exostoses in a cat. Vet Pathol 1972;9: 350–9.
38. Doige CE, Pharr JW, Withrow SJ. Chondrosarcoma arising in multiple cartilaginous exostoses in a dog. J Am Anim Hosp Assoc 1978;14:605–11.
39. Owen LN, Bostock DE. Multiple cartilaginous exostoses with development of a metastasizing osteosarcoma in a Shetland sheepdog. J Soc Adm Pharm 1971;12:507–12.
40. Brehm DM, Vite CH, Steinberg HS, et al. A retrospective evaluation of 51 cases of peripheral nerve sheath tumors in the dog. J Am Anim Hosp Assoc 1995;31:349–59.
41. Bradley RL, Withrow SJ, Snyder SP. Nerve sheath tumors in the dog. J Am Anim Hosp Assoc 1982;18:915–21.
42. Fingeroth JM, Prata RG, Patnaik AK. Spinal meningiomas in dogs: 13 cases (1972–1987). J Am Vet Med Assoc 1987;191:720.
43. Raskin RE. An atypical spinal meningioma in a dog. Vet Pathol 1984;27:538–40.

44. Targett MP, Dyce J, Houlton JEF. Tumours involving the nerve sheaths of the forelimb in dogs. J Small Anim Pract 1993;34:221.
45. Yoshioka MM. Meningioma of the spinal cord in a cat. Comp Cont Educ Pract 1987;9:34–8.
46. Blass CE, Kirby BM, Kreeger JM, et al. Teratomatous medulloepithelioma in the spinal cord of a dog. J Am Anim Hosp Assoc 1988;24:51–4.
47. Ferretti A, Scanziani E, Colombo S. Surgical treatment of a spinal cord tumor resembling nephroblastoma in a young dog. Prog Vet Neurol 1993;4:84–7.
48. Moissonnier P, Abbott DP. Canine neuroepithelioma: case report and literature review. J Am Anim Hosp Assoc 1993;29:397–401.
49. Summers BA, deLahunta A, McEntee M, et al. A novel intradural extramedullary spinal cord tumor in young dogs. Acta Neuropathol 1988;75:402–10.
50. De Vries-Chalmers Hoynk van Paperdrecht HR, Vos JH, van Nes JJ. Spinal cord ependymoma in two young dogs. Vet Q 1988;10:205–10.
51. Morita T, Kondo H, Okamoto M, et al. Periventricular spread of primary central nervous system T-cell lymphoma in a cat. J Comp Pathol 2009;140(1):54–8.
52. Shell L, Dallman M, Sponenburg P. Chondrosarcoma in a cat presenting with forelimb monoparalysis. Comp Cont Educ Pract 1987;9:391–7.
53. Steinberg HS. Brachial plexus injuries and dysfunction. Vet Clin North Am 1988;18:565–80.
54. Flatland B, Fry MM, Newman SJ, et al. Large anaplastic spinal B-cell lymphoma in a cat. Vet Clin Pathol 2008;37(4):389–96, 3.
55. McCarthy RJ, Feeney DA, Lipowitz AJ. Preoperative diagnosis of tumors of the brachial plexus by use of computed tomography in three dogs. J Am Vet Med Assoc 1993;202:291–4.
56. Morgan JP, Ackerman N, Bailey CS, et al. Vertebral tumors in the dog: a clinical radiologic and pathologic study of 61 primary and secondary lesions. Vet Radiol Ultrasound 1980;21:197–212.
57. Bagley RS, Tucker RL. Specialty Board Review, neuroradiology. Prog Vet Neurol 1996;7:62.
58. Gambardella PC, Osborne CA, Stevens JB, et al. Multiple cartilaginous exostoses in the dog. J Am Vet Med Assoc 1975;166:761.
59. Kippenes H, Gavin PR, Bagley RS, et al. Magnetic resonance imaging features of tumors of the spine and spinal cord. Vet Radiol Ultrasound 1999;40:627–33.
60. Bailey CS. Long-term survival after surgical excision of a schwannoma of the sixth cervical spinal nerve in a dog. J Am Vet Med Assoc 1990;196:754.
61. Bell FW, Fenney DA, O'Brien TJ, et al. External beam radiation therapy for recurrent intraspinal meningioma in a dog. J Am Anim Hosp Assoc 1992;28:318–22.
62. Dernell WS, Van Vechten BJ, Straw RC, et al. Outcome following treatment of vertebral tumors in 20 dogs (1986–1995). J Am Anim Hosp Assoc 2000;36:245–51.
63. Jeffery ND. Treatment of epidural haemangiosarcoma in a dog. J Small Animal Practice 1991;32:359–62.
64. Parker AJ, Park RD. Successful removal of a spinal cord tumor. Canine Pract 1974;1:35–7.
65. Yturraspe DJ, Lumb WV, Young S, et al. Neurologic and pathological effects of second lumbar spondylectomy and spinal column shortening in the dog. J Neurosurg 1975;42:47–58.
66. Lipsitz D, Bailey CS. Lateral approach for cervical spinal cord decompression. Prog Vet Neurol 1992;3:39–44.

67. Piermattei DL, Greely RG. An atlas of surgical approaches to the bones of the dog and cat. 4th edition. Philadelphia: WB Saunders; 2004.
68. Sharp NJH. Craniolateral approach to the canine brachial plexus. Vet Surg 1988; 17:18–21.
69. Powers BE, Beck ER, Gillette EL, et al. Pathology of radiation injury to the canine spinal cord. Int J Radiat Oncol Biol Phys 1992;23:539–49.
70. Clemmons RM, Gorman NT, Calderwood Mays MB. Lumbar epidural chondrosarcoma in a dog treated by excision and chemotherapy. J Am Vet Med Assoc 1983; 183:1006–7.
71. Seppälä MT, Haltia MJJ, Sankila RJ, et al. Long-term outcome after removal of spinal schwannoma: a clinicopathological study of 187 cases. J Neurosurg 1995;83:621.

Canine Degenerative Myelopathy

Joan R. Coates, DVM, MS*, Fred A. Wininger, VMD, MS

KEYWORDS

- Dog • Spinal cord • Amyotrophic lateral sclerosis
- Axonopathy • Neurodegeneration • Superoxide dismutase 1
- Genome-wide association mapping • Degenerative myelopathy

Canine degenerative myelopathy (DM) was first described in 1973 by Averill[1] as an insidious, progressive, general proprioceptive (GP) ataxia and upper motor neuron (UMN) spastic paresis of the pelvic limbs beginning in late adulthood, ultimately leading to paraplegia and necessitating euthanasia. Until recently, presence of primary axonal degeneration and nerve fiber loss that was restricted to spinal cord white matter and most severe in the mid to caudal thoracic region was compatible with a diagnosis of DM. The disease was termed "degenerative myelopathy" because of its histopathologic nature as a nonspecific degeneration of spinal cord tissue of undetermined cause. In 1975, Griffiths and Duncan[2] published a series of cases with similar clinical signs and histologic changes in the white matter; they also reported hyporeflexia and nerve root involvement, and termed the condition chronic degenerative radiculomyelopathy. Although most of the dogs in these initial reports were German Shepherd dogs (GSD), other breeds were represented. Nonetheless, for many years DM was considered a UMN and GP disease in the GSD.[3] More recently DM has been recognized as a common problem in several breeds, with an overall prevalence of 0.19%.[4] In addition, the clinical spectrum of DM has been broadened to involve both the UMN and lower motor neuron (LMN) systems.[5] This article reviews the current knowledge of canine DM with regard to its signalment, clinical spectrum, diagnostic approach, histopathology, and treatment. A recent advance in the molecular genetics of DM indicates that this canine disease may share pathogenic mechanisms with some forms of human amyotrophic lateral sclerosis (ALS or Lou Gehrig disease).[5] The implications of this finding on both diseases are also discussed.

SIGNALMENT

There is no sex predilection. Age of onset of neurologic signs is usually 5 years or older, with a mean age of 9 years in large dog breeds with DM.[1,2,6,7] Most dogs are

This work was supported by Grant Numbers 2220, 821, 1212, and 1213 from the AKC Canine Health Foundation, and participating breed clubs and foundations.
Department of Veterinary Medicine and Surgery, College of Veterinary Medicine, University of Missouri, 900 East Campus Drive, Clydesdale Hall, Columbia, MO 65211, USA
* Corresponding author.
E-mail address: coatesj@missouri.edu

Vet Clin Small Anim 40 (2010) 929–950
doi:10.1016/j.cvsm.2010.05.001 **vetsmall.theclinics.com**
0195-5616/10/$ – see front matter

at least 8 years of age at onset of clinical signs. A study in Pembroke Welsh Corgis (PWC) reported a mean age of onset of 11 years.[4] Histopathologically confirmed cases of DM have been reported in the following dog breeds: GSD,[1–3,5,6] Siberian Husky,[8] Miniature Poodle,[9] Boxer,[5,10] PWC,[4,11] Chesapeake Bay Retriever,[5,12] Rhodesian Ridgeback,[5] and mixed breed.[1] Other previously reported breeds presumptively diagnosed without histopathologic confirmation include the Irish Terrier,[2] Kerry Blue Terrier,[2] Labrador Retriever,[7] Bernese Mountain dog,[7] Hovawart,[7] Kuvasz,[7] Collie,[7] Belgian Shepherd,[7] Giant Schnauzer,[7] Soft-coated Wheaten Terrier,[7] Mastiff,[7] Borzoi,[7]and Great Dane.[13] As part of their ongoing studies, the authors have been able to histopathologically confirm DM in the Bernese Mountain Dog, Standard Poodle, Kerry Blue Terrier, Cardigan Welsh Corgi, Golden Retriever, Wire Fox Terrier, American Eskimo dog, Soft-coated Wheaten Terrier, and Pug.

CLINICAL SPECTRUM

Progressive, asymmetric UMN paraparesis, pelvic limb GP ataxia, and lack of paraspinal hyperesthesia are key clinical features of DM. The original clinical descriptions of DM were from the GSD and other large dog breeds that are euthanized early in the course of the disease.[1–3] The predominant clinical signs in dogs of these earlier reports were UMN spastic paraparesis and pelvic limb GP ataxia with a T3 to L3 neuroanatomic localization. With longer disease duration, clinical signs will progress to LMN paralysis in the pelvic limbs and eventually affect the thoracic limbs.[1,4,5,7,9] This scenario has been described in a Miniature Poodle and the PWCs.[4,5,9]

The clinical course of DM can vary after the presumptive diagnosis, with a mean time for disease duration of 6 months in larger dog breeds (**Fig. 1**).[1,3,6] Most large dogs progress to nonambulatory paraparesis within 6 to 9 months from onset of clinical signs. Pet owners usually elect euthanasia when the dogs can no longer support weight in their pelvic limbs and need walking assistance. Smaller dog breeds can be cared for by the pet owner over a longer time.[4,9] The median disease duration in the PWC was 19 months.[4] The PWCs often have signs of thoracic limb paresis at the time of euthanasia.

Early Disease

The earliest clinical signs of DM are GP ataxia and mild spastic paresis in the pelvic limbs (**Fig. 2**). Worn nails and the appearance of asymmetric pelvic limb lameness can be seen on physical examination. Asymmetry of signs at disease onset is frequently reported.[1,4,7,9] At disease onset, spinal reflex abnormalities are consistent with UMN paresis localized in the T3 to L3 spinal cord segments.[1] Patellar reflexes may be normal or exaggerated to clonic; however, hyporeflexia of the patellar reflex has also been described in dogs at similar disease stage.[2] Involvement of the dorsal roots of the femoral nerve may inhibit sensory impulses from stretch receptors located in the quadriceps muscle. Patellar hyporeflexia in older dogs has also been associated with a normal age-dependent decline in patellar reflex magnitude.[14] Flexor (withdrawal) reflexes may also be normal or show crossed extension (suggestive of chronic UMN dysfunction). Often, dogs progress to nonambulatory paraparesis and are euthanized during this disease stage.

Late Disease

If the dog is not euthanized early, clinical signs will progress to LMN paraplegia and ascend to affect the thoracic limbs (**Fig. 2**).[1,4,7,9] Flaccid tetraplegia occurs in dogs

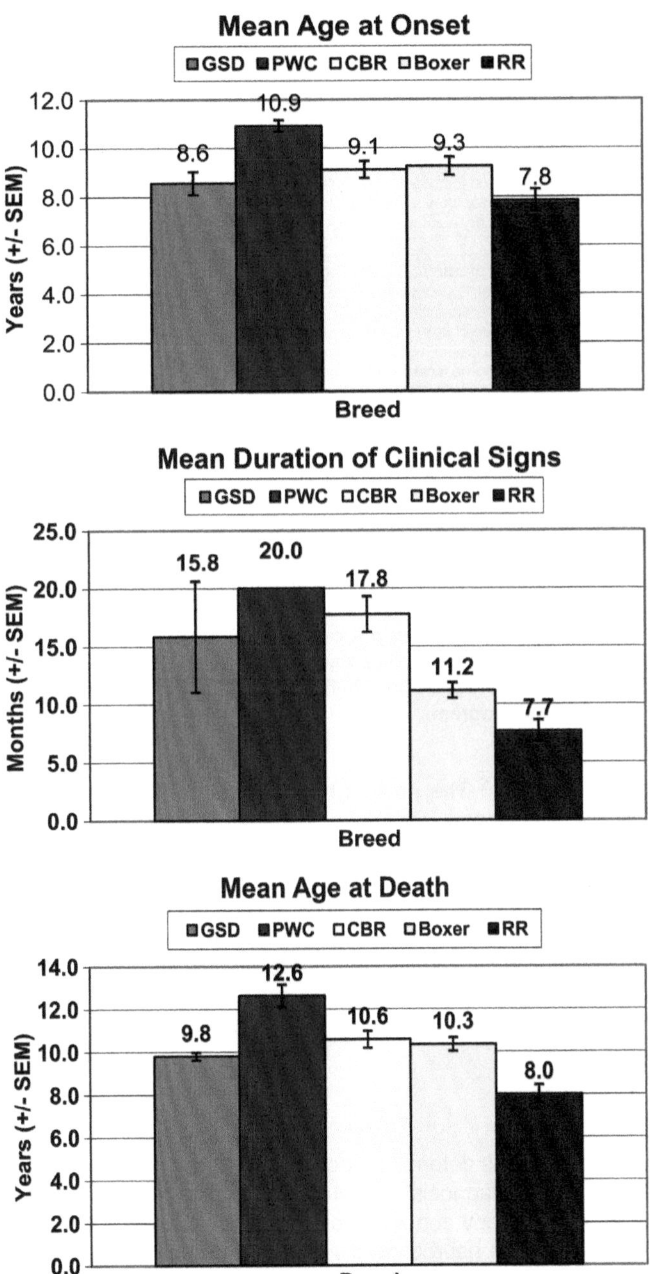

Fig. 1. Mean age at disease onset, mean disease duration, and mean age at death for degenerative myelopathy (DM) affected German Shepherd dog (GSD), Pembroke Welsh Corgi (PWC), Chesapeake Bay Retriever (CBR), Boxer, and Rhodesian Ridgeback (RR).

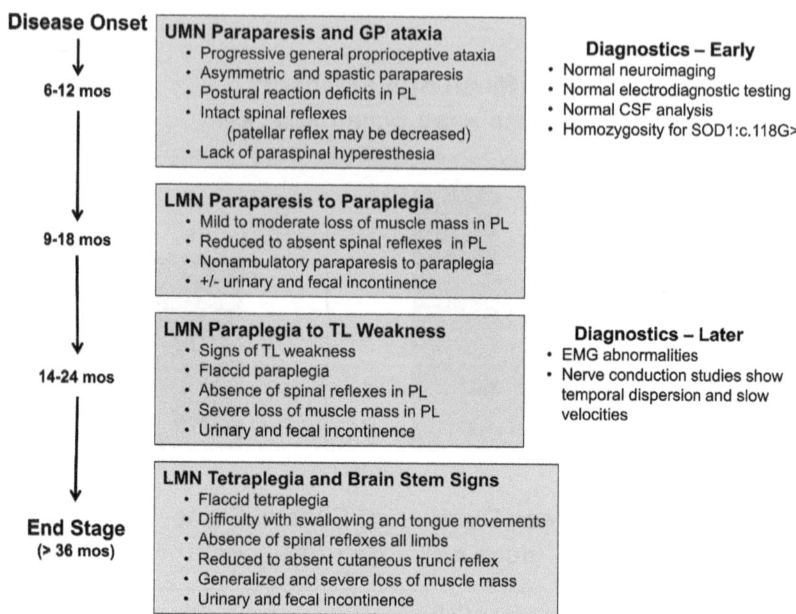

Fig. 2. Classification scheme of clinical signs for *SOD1*-associated canine DM. Dogs with DM follow a pattern of clinical signs, which initially begins with upper motor neuron (UMN) pelvic limb (PL) paresis and general proprioceptive (GP) ataxia to progress to lower motor neuron (LMN) weakness and then involve the thoracic limbs (TL). Smaller breeds with DM may have a slower disease progression when compared with larger breeds. CSF, cerebrospinal fluid; EMG, electromyogram.

with advanced disease.[4,5,9] The paresis becomes more symmetric as the disease progresses.

LMN signs emerge as hyporeflexia of the patellar and withdrawal reflexes, flaccid paralysis, and widespread muscle atrophy beginning in the pelvic limbs as the dogs become nonambulatory.[5,9] Widespread and severe loss of muscle mass occurs in the appendicular muscles in the late stage of DM. Most reports attributed loss of muscle mass to disuse[1,2,4,8,9] but flaccidity in dogs with protracted disease suggests denervation.[5,8,9] Cranial nerve signs include swallowing difficulties and inability to bark.[4,5,9] Urinary and fecal continence usually are spared also until the latter disease stage with paraplegia.[1,4,7,8]

DIFFERENTIAL DIAGNOSIS

Definitive diagnosis of DM is determined post mortem by histopathologic examination of the spinal cord. The diagnosis of DM can be challenging because the clinical presentation can mimic many acquired spinal cord diseases. Older dogs often have concurrent orthopedic and neurologic disease that can confound the interpretation of the neurologic examination.[15] Disorders that often mimic and coexist with DM include degenerative lumbosacral syndrome, intervertebral disc disease, spinal cord neoplasia, and degenerative joint diseases such as hip dysplasia or cranial cruciate ligament rupture.[16] The PWC is a chondrodystrophic breed and is prone to Hansen type I intervertebral disc disease. Hansen type II intervertebral disc disease can be an incidental or clinically significant finding more common in the older large, nonchondrodystrophic breeds.[17] Pelvic limb dysfunction can present prior to thoracic limb paresis in cervical spinal cord disease (eg, caudal cervical spondylomyelopathy), and in generalized neuromuscular diseases. Paw replacement (proprioceptive positioning) is a very useful test that distinguishes between orthopedic and neurologic diseases because it does not require weight bearing. Animals with orthopedic disease will not have paw replacement deficits.

Descriptions of the other degenerative spinal cord disorders of dogs are beyond the scope of this review, and the reader is referred to other articles for further discussions.[18] These disorders differ in anatomic distribution, clinical signs and age of onset. Their signalment often indicates a breed predisposition that may have an inherited basis. Definitive diagnosis of these diseases is usually determined by histopathology of the central nervous system (CNS) and peripheral nervous system.

HISTOPATHOLOGY

DM has been described as primary central axonopathy restricted to the spinal cord.[1,3] Axon and myelin degeneration of the spinal cord occurs in all funiculi and involves the somatic sensory, GP sensory, and motor tracts in the absence of observable neuronal cell body degeneration or loss. Hence the lesion description is best denoted as a segmental degeneration of the axon and associated myelin rather than Wallerian degeneration.[18] In the purest sense, Wallerian degeneration is defined as fragmentation and dissolution of the part of the axon distal to the primary injury of the axon, and active digestion and removal of the collapsed myelin by macrophages.[18] The pathology of DM involves segments of the axons within the various tracts that would be consistent with either a defect in cells supporting axon maintenance (astrocytes and/or oligodendrocytes) or defects in both anterograde and retrograde axoplasmic transport.[11] However, the paucity of spheroids does not support DM to be categorized as a neuroaxonal dystrophy. Neuroaxonal dystrophies can be histopathologically distinguished from other diseases by presence of spheroids (swellings) that involve distal or preterminal parts of the axon and are found in gray matter with proximity to the neuronal cell bodies.[19,20]

The recent discovery of a mutation in the superoxide dismutase 1 (*SOD1*) gene in affected dogs has provided a better understanding of the clinical spectrum for DM, which is more akin to ALS or Lou Gehrig disease.[5] Common pathologies shared amongst the types of ALS in humans include aggregation of misfolded protein, motor neuron loss, altered RNA metabolism, and abnormalities of axonal transport.[21,22] Motor neuronopathies are characterized by degeneration and loss of the somatic motor (LMN) neuronal cell body and its axon in the brainstem and spinal cord.[18,23] Inherited forms of motor neuron disease closely related to spinal muscular atrophy have been described for dogs.[23] However, to date no light microscopic lesions have been identified in these neurons in dogs with DM. Neuronopathy is also part of the pathologic spectrum for multisystem degeneration disorders that also exhibit axonopathy throughout the CNS and may include neuropathy. Because ALS affects the UMN and LMN systems, this has led to further clinical studies of the peripheral nervous system in DM-affected dogs.[5] Canine DM may be most accurately classified as a multisystem central and peripheral axonopathy. Studies are underway to further describe the neuronal cell body, nerve root, and spinal nerve pathology associated with DM.

Spinal Cord Pathology

In general, the spinal cord pathology of DM is consistent with a noninflammatory axonal degeneration (**Fig. 3**).[1–3] Dogs with DM have characteristic patterns of axon

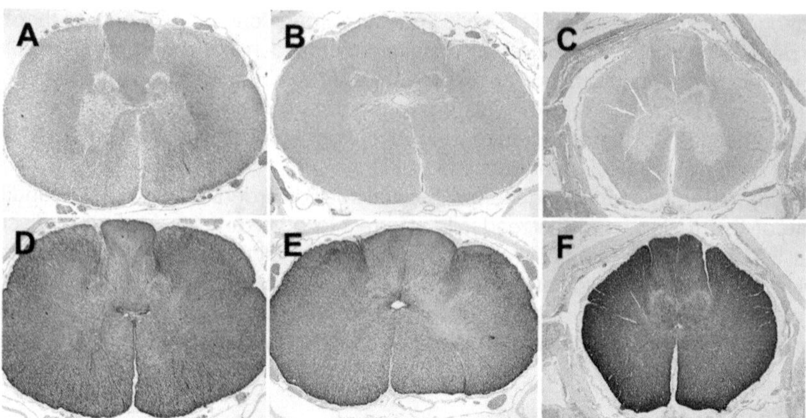

Fig. 3. Histopathology of the thoracic spinal cord. Comparison of Luxol fast blue with a periodic acid-Schiff couterstain (LFB/PAS) staining (*A–C*) and immunohistochemistry detecting glial fibrillary acidic protein (*D–F*) from a normal unaffected 14.5-year-old Pembroke Welsh Corgi (PWC) (*A, D*), a 10-year-old PWC with clinical signs of DM for 6 months and mild paraparesis and pelvic limb ataxia (*B, E*), and a 14-year-old PWC with clinical signs of DM for 48 months and flaccid tetraplegia (*C, F*). Myelin loss in the white matter is depicted by loss of blue color with LFB (*B, C*). Note the severity of pallor in the white matter and increased areas of astrogliosis in the PWC with longer disease duration. (*Courtesy of* Gayle C. Johnson, DVM, PhD, Columbia, MO.)

cylinder vacuolization and dropout. Regional axonal loss is severe in many DM-affected dogs with complete loss of axonal and myelin profiles and replacement by large areas of astrogliosis.[1,2,6,11] Macrophages can be occasionally identified around areas of axonal and myelin debris.[1,11] March and colleagues[11] showed that CD18-positive macrophages were moderately increased where lesion severity was pronounced in DM-affected dogs. The presence of macrophages was presumed to be a secondary response of the neurodegenerative process involving fragmentation and phagocytosis of axonal and myelin debris. Another study provided immunohistochemical evidence for immunoglobulin and complement deposition in the spinal cord of DM dogs, but control dogs were lacking.[24] By contrast, there is absence of T and B lymphocytes and minimal to absence of immunoreactivity for the complement component C3 in spinal cords of DM-affected PWCs.[11] Lesion distribution involves the spinal cord myelin and axons in all funiculi but affects the mid to caudal thoracic region most extensively.[1–3,11]

The longitudinal distribution of the lesions appears to vary as the disease progresses. Longitudinal lesion distribution in GSDs was described as being discontinuous, with multifocal areas of fibers showing myelin loss and axonal degeneration.[3,6] In the PWC, the overall distribution of white matter lesions is similar.[11] In contrast to the large dog breeds, PWCs and smaller dogs are often maintained longer with DM and have longitudinally continuous lesions within more clearly defined funicular areas.[9,11] The transverse and longitudinal extent of spinal cord lesions also parallel the more severe neurologic deficits found in the PWC as compared with large dog breeds with DM.[11] The more severely affected dogs show significantly greater axonal degeneration and loss in the thoracic spinal cord segments, and progression to the cervical and lumbar spinal cord.[11] Averill[1] suggested that neuronal vulnerability in the thoracic spinal cord may contribute to the pathogenesis of DM. The putative increased vulnerability may be caused by decreased perfusion from radicular arteries, which are smaller in diameter in the thoracic spinal cord than those in other spinal cord regions.[25] This paucity of vessels creates a "watershed" effect that may predispose neural tissue to ischemic processes associated with oxidative stress and excitotoxicity. Nonetheless, lesion variability between and within breeds affected by DM raises the possibility of whether there are different phenotypic variants of DM.[11]

There was tendency for increased lesion severity within the dorsal portion of the lateral funiculus involving the peripheral and deeper white matter tracts[1–3,11] and in the dorsal funiculus in some dogs.[1,11] The area in the dorsal portion of the lateral funiculus comprises the ascending dorsal spinocerebellar and descending rubrospinal, medullary reticulospinal, and lateral corticospinal tracts (**Fig. 4**). The dorsal spinocerebellar tract relays information to the cerebellum from the spinal ganglia of the spinal nerves serving the muscle spindles of the pelvic limbs.[26] Lesions in the dorsal funiculus tend to localize medially within the fasciculus gracilis.[1,2,11] Impulses from the thoracic and pelvic regions related to conscious perception for touch, pressure, and joint proprioception are transmitted through the fasciculus cuneatus (for thoracic limbs) and gracilis (for pelvic limbs) within the dorsal funiculus (see **Fig. 4**). These fibers ascend and synapse in the nucleus gracilis or cuneatus in the medulla. Involvement of the dorsal funiculi caudal to L3 also suggests involvement of not only the fasciculus gracilis but also the unconscious proprioceptive fibers ascending to Clarke's column (nucleus thoracicus–nucleus of the dorsal spinocerebellar tract) located in the base of the dorsal funiculus between the T3 and L3 spinal cord segments (see **Fig. 4**).[26,27] Other proprioceptive and motor tracts are variably affected in the cervical, thoracic, and lumbar regions.

Lesions in the ascending and descending pathways within the dorsal portion of the lateral funiculus and the ascending pathways within the dorsal funiculus would explain the loss of general proprioception and paraparesis (see **Figs. 3** and **4**). The spread of lesions in the ascending GP pathways and the descending UMN pathways to the cranial thoracic and cervical spinal cord explains the clinical progression to

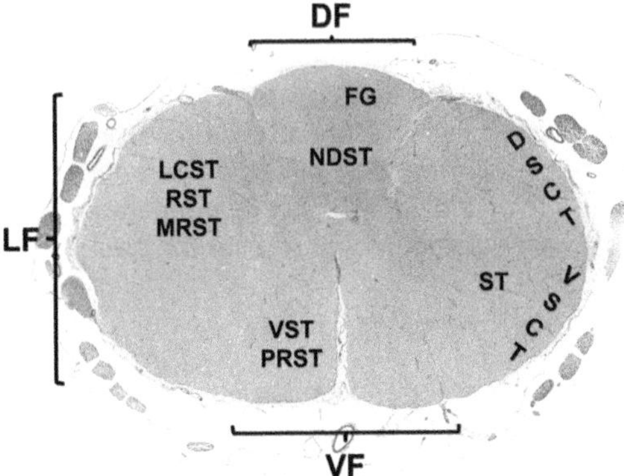

Fig. 4. Luxol fast blue stain of a transverse section of a normal mid-thoracic spinal cord labeled for the white matter regions (DF, dorsal funiculus; LF, lateral funiculus; VF, ventral funiculus), containing the ascending (FG, fasciculus gracilis; DSCT, dorsal spinocerebellar tract; VSCT, ventral spinocerebellar tract; ST, spinothalamic tract; NDST, nucleus of the dorsal spinocerebellar tract) fibers and descending (LCST, lateral corticospinal tract; RST, rubrospinal tract; MRST, medullary reticulospinal tract; VST, vestibulospinal tract; PRST, pontine reticulospinal tract) UMN pathways.

tetraparesis and ataxia. Fecal and urinary incontinence in some dogs may be associated with lesions in the dorsal funiculus of the thoracolumbar and lumbosacral spinal cord, which comprise the sensory pathways signaling colorectal and urinary bladder distension.[26,28] Disruption in these pathways may also contribute to a lack of visceral sensory feedback to the brain centers, resulting in loss of recognition of rectal and/or bladder distension and eventual involuntary evacuation of feces or urine. However, clinical observation of the urinary incontinence may also reflect an LMN abnormality in the micturition pathway. Further studies of the sacral segments and nerve roots need to be pursued.

Brain Pathology

Characterization of the brain pathology of DM-affected dogs has been limited. Johnston and colleagues[6] described abnormalities in the red nucleus and lateral vestibular nucleus of the brainstem, and in the lateral (dentate) and fastigial nucleus of the cerebellum. Others who examined brains from DM-affected dogs by light microscopy did not find lesions in the brain.[1,3,11]

Nerve and Muscle Pathology

With DM, the nerve pathology and LMN signs do not become evident until later in the disease progression. Chromatolysis has been reported in the intermediate gray matter,[6] but motor neuron loss has not been recognized as a pathologic feature of canine DM.[1,11] Although the neuronal population in the ventral horn neurons appears normal, quantitative changes may have gone undetected as neuronal morphometry has not been reported. When examined, nerves have been described as normal or exhibiting sporadic axonal loss.[1,11] Griffiths and Duncan[2] described pathologic changes in the dorsal roots.

A recent study documented neuromuscular pathology in DM-affected dogs manifesting LMN signs.[5] Nerve specimens showed nerve fiber loss resulting from axonal degeneration, endoneurial fibrosis, numerous inappropriately thinly myelinated fibers, and secondary demyelination (**Fig. 5**).[5] Preliminary studies of the common fibular (peroneal) nerve showed that these changes vary in severity according to the disease stage with more severe changes later in the disease course.[29] Nonetheless, nerve pathology of DM-affected dogs must be distinguished from normal age-related ballooning and segmental demyelination with remyelination.[30]

Muscle specimens from dogs with advanced DM show excessive variability in myofiber size, with large and small groups of atrophic fibers typical of denervation (see **Fig. 5**). Myofiber-type grouping indicative of nerve regeneration may vary with disease chronicity and possibly with genetic background or the size of the dog.[29]

PATHOGENESIS OF DEGENERATIVE MYELOPATHY

Many past investigators have sought to understand pathophysiologic mechanisms underlying DM. The pattern of concurrent axonal and myelin degeneration of the spinal cord with presence of a macrophage response is similar to that found in Wallerian type degeneration.[1,11] Although Wallerian degeneration has been described in the dorsal roots,[2] the topography of the spinal cord lesion does not support Wallerian degeneration. Griffiths and Duncan[2] suggested a toxic etiology and hypothesized that DM is a "dying-back disease" confined to the CNS based on degeneration of the lateral corticospinal tract. The degenerative process in dying-back disease first occurs in the distal portion of the longest and largest diameter fibers with gradual degeneration toward the cell body.[31] It has been established that in many dying-back neuropathies

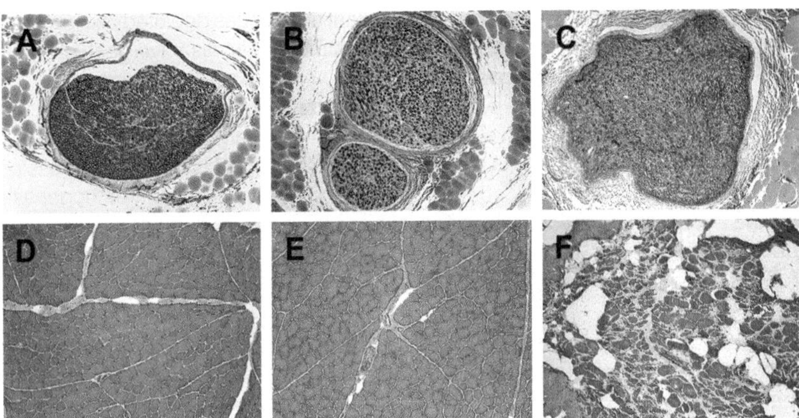

Fig. 5. Peripheral nerve and skeletal muscle histopathology in an aged normal unaffected Boxer (*A, D*), an 11-year-old Boxer with clinical signs of DM for 12 months and nonambulatory paraparesis (*B, E*), and a 10-year-old Boxer with clinical signs for 36 months and flaccid tetraplegia (*C, F*). (*A–C*) Toluidine blue stained resin embedded sections of the fibular (peroneal) nerve. Note the myelinated fiber loss, endoneurial fibrosis, and secondary demyelination in the Boxer with longer disease duration. (*D–F*) Hematoxylin and eosin–stained paraffin sections of the gastrocnemius muscle. Note the mild evidence of fiber atrophy in the less severely affected Boxer (*E*) compared with the excessive variability in myofiber size with large and small groups of atrophic fibers, and myofiber loss and fibrosis consistent with end-stage denervation in the severely affected Boxer (*F*) (original magnification ×100). (*Courtesy of* G. Diane Shelton, DVM, PhD, San Diego, CA.)

that there is combined central and peripheral nervous system involvement, constituting a central-peripheral distal axonopathy.[32] Braund and Vandevelde[3] refuted this hypothesis based on morphometric data in DM-affected GSDs showing that the lesions were discontinuous, not restricted to specific tracts, and not bilaterally symmetric. Moreover, this distal-to-proximal pattern may explain the involvement of the UMN tracts of the motor systems, but does not explain the lesions in the axons of the proprioceptive pathways in the thoracic spinal cord and the paucity of lesions of these pathways in their distal fiber terminations in the brainstem and cerebellum.[11] Later studies by Johnston and colleagues[6] on the brainstem of DM-affected dogs have shown neuronal degeneration and loss. In addition, astrogliosis was found in the dorsal horn region that gives rise to the dorsal spinocerebellar tracts.[6] These investigators hypothesized that DM might result from a defect in the neuronal cell body that leads to an axon transport defect, as has also been proposed for ALS. However, light microscopic lesions in the neurons of the brainstem have not been detected by others.[1,11]

Immunologic,[24,33,34] metabolic or nutritional,[35–40] oxidative stress,[4] excitotoxic,[41] and genetic mechanisms have been explored as underlying the pathogenesis of DM. A role for the immune system in the pathogenesis for degenerative myelopathy in GSDs has been based on observations by Waxman and colleagues[33] of depressed responses to thymus-dependent mitogens and increased concentrations of circulating immune complexes.[34] These investigators hypothesized that immune-mediated events lead to chronic demyelinating disease similar to multiple sclerosis or experimental allergic encephalomyelitis.[33] The role of neuroinflammation in the pathophysiology of DM needs continued exploration because of its importance in the pathogenesis of ALS and other neurodegenerative diseases.[42]

Vitamin E (α-tocopherol) functions as an antioxidant and tissues depleted of α-tocopherol are susceptible to free radical damage. Low vitamin E blood levels have been associated with degenerative myeloencephalopathy and motor neuron disease in horses.[43–45] Other studies in DM-affected GSDs, however, have reported no significant differences in serum vitamin E levels and expression levels of the α-tocopherol transfer protein mRNA.[38,39,46] Furthermore, supplementation with vitamin E does not affect disease progression in DM-affected dogs.[39] Discussion of other underlying mechanisms of pathogenesis is beyond the scope of this article, which focuses more on recent findings on the genetics of the disease.

Genetics

The uniformity of clinical signs, histopathology, age, and breed predilections suggest an inherited basis for DM; however, the late onset of disease has made it difficult to collect data from parents and siblings to substantiate this theory. Segregation of DM in families has been reported in the Siberian Husky,[8] PWC,[4] and Chesapeake Bay Retriever.[12] Familial DM also occurs in the Rhodesian Ridgeback and Boxer (Coates, unpublished data, 2010). Clemmons and colleagues[47] reported a point mutation in hypervariable region 2 of *DLA-DRB1* in GSD with DM, and have offered a DNA test for DM based on this allele. Others were unable to confirm a correlation between this mutation and DM in GSDs.[48]

There are several approaches that can be used to identify disease-related genes including candidate gene sequencing, linkage mapping, and genome-wide association. Genome-wide association analysis using a single nucleotide polymorphism (SNP) arrays is a cost-effective, highly automated, and accurate approach.[49,50] Association mapping uses cases and controls, removing the need of identifying multigeneration families typically used in linkage. Awano and colleagues[5] used genome-wide association and DNA from PWCs to map the DM locus (**Fig. 6**). The SNPs of highest association with DM were clustered in a region of chromosome 31, which contained the *SOD1* gene. Clinical similarities between DM and ALS made *SOD1* a viable candidate gene, and a mutation in the gene was subsequently identified. Resequencing *SOD1* from normal and DM-affected PWCs revealed a G to A transition in exon 2, which corresponds to nucleotide 118 of the cDNA, and predicted a glutamic acid to lysine missense mutation at amino acid 40. All representatives of the 5 breeds in this study, which included Boxers, Chesapeake Bay Retrievers, GSDs, PWCs, and Rhodesian Ridgebacks with histopathologically confirmed DM, were homozygous for the *SOD1* mutation.[5] Some dogs were homozygous for the mutation but free of clinical signs, suggesting age-related incomplete penetrance.

Before the discovery of an *SOD1* mutation in canine DM, there were no previous reports of spontaneously occurring *SOD1*-linked ALS in animals. Equine motor neuron disease is a naturally occurring disease of the horse in which the distribution and nature of pathologic lesions resembles the progressive muscular atrophy form of ALS in humans, and its epidemiology is similar to sporadic ALS.[44,51,52] There has been no conclusive evidence for *SOD1* mutations in equine motor neuron disease.[53] Although the clinical signs, disease progression, and genetic analysis are provocative for considering DM as a canine model of ALS, there remain significant pathologic and clinical differences. These variations include the absence of any evidence of neuronal cell body degeneration or loss in the ventral horn of the spinal cord, and the diffuse nature of the axonopathy that involves sensory tracts as well as the UMN tracts.

SUPEROXIDE DISMUTASE 1

The SOD-1 protein, one of the most abundant proteins in the CNS, is 153 amino acids in length and functions as a free radical scavenger. Rosen and colleagues[54] discovered the first ALS causative genetic mutations in SOD-1 in 1973. More than 140 different *SOD1* mutations have been identified in ALS patients (http://alsod.iop.kcl.ac.uk), accounting for approximately 20% of the familial ALS (FALS) cases and about 6% of all cases.[55] Mutations in *SOD1* of ALS patients are distributed in all 5 exons of the gene, resulting in alteration of amino acids throughout the SOD-1 protein. Mutations of *SOD1* do not lead to disease by loss of normal enzyme function. Studies in transgenic rodents have determined instead that neurodegeneration results from a toxic gain of function.[22] These mutations lead to misfolded protein, which accumulates in the neurons and glia. The misfolding of mutant SOD-1 may induce neurodegeneration by forming insoluble aggregates that alter intracellular function or alter the enzyme substrate specificity, and generate toxic by-products.[56,57] The canine SOD-1 amino acid position 40 lies within the short "Greek key" connecting loop that stabilizes the alignment between the 2 sets of β-strands comprising the β-barrel.[58,59] The canine E40K mutation and several other ALS-associated *SOD1* mutations reduce the net negative charge of SOD-1.[60,61] The SOD-1 isoforms with reduced net negative charge may be prone to aggregation because of reduced repulsive Coulombic forces or because of increased interaction with anionic membrane surfaces.[61] Still it remains to be established whether SOD-1aggregates are directly toxic or a neutral by-product of the disease process, or even have a beneficial effect by sequestering misfolded SOD-1.[62]

In vivo neuropathologic evidence of SOD-1 misfolding lies in the presence of aggregates containing the SOD-1 antigen.[63,64] Light microscopic evaluation of spinal cords from some patients with ALS contain cytoplasmic inclusions known as Lewy body–like hyaline inclusions (LBHIs) if in neurons[65] or astrocytic hyaline inclusions (Ast-HIs) if in astrocytes.[66] Light microscopic evaluation of hematoxylin and eosin–stained spinal cords from DM-affected dogs have shown no evidence of LBHIs or Ast-HIs, but cytoplasmic aggregates in spinal cords from these dogs were consistently stained with anti-SOD-1 antibodies (**Fig. 7**).[5] The SOD-1–containing aggregates were consistently absent from spinal cord neurons from normal homozygous dogs. It is interesting that some asymptomatic heterozygotes had lightly stained SOD-1 aggregates, which may reflect subclinical disease.

AMYOTROPHIC LATERAL SCLEROSIS

ALS is the most common adult motor neuron disease, first described in 1869 by Jean-Martin Charcot.[67] *Amyotrophy* refers to atrophy of muscle fibers that are denervated as a result of motor neuron degeneration. *Lateral sclerosis* refers to "hardening" of the posterior and lateral tracts and replacement by gliosis. Amyotrophic lateral sclerosis is a heterogeneous disease in its clinical presentation, onset of clinical signs, and survival.[68,69] The disease usually affects people in their fourth to sixth decade of life. The overall survival is 3 to 5 years for more than 50% of ALS patients, although this can vary between 1 and 20 years.[70] Approximately 5% to10% of ALS cases are familial; the rest appear as isolated cases or sporadic ALS (SALS).[68] The mode of inheritance for FALS is usually autosomal dominant, but autosomal recessive ALS has also been reported.[71]

The major hallmark clinical signs of ALS include UMN and LMN systems degeneration and the progressive spread of these signs within a region or to other regions. Some ALS patients exhibit cognitive abnormalities that may precede or occur after the onset of symptoms, a pathologic continuum underlying this multisystem disorder.[72] At disease onset, an ALS patient usually presents with only upper or LMN signs that involve mainly muscles innervated by bulbar (brainstem) neurons or limb muscles. Thus, these forms of ALS are termed

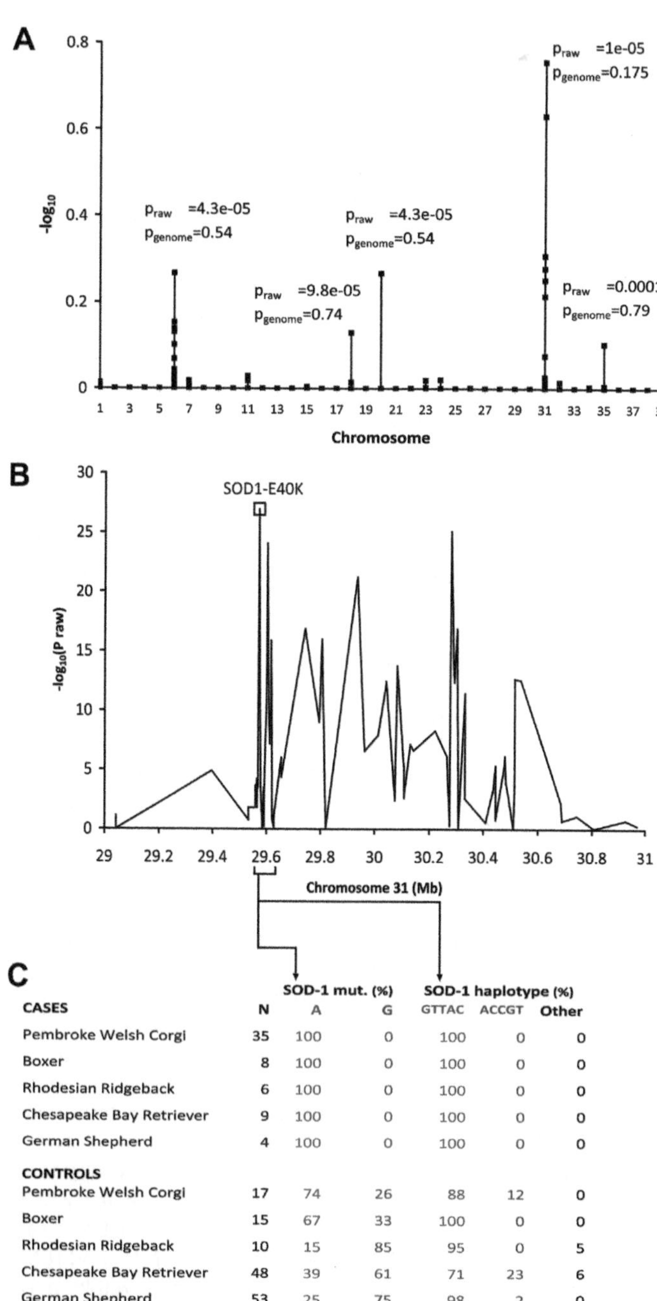

CASES	N	SOD-1 mut. (%) A	SOD-1 mut. (%) G	SOD-1 haplotype (%) GTTAC	ACCGT	Other
Pembroke Welsh Corgi	35	100	0	100	0	0
Boxer	8	100	0	100	0	0
Rhodesian Ridgeback	6	100	0	100	0	0
Chesapeake Bay Retriever	9	100	0	100	0	0
German Shepherd	4	100	0	100	0	0
CONTROLS						
Pembroke Welsh Corgi	17	74	26	88	12	0
Boxer	15	67	33	100	0	0
Rhodesian Ridgeback	10	15	85	95	0	5
Chesapeake Bay Retriever	48	39	61	71	23	6
German Shepherd	53	25	75	98	2	0

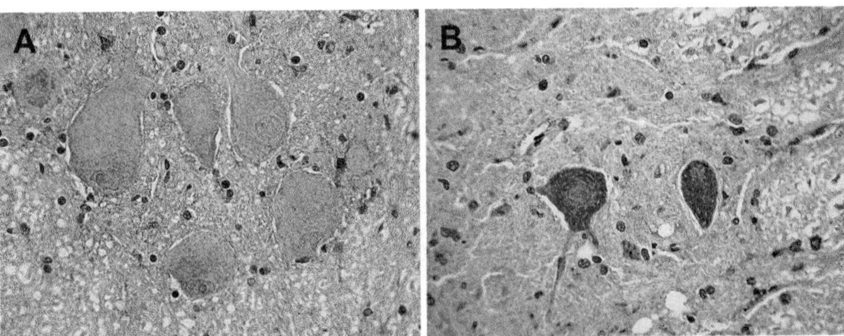

Fig. 7. Immunohistochemical staining with anti-SOD1 antibody from the spinal cords from a G/G homozygous normal 12-year-old Rhodesian Ridgeback (*A*) and an A/A homozygous DM-affected 14-year-old Pembroke Welsh Corgi (*B*). Note the neurons containing cytoplasmic aggregates, which when stained with anti-SOD1 antibodies appear as well-defined dark clumps (*B*). (*Courtesy of* Martin L. Katz, PhD, Columbia, MO.)

UMN onset, LMN onset, or bulbar onset (**Fig. 8**). About two-thirds of patients with typical ALS have a spinal form of the disease related to focal muscle weakness that may start distally or proximally in the upper or lower limbs.[69] Most of these patients go on to develop bulbar and respiratory symptoms. Canine DM is similar in its clinical spectrum to UMN-onset ALS (see **Fig. 8**).

DIAGNOSTIC APPROACH

Accurate antemortem diagnosis is based on pattern recognition of the progression of clinical signs followed by the completion of a series of diagnostic steps to exclude other disorders.[15,16] Neurodiagnostic techniques for evaluation of spinal cord disease include cerebrospinal fluid (CSF) analysis, electrodiagnostic testing, and spinal cord imaging procedures (see **Fig. 2**). A presumptive diagnosis of DM often is made based on lack of clinically relevant compressive myelopathy as determined by myelography or magnetic resonance imaging (MRI).

A study using computed tomography/myelography in confirmed and presumptively diagnosed DM dogs identified other concurrent spinal cord disorders: stenosis, spinal cord atrophy, and focal attenuation of subarachnoid space.[73] MRI is especially useful for identifying early intramedullary spinal cord neoplasia and evidence of extradural

Fig. 6. Mapping of a major DM locus. (*A*) Genome-wide association of 49,663 single nucleotide polymorphisms (SNPs) by using 38 cases (phenotypic stringencies 1–4) and 17 controls from Pembroke Welsh Corgis identified a major locus on CFA31 (P_{genome} = 0.18) and weaker signals on other chromosomes by using 10,000 permutations in PLINK. (*B*) The CFA31 region of association spans approximately 1.5 Mb and includes *SOD1*. *P* values from fine-mapping with 90 SNPs in 63 cases (phenotypic stringency levels 1–3) and 144 controls from 5 breeds (Boxer, 8/15 [Case/Control]; Chesapeake Bay Retriever, 9/48; German Shepherd dog, 4/54; Pembroke Welsh Corgi, 35/17; and Rhodesian Ridgeback, 7/8) are shown as well as the association for the missense mutation, which was separately assayed. (*C*) Fine-mapping data show that a 195-kb haplotype surrounding the *SOD1* mutation is associated in all 5 breeds and that this haplotype is older than the *SOD1* mutation. (*From* Awano T, Johnson GS, Wade CM, et al. Genome-wide association analysis reveals a SOD1 mutation in canine degenerative myelopathy that resembles amyotrophic lateral sclerosis. Proc Natl Acad Sci U S A 2009;106:2795; with permission.)

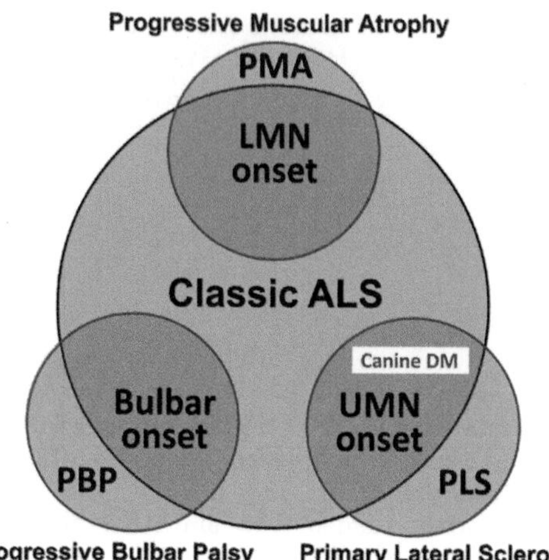

Fig. 8. Clinical spectrum of amyotrophic lateral sclerosis (ALS) in humans. Clinical signs of classic ALS manifest generalized UMN and LMN involvement. At onset, ALS may present only with UMN, LMN, or brainstem (bulbar) signs. Thus, these forms of ALS are termed UMN onset, LMN onset, or bulbar onset. The clinical spectrum of ALS can overlap with separate disease subtypes: progressive muscle atrophy (PMA), progressive bulbar palsy (PBP), and primary lateral sclerosis (PLS). Canine degenerative myelopathy has similarities in its clinical spectrum to UMN-onset ALS.

compressive myelopathy. Imaging often reveals disc protrusions that can confound a diagnosis of DM. The clinician must be guided by clinical experience to evaluate for rapidity of disease progression, presence of paraspinal hyperesthesia, and amount of spinal cord compression to account for the severity of the myelopathy.

CSF analysis can help rule out meningitis but also may be a potential source for biomarker identification. No cytologic or protein abnormalities are seen in the CSF of dogs with DM.[4] Biomarkers are useful for diagnosis, establishing prognosis and mechanism of disease, and monitoring of disease progression for therapeutic trials. Various biologic changes have been described from the analysis of body fluids, and neuroimaging and neurophysiologic studies of ALS patients.[74,75] Recently, the CSF in DM-affected dogs has been evaluated for markers of immune responses with intrathecal formation of immunoglobulins by detecting the presence of oligoclonal banding,[76,77] for demyelination by detecting increased concentrations of myelin basic protein, and for oxidative stress.[78] Although oligoclonal immunoglobulin banding has been reported in the CSF from DM-affected dogs, the significance of these bands is questionable because similar bands were detected in control samples.[76,77] Cerebrospinal fluid concentrations of 8-isoprostane, a stable marker of oxidative stress derived from the peroxidation of arachidonic acid, were not elevated in DM-affected PWCs when compared with normal older dogs.[4] A plausible explanation for lack of differences may be that the quantities of 8-isoprostane did not reflect the active or actual disease process. DM is a disease of insidious onset, which may make detection of biochemical mediators in CSF difficult.

Abnormalities in electrodiagnostic testing have been reported, but still need characterization at various disease stages.[2,4,5,7] Early in the progression of DM, no spontaneous activity is detected by electromyography (EMG) and nerve conduction velocities are within normal limits.[5] Later in the disease, EMG reveals multifocal spontaneous activity in the distal appendicular musculature. Fibrillation potentials and sharp waves are the more common waveforms recorded. Recordings of compound muscle action potentials (M waves) from stimulation of the tibial and ulnar nerves have shown temporal dispersion and decreases in amplitudes. The proximal and distal motor nerve conduction velocities were decreased when compared with the normal reference range.[5] These findings provide evidence of motor axonopathy and demyelination in the late disease stage of DM.

Genetic Testing

A DNA test based on the *SOD1* mutation is commercially available. The dogs homozygous for the mutation are at risk of developing DM and will contribute one chromosome with the mutant allele to all of their offspring. The heterozygotes are DM carriers that are unlikely to develop clinical DM but could pass on a chromosome with the mutant allele to half of their offspring. The normal homozygotes are unlikely to develop DM and will provide all of their offspring with a protective normal allele. Thus, the *SOD1* DNA test is of potential use to dog breeders wishing to reduce the incidence of DM in the breed or line.

The authors have detected the DM-associated SOD1:c.118A allele in at least 91 different dog breeds. It remains to be seen whether mutant homozygotes are at risk of developing DM on all of these different genetic backgrounds. The mutant allele appears to be very common in some breeds. Overly aggressive breeding programs to remove the mutant allele may further create a “bottleneck” effect, possibly selecting for other diseases and eliminating other desirable qualities of the breed. A realistic approach when considering which dogs to select for breeding would be to treat the test results as one would treat any other undesirable trait or fault. Dogs testing as at-risk should be considered to have a more serious fault than those testing as carriers. Using this approach and factoring the DM test results into the breeding decisions should reduce the prevalence of DM in the subsequent generations while continuing to maintain and improve on positive, sought-after traits. In addition, it will be important to continue the histopathologic examination of spinal cords from DM suspects of various breeds to confirm the diagnosis and identify breeds that are susceptible to DM.

MANAGEMENT STRATEGIES FOR CANINE DEGENERATIVE MYELOPATHY

Treatment regimens have been empiric, with a lack of evidence-based medicine approaches. Although it is hypothesized that DM is an immune-mediated neurodegenerative disease, immunosuppressive therapies using corticosteroids have shown no long-term benefits in halting the progression of DM.[13,79] An antiprotease agent, ε-aminocaproic acid, has been advocated for long-term management of DM.[80,81] A recent study evaluated a combined therapy of ε-aminocaproic acid and *N*-acetylcysteine with vitamins B, C, and E, and found no beneficial effects.[13] Therapy with parenteral cobalamin or oral tocopherol also did not affect neurologic progression in a study of DM-affected dogs; moreover, serum concentrations of α-tocopherol in DM-affected GSDs did not yield significant differences when compared with unaffected DM dogs.[35,37,39] Kathmann and colleagues[7] reported survival data from 22 DM-affected dogs that received varying degrees of physiotherapy. Dogs that received intensive physiotherapy had significantly longer survival times (mean = 255 days) than dogs that received moderate (mean = 130 days) or no physiotherapy (mean = 55 days). Limitations of this study include lack of randomization and definitive diagnosis, small group size, and bias from owner perception, which warrant further investigation into the efficacy of physiotherapy in DM-affected dogs. Still, physiotherapy and principles of physical rehabilitation may improve the quality of life for the DM-affected pet and pet owner.[82] Overall, the long-term prognosis of DM is poor.

At present, there exists no prophylactic or curative treatment for humans with ALS. The antiglutaminergic drug riluzole can extend life by a few months.[83] In addition, a multidisciplinary approach to care with assisted ventilation and nutritional support has yielded a 45% relative survival benefit.[84] Delivery of small molecule therapies to the spinal cord of ALS mice with viral vectors has yielded the greatest rescue to date.[85] Other therapies on the horizon include targeted stem cell therapy[86] and immunotherapy.[87] ALS is a heterogeneous disease that will require a multitherapeutic approach.[84] Thus, the need for significant disease-modifying therapies is paramount.

SOD1-ASSOCIATED CANINE DEGENERATIVE MYELOPATHY AND TRANSLATION TO HUMAN ALS

Canine diseases can play a key role in the translation of basic science knowledge to clinical applications. The transgenic rodent ALS models have been used as a tool to study the pathogenesis of ALS and to evaluate more than 150 potential therapeutic agents.[88] The choice of therapeutic agents in clinical trials of human ALS has been predicated on the efficacy of these drugs when studied in transgenic mice. One of the disappointments with the rodent models is that many drugs that have shown a positive effect in rodents have failed to be efficacious in human ALS trials.[89,90] The primitive nervous system and limited cognitive capacity of mice also may restrict their usefulness in evaluating the efficacy of therapeutic interventions to treat neurodegenerative diseases.[91] Compared with those of rodents, the nervous system and cognition in dogs more closely resemble those of humans. Advances in drug delivery technologies and the larger size of the dog, with a brain and spinal cord volume more closely approximating humans, will facilitate potential treatment strategies. Intraventricular or intrathecal injections of therapeutic agents may be more relevant in the dog disease than in the mouse or rat model, especially with respect to CSF dynamics and the pharmacologic properties of drugs penetrating into a larger brain and spinal cord.[91]

The *SOD1*-associated canine DM disease may offer several advantages over the current rodent ALS models. Dogs have a spontaneous mutation and are unlikely to possess the very high levels of mutant *SOD1* expression that occur in many of the transgenic rodent models.[92] These high expression levels may induce pathologic processes distinct from those affecting ALS patients.[93] The pattern of clinical progression of canine DM is relatively homogeneous in comparison with the phenotypic heterogeneity in human ALS. The spontaneous canine disease also offers a ready clinical population for which therapies can be evaluated in an environment closely mimicking human clinical trials. This approach has proven successful in developing chemotherapies in canine patients that have then been applied to humans as well as animals.[94] Thus, the results from clinical trials conducted with DM-affected dogs may better predict the efficacies of therapeutic interventions for treating ALS.

SUMMARY

- DM is a progressive, adult-onset neurodegenerative disease that occurs in many dog breeds.
- Clinical signs initially are characterized by GP ataxia and UMN spastic paraparesis. Later in the disease course, clinical signs will ascend causing flaccid tetraparesis and other LMN signs.

- Definitive diagnosis of DM is based on histopathologic examination. Histopathologic changes include degeneration and nerve fiber loss of ascending sensory and descending motor pathways that are most severe in the mid to caudal thoracic spinal cord. In dogs with advanced DM, nerve specimens show fiber loss resulting from axonal degeneration and secondary demyelination. Muscle specimens have changes typical of denervation atrophy.
- Absence of any evidence of neuronal cell body degeneration or loss in the ventral horn of the spinal cord is not a prominent histopathologic finding. Canine DM is most accurately classified as a multisystem central and peripheral axonopathy.
- Genome-wide association mapping of DM produced strongest associations with markers on CFA31 in a region containing the candidate gene *SOD1*. Resequencing of *SOD1* in DNA from normal and DM-affected dogs revealed a missense mutation in exon 2. Spinal cords from DM-affected dogs contain cytoplasmic aggregates that stain with anti-SOD1 antibodies. Homozygosity for the SOD1:c.118G>A allele is a major risk factor for canine DM. However, many dogs homozygous for this mutation do not develop clinical signs, suggesting an age-related incomplete penetrance.
- Mutations in *SOD1* are an underlying cause for some forms of human ALS (Lou Gehrig disease), an adult-onset fatal paralytic neurodegenerative disease. Canine DM associated with this *SOD1* mutation resembles a UMN-onset form of human ALS.
- DM is a spontaneous disease with uniformity in onset of clinical signs and disease progression. Dogs affected with DM could be used to investigate processes underlying motor neuron degeneration, evaluate potential therapeutic interventions, and map modifier loci.

ACKNOWLEDGMENTS

The authors would like to thank Drs Alexander de Lahunta, Gary S. Johnson, and Dennis P. O'Brien for their helpful advice and meticulous review of this article, and Howard A. Wilson for preparing the figures. A special acknowledgment is given to Liz Hansen who coordinates the sample collections and has provided sound advice from a breeder's and dog owner's perspective. In addition, the authors sincerely thank the pet owners, ACVIM Diplomates, other specialists, and general practitioners for their assistance with the study of canine degenerative myelopathy over the years.

REFERENCES

1. Averill DR. Degenerative myelopathy in the aging German shepherd dog: clinical and pathologic findings. J Am Vet Med Assoc 1973;162(12):1045–51.
2. Griffiths IR, Duncan ID. Chronic degenerative radiculomyelopathy in the dog. J Small Anim Pract 1975;16(8):461–71.
3. Braund KG, Vandevelde M. German shepherd dog myelopathy—a morphologic and morphometric study. Am J Vet Res 1978;39(8):1309–15.
4. Coates JR, March PA, Oglesbee M, et al. Clinical characterization of a familial degenerative myelopathy in Pembroke Welsh Corgi dogs. J Vet Intern Med 2007;21(6):1323–31.
5. Awano T, Johnson GS, Wade CM, et al. Genome-wide association analysis reveals a SOD1 mutation in canine degenerative myelopathy that resembles amyotrophic lateral sclerosis. Proc Natl Acad Sci U S A 2009;106:2794–9.

6. Johnston PEJ, Barrie JA, McCulloch MC, et al. Central nervous system pathology in 25 dogs with chronic degenerative radiculomyelopathy. Vet Rec 2000;146(22):629–33.
7. Kathmann I, Cizinauskas S, Doherr MG, et al. Daily controlled physiotherapy increases survival time in dogs with suspected degenerative myelopathy. J Vet Intern Med 2006;20:927–32.
8. Bichsel P, Vandevelde M, Lang J, et al. Degenerative myelopathy in a family of Siberian husky dogs. J Am Vet Med Assoc 1983;183(9):998–1000.
9. Matthews NS, de Lahunta A. Degenerative myelopathy in an adult miniature poodle. J Am Vet Med Assoc 1985;186(11):1213–5.
10. Miller AD, Barber R, Porter BF, et al. Degenerative myelopathy in two boxer dogs. Vet Pathol 2009;46(4):684–7.
11. March PA, Coates JR, Abyad RJ, et al. Degenerative myelopathy in 18 Pembroke Welsh Corgi dogs. Vet Pathol 2009;46:241–50.
12. Long SN, Henthorn PS, Serpell J, et al. Degenerative myelopathy in Chesapeake Bay retrievers. J Vet Intern Med 2009;23:401–2.
13. Polizopoulou ZS, Koutinas AF, Patsikas MN, et al. Evaluation of a proposed therapeutic protocol in 12 dogs with tentative degenerative myelopathy. Acta Vet Hung 2008;56(3):293–301.
14. Levine JM, Hillman RB, Erb HN, et al. The influence of age on patellar reflex response in the dog. J Vet Intern Med 2002;16:244–6.
15. Braund KG. Hip dysplasia and degenerative myelopathy: making the distinction in dogs. Vet Med 1987;82:782–9.
16. Kneller SK, Oliver JE, Lewis RE. Differential diagnosis of progressive caudal paresis in an aged German shepherd dog. J Am Anim Hosp Assoc 1975;11:414–7.
17. Hoerlein BF. Intervertebral disc disease. In: Oliver JE, Hoerlein BF, Mayhew IG, editors. Veterinary neurology. Philadelphia: W.B. Saunders; 1987. p. 321–41.
18. Summers BA, Cummings JF, de Lahunta A. Veterinary neuropathology. St. Louis (MO): Mosby; 1995. p. 189–207.
19. Cork LC, Troncoso JC, Price DL, et al. Canine neuroaxonal dystrophy. J Neuropathol Exp Neurol 1983;42(3):286–96.
20. Chrisman CL, Cork LC, Gamble DA. Neuroaxonal dystrophy of Rottweiler dogs. J Am Vet Med Assoc 1984;184(4):464–7.
21. Bruijn LI, Miller TM, Cleveland DW. Unraveling the mechanisms involved in motor neuron degeneration in ALS. Annu Rev Neurosci 2004;27:723–49.
22. Boillee S, Vande Velde C, Cleveland DW. ALS: a disease of motor neurons and their nonneuronal neighbors. Neuron 2006;52(1):39–59.
23. Olby N. Motor neuron disease: inherited and acquired. Vet Clin North Am Small Anim Pract 2004;34:1403–18.
24. Barclay KB, Haines DM. Immunohistochemical evidence for immunoglobulin and complement deposition in spinal cord lesions in degenerative myelopathy in German shepherd dogs. Can J Vet Res 1994;58(1):20–4.
25. Caulkins SE, Purinton PT, Oliver JE. Arterial supply to the spinal cord of dogs and cats. Am J Vet Res 1989;50(3):425–30.
26. de Lahunta A, Glass E. Veterinary neuroanatomy and clinical neurology. St. Louis (MO): Saunders Elsevier; 2009.
27. Grant G, Rexed B. Dorsal spinal afferents to Clarke's column. Brain 1958;81:567–76.
28. Al-Chaer ED, Lawand NB, Westlund KN, et al. Pelvic visceral input into the nucleus gracilis is largely mediated by the postsynaptic dorsal column pathway. J Neurophysiol 1996;76:2675–90.

29. Shelton GD, Johnson GC, Johnson GS, et al. Peripheral nerve pathology in canine degenerative myelopathy with mutation in superoxide dismutase 1 gene. J Vet Intern Med 2009;23:710–1.
30. Griffiths IR, Duncan ID. Age changes in the dorsal and ventral lumbar nerve roots of dogs. Acta Neuropathol 1975;32(1):75–85.
31. Cavanagh JB. The significance of the "dying back" process in experimental and human neurological disease. Int Rev Exp Pathol 1964;3:219–67.
32. Spencer PS, Schaumburg HH. Central peripheral distal axonopathy—the pathology of dying-back polyneuropathies. Prog Neuropathol 1976;3:253–95.
33. Waxman FJ, Clemmons RM, Johnson G, et al. Progressive myelopathy in older German shepherd dogs. I. Depressed response to thymus-dependent mitogens. J Immunol 1980;124(3):1209–15.
34. Waxman FJ, Clemmons RM, Hinrichs DJ. Progressive myelopathy in older German shepherd dogs. II. Presence of circulating suppressor cells. J Immunol 1980;124(3):1216–22.
35. Williams DA, Sharp NJH, Batt RM. Enteropathy associated with degenerative myelopathy in German shepherd dogs. In: Proceedings of the First ACVIM Forum. 1983. p. 40.
36. Williams DA, Batt RM, Sharp NJH. Degenerative myelopathy in German shepherd dogs: an association with mucosal biochemical changes and bacterial overgrowth in the small intestine. Clin Sci 1984;66:25.
37. Williams DA, Prymak C, Baughan J. Tocopherol (vitamin E) status in canine degenerative myelopathy. In: Proceedings 3rd ACVIM Forum. 1985. p. 154.
38. Fechner H, Johnston PE, Sharp NJH, et al. Molecular genetic and expression analysis of alpha-tocopherol transfer protein mRNA in German shepherd dogs with degenerative myelopathy. Berl Munch Tierarztl Wochenschr 2003;11:631–6.
39. Johnston PEJ, Knox K, Gettinby G, et al. Serum α-tocopherol concentrations in German shepherd dogs with chronic degenerative radiculomyelopathy. Vet Rec 2001;148:403–7.
40. Sheahan BJ, Caffrey JF, Gunn HM, et al. Structural and biochemical changes in a spinal myelinopathy in twelve English foxhounds and two harriers. Vet Pathol 1991;28(2):117–24.
41. Olby NJ, Sharp NJH, Muñana KR, et al. Chronic and acute compressive spinal cord lesions in dogs are associated with increased lumbar CSF glutamate levels. J Vet Intern Med 1999;13(3):240.
42. Appel SH. CD4+ T cells mediate cytotoxicity in neurodegenerative diseases. J Clin Invest 2009;119(1):13–5.
43. Blythe LL, Craig AM, Lassen ED, et al. Serially determined plasma α-tocopherol concentrations and results of the oral vitamin E absorption test in clinically normal horses and in horses with degenerative myeloencephalopathy. Am J Vet Res 1991;52(6):908–11.
44. Cummings JF, de Lahunta A, Mohammed HO, et al. Equine motor neuron disease: a new neurologic disorder. Equine Pract 1991;13(9):15–8.
45. Divers TJ, Cummings JE, de Lahunta A, et al. Evaluation of the risk of motor neuron disease in horses fed a diet low in vitamin E and high in copper and iron. Am J Vet Res 2006;67(1):120–6.
46. Flegel T, Sharp N, Olby N, et al. Analysis of the canine αTTP gene—a candidate gene for degenerative myelopathy? J Vet Intern Med 1999;13(3):240.
47. Clemmons RM, Cheeseman JA, Kamishina H, et al. Genetic analysis of a spontaneous canine model of primary multiple sclerosis. FASEB J 2006;20:A1417.

48. Clark LA, Tsai KL, Murphy KE. Alleles of DLA-DRB1 are not unique in German shepherd dogs having degenerative myelopathy. Anim Genet 2008;39(3):332.
49. Karlsson EK, Baranowska I, Wade CM, et al. Efficient mapping of mendelian traits in dogs through genome-wide association. Nat Genet 2007;39:1321–8.
50. Lindblad-Toh K, Wade CM, Mikkelsen TS, et al. Genome sequence, comparative analysis and haplotype structure of the domestic dog. Nature 2005;438:803–19.
51. Divers TJ, Mohammed HO, Cummings JF, et al. Equine motor neuron disease: findings in 28 horses and proposal of a pathophysiological mechanism for the disease. Equine Vet J 1994;26(5):409–15.
52. Valentine BA, de Lahunta A, George C, et al. Acquired equine motor neuron disease. Vet Pathol 1994;31(1):130–8.
53. de la Rúa-Domenèch R, Wiedmann M, Mohammed HO, et al. Equine motor neuron disease is not linked to Cu/Zn superoxide dismutase mutations: sequence analysis of the equine Cu/Zn superoxide dismutase cDNA. Gene 1996;178:83–8.
54. Rosen DR, Siddique T, Patterson D, et al. Mutations in Cu/Zn superoxide dismutase gene are associated with familial amyotrophic lateral sclerosis. Nature 1993; 362(6415):59–62.
55. Dion PA, Daoud H, Rouleau GA. Genetics of motor neuron disorders: new insights into pathogenic mechanisms. Nat Rev Genet 2009;10(11):769–82.
56. Rakhit R, Chakrabartty A. Structure, folding, and misfolding of Cu, Zn superoxide dismutase in amyotrophic lateral sclerosis. Biochim Biophys Acta 2006; 1762(11–12):1025–37.
57. Bruijn LI, Houseweart MK, Kato S, et al. Aggregation and motor neuron toxicity of an ALS-linked SOD1 mutant independent from wild-type SOD1. Science 1998; 281(5384):1851–4.
58. Green SL, Tolwani RJ, Varma S, et al. Structure, chromosomal location, and analysis of the canine Cu/Zn superoxide dismutase (SOD1) gene. J Hered 2002; 93(2):119–24.
59. Boissinot M, Karnas S, Lepock JR, et al. Function of the Greek key connection analysed using circular permutants of superoxide dismutase. EMBO J 1997; 16(9):2171–8.
60. Deng HX, Hentati A, Tainer JA, et al. Amyotrophic lateral sclerosis and structural defects in Cu, Zn superoxide dismutase. Science 1993;261(5124):1047–51.
61. Sandelin E, Nordlund A, Andersen PM, et al. Amyotrophic lateral sclerosis-associated copper/zinc superoxide dismutase mutations preferentially reduce the repulsive charge of the proteins. J Biol Chem 2007;282(29):21230–6.
62. Shaw BF, Valentine JS. How do ALS-associated mutations in superoxide dismutase 1 promote aggregation of the protein? Trends Biochem Sci 2007;32:78–85.
63. Jonsson PA, Ernhill K, Andersen PM, et al. Minute quantities of misfolded mutant superoxide dismutase-1 cause amyotrophic lateral sclerosis. Brain 2004;127(Pt 1):1–88.
64. Wang J, Slunt H, Gonzales V, et al. Copper-binding-site-null SOD1 causes ALS in transgenic mice: aggregates of non-native SOD1 delineate a common feature. Hum Mol Genet 2003;12(21):2753–64.
65. Hirano A, Kurland LT, Sayre GP. Familial amyotrophic lateral sclerosis. A subgroup characterized by posterior and spinocerebellar tract involvement and hyaline inclusions in the anterior horn cells. Arch Neurol 1967;16(3):232–43.
66. Kato S, Hayashi H, Nakashima K, et al. Pathological characterization of astrocytic hyaline inclusions in familial amyotrophic lateral sclerosis. Am J Pathol 1997; 151(2):611–20.

67. Charcot J-M, Joffroy A. Deux cas d'atrophie musculaire progressive avec lésions de l substance grise et de faisceaux antérolatéraux de la moelle épinière. Arch Physiol Norm Pathol 1869;I:354–7.
68. Leigh PN. Amyotrophic lateral sclerosis. In: Eisen AA, Shaw PJ, editors, Motor neuron disorders and related diseases, vol. 82. Amsterdam: Elsevier; 2007. p. 249–68.
69. Wijesekera LC, Leigh PN. Amyotrophic lateral sclerosis. Orphanet J Rare Dis 2009;4:1–22. Available at: http://www.orjrd.com/content/4/1/3. Accessed May 18, 2010.
70. Magnus T, Beck M, Giess R, et al. Disease progression in amyotrophic lateral sclerosis: predictors of survival. Muscle Nerve 2002;25(5):709–14.
71. Andersen PM. Amyotrophic lateral sclerosis associated with mutations in the CuZn superoxide dismutase gene. Curr Neurol Neurosci Rep 2006;6(1):37–46.
72. Wilson CM, Grace GM, Munoz DG, et al. Cognitive impairment in sporadic ALS: a pathologic continuum underlying a multisystem disorder. Neurology 2001;57(4): 651–7.
73. Jones JC, Inzana KD, Rossmeisl JH, et al. CT myelography of the thoraco-lumbar spine in 8 dogs with degenerative myelopathy. J Vet Sci 2005;6:341–8.
74. Pradat PF, Dib M. Biomarkers in amyotrophic lateral sclerosis: facts and future horizons. Mol Diag Ther 2009;13(2):115–25.
75. Turner MR, Kiernan MC, Leigh PN, et al. Biomarkers in amyotrophic lateral sclerosis. Lancet Neurol 2009;8(1):94–109.
76. Ruaux CG, Coates JR, March PA, et al. Analysis of oligoclonal banding in CSF and serum from dogs with degenerative myelopathy. J Vet Intern Med 2003;17:401.
77. Kamishina H, Oji T, Cheeseman JA, et al. Detection of oligoclonal bands in cerebrospinal fluid from German shepherd dogs with degenerative myelopathy by isoelectric focusing and immunofixation. Vet Clin Pathol 2008;37(2):217–20.
78. Oji T, Kamishina H, Cheeseman JA, et al. Measurement of myelin basic protein in the cerebrospinal fluid of dogs with degenerative myelopathy. Vet Clin Pathol 2007;36(3):281–4.
79. Clemmons RM. Degenerative myelopathy. In: Kirk RW, editor. Current veterinary therapy X. Small animal practice. Philadelphia: W.B. Saunders Company; 1989. p. 830–3.
80. Clemmons RM. Therapeutic considerations for degenerative myelopathy of German shepherds. In: Proceedings 9th ACVIM Forum. New Orleans (LA), 1991. p. 773–5.
81. Clemmons RM. Degenerative myelopathy. Vet Clin North Am Small Anim Pract 1992;22(4):965–71.
82. Sherman J, Olby NJ. Nursing and rehabilitation of the neurological patient. In: Platt SR, Olby NJ, editors. BSAVA manual of canine and feline neurology. 3rd edition. Gloucester (UK): BSAVA; 2004. p. 394–407.
83. Bensimon G, Lacomblez L, Meininger V. A control trial of riluzole. N Engl J Med 1994;330:585–91.
84. Van Damme P, Robberecht W. Recent advances in motor neuron disease. Curr Opin Neurol 2009;22:486–92.
85. Smith RA, Miller TM, Yamanaka K, et al. Antisense oligonucleotide therapy for neurodegenerative disease. J Clin Invest 2006;116(8):2290–6.
86. Nayak MS, Kim YS, Goldman M, et al. Cellular therapies in motor neuron diseases. Biochim Biophys Acta 2006;1762(11–12):1128–38.
87. Urushitani M, Ezzi SA, Julien JP. Therapeutic effects of immunization with mutant superoxide dismutase in mice models of amyotrophic lateral sclerosis. Proc Natl Acad Sci U S A 2007;104(7):2495–500.

88. Turner BJ, Talbot K. Transgenics, toxicity and therapeutics in rodent models of mutant SOD1-mediated familial ALS. Prog Neurobiol 2008;85(1):94–134.
89. Benatar M. Lost in translation: treatment trials in the SOD1 mouse and in human ALS. Neurobiol Dis 2007;26(1):1–13.
90. DiBernardo AB, Cudkowicz ME. Translating preclinical insights into effective human trials in ALS. Biochim Biophys Acta 2006;1762(11–12):1139–49.
91. Ellinwood NM, Vite CH, Haskin ME. Gene therapy for lysosomal storage diseases: the lessons and promise of animal models. J Gene Med 2004;6:481–506.
92. Rakhit R, Cunningham P, Furtos-Matei A, et al. Oxidation-induced misfolding and aggregation of superoxide dismutase and its implications for amyotrophic lateral sclerosis. J Biol Chem 2002;277(49):47551–6.
93. Wong PC, Pardo CA, Borchelt DR, et al. An adverse property of a familial ALS-linked SOD1 mutation causes motor neuron disease characterized by vacuolar degeneration of mitochondria. Neuron 1995;14(6):1105–16.
94. Paoloni M, Khanna C. Translation of new cancer treatments from pet dogs to humans. Nat Rev Cancer 2008;8:147–56.

Congenital Spinal Malformations in Small Animals

Diccon R. Westworth, BVSc (Hons)[a,b,*], Beverly K. Sturges, DVM, MS[b]

KEYWORDS

- Spine • Anomaly • Congenital • Deformity • Malformation
- Congenital

Congenital spinal malformations are commonly identified in small animals and may cause pain, myelopathy, radiculopathy, and gross spinal deformities. However, many spinal malformations do not produce overt neurologic dysfunction, and it is the responsibility of the clinician to investigate and determine whether the malformation is an incidental finding or the underlying cause of the clinical signs. The clinical examination of an animal suspected of having a neurologic disorder includes assessment of signalment and history combined with a thorough physical and neurologic examination. The end point of this assessment is to determine whether a neurologic problem exists, and if so, the location along the neuraxis. Spinal malformations occurring within the region of localization are considered a differential diagnosis for the cause of the neurologic signs.

The underlying cause of most congenital spinal anomalies is not known; however, a genetic predisposition or mutation has been identified in some cases. Many potential causes have been postulated including metabolic disease, particularly the role of folate, teratogenous drugs, and toxin exposure.[1,2]

Dogs and cats with congenital spinal malformations may have concurrent congenital anomalies affecting other systems or other regions of the central nervous system. A thorough review of all systems should be done to fully identify all possible anomalies and document their clinical significance in order to mitigate unforeseen complications, particularly when considering anesthesia or surgery. Review of pedigree for possible heritability should also be attempted in clinically significant conditions, and caution raised against continued breeding of such animals.

To promote further understanding of the development, structural change, and clinical significance of an anomaly, emphasis is placed on the correct use of terminology

[a] VCA Animal Care Center of Sonoma County, 6470 Redwood Drive, Rohnert Park, CA 94928, USA
[b] Department of Surgical and Radiological Sciences, School of Veterinary Medicine, University of California Davis, 1 Shields Avenue, Davis, CA 95616, USA
* Corresponding author. Department of Surgical and Radiological Sciences, School of Veterinary Medicine, University of California Davis, 1 Shields Avenue, Davis, CA 95616.
E-mail address: dwestworth@ucdavis.edu

Vet Clin Small Anim 40 (2010) 951–981
doi:10.1016/j.cvsm.2010.05.009
0195-5616/10/$ – see front matter

and classification systems. Classification of congenital spinal anomalies has not been clearly defined in domestic animals and appropriate terminology is not uniformly applied, this being partly due to the relative lack of neuroradiological and neuropathological data that are needed for accurate categorization of anomalies. In this article congenital spinal anomalies are grouped into either the (1) originating developmental stage or (2) anatomic region/structures involved. Modified accepted human classification schemes were applied where considered apposite. Often, malformations are complex and placement into a single category is difficult. Although classification remains somewhat arbitrary in such cases, the authors have attempted to use the most clinically useful classification systems for the reported spinal anomalies in dogs and cats.

In this article neural tube defects (abnormalities of neural and mesenchymal structures) are discussed first, followed by vertebral column malformations (purely mesenchymal structures), vascular malformations, and arachnoid diverticulae. Definitions of terminology frequently used when discussing congenital spinal anomalies is provided in **Box 1**.

SPINAL DYSRAPHISM

Spinal neural tube defects are congenital malformations of the vertebral column and spinal cord that occur secondary to abnormal closure of the caudal neuropore of the developing neural tube. This results in a defective neural arch through which meninges or neural elements may herniate. The term spinal dysraphism includes the overall group of dorsal midline defects derived from the secondary maldevelopment of ectoderm, mesoderm, and neurectoderm layers of tissue, and encompasses a variety of malformations including spina bifida, meningocele, meningomyelocele, syringomyelia, split cord anomalies (diastematomyelia), and others. In humans spinal dysraphisms are categorized clinically into open and closed, based on whether the abnormal nervous tissue is exposed to the environment or covered by skin (**Box 2**).[3]

Open Spinal Dysraphism

Spina bifida manifesta, cystica, and aperta are synonymous terms that have been applied to open spinal dysraphism (OSD) based on imaging findings, pathologic findings, or both. OSDs include myeloceles and meningomyeloceles, whereby the spinal cord fails to fuse dorsally, remaining as a plate, and is open to the environment because it is not covered by skin. These severe dysraphisms often are considered surgical emergencies in human neonates and, in animal neonates, usually result in death or early termination. Such entities have rarely been reported in dogs[4,5] or cats.[6]

Closed Spinal Dysraphism

Closed spinal dysraphism (CSD), also known as spina bifida occulta, includes various malformations that are covered by skin (with or without other structures) and are periodically seen in dogs. In the individual, multiple anomalies may be present. The simplest form of CSD is dorsal spina bifida, a simple fusion defect of the posterior neural arch (single or multiple), and is usually clinically insignificant, with no or minor neural anomalies (**Fig. 1**). Occasionally a subcutaneous mass may be present in CSD, that is, a meningocele (and/or lipoma), in dogs[7,8] and Manx cats.[9] Intradural lipomas and filum terminale lipomas are rarely reported in the dog[10] and cat.[11] In most cases of CSD there is no apparent mass. Dermal sinus tracts are a well-recognized form of CSD.[12] Complex dysraphic states include anomalies such as

Box 1
Definition of terms

Neural tube defect: Any one of various congenital anomalies caused by incomplete closure of the neural tube during the early stages of embryonic development, eg, spina bifida (spinal cord), anencephaly (brain).

Spina bifida: A neural tube defect marked by a congenital (dorsal) cleft of the spinal column with or without hernial protrusion of the meninges and sometimes the spinal cord.

Spinal dysraphism: Defective closure of the neural tube.

Open spinal dysraphism: A form of spinal dysraphism whereby nervous tissue is exposed to the environment; usually seen as a protruding cyst made up of either spinal cord (myelocele) or meninges in combination with spinal cord tissue (meningomyelocele). This term is synonymous with several older terms that were used based on imaging and/or pathologic findings: *spina bifida aperta, spina bifida cystica, spinal bifida manifesta*.

Closed spinal dysraphism: A form of spinal dysraphism whereby nervous tissue is protected from exposure to the environment by one or more layers of tissue coverings. This term is synonymous with the older term *spina bifida occulta*.

Meningocele: A protrusion of meninges through a laminar defect in the spinal column (as in spina bifida) forming a dural sac filled with cerebrospinal fluid.

Myelocele: Failure of the spinal cord to fuse dorsally, remaining as a plate open to the environment.

Meningomyelocele: A protrusion of meninges and spinal cord through a defect in the spinal column.

Diastomatomyelia: Congenital sagittal division (split) of the spinal cord. The 2 cords may be contained within the same meningeal sheath, or separate, often divided by a fibrous sheath or bone. Diplomyelia is the term used if the 2 hemicords do not reunite caudally and remain as 2 separate spinal cords.

Myelodysplasia: A general term for a neural tube defect causing a developmental anomaly of the spinal cord; the term "spinal dysraphism" has largely replaced this term.

Dermal sinus tract: Incomplete neural tube closure resulting from failure of surface ectoderm and dermal elements to separate. Four types are typically described, all originating at the level of the skin and extending ventrally to varying depths.

Myeloschisis: Dorsal spinal cord cleft.

Hydromyelia: Widening or enlargement of the central canal of the spinal cord.

Data from Medline plus online medical dictionary (Merriam Webster): Bethesda (MD): US National Library of Medicine and the NIH; 20894; and Stedman's Electronic Medical Dictionary, v7.0 for Windows.

sacrocaudal dysgenesis in Manx cats,[9] hydromyelia, and rare anomalies such as diastematomyelia (split cord).

Meningocele

Meningoceles are reported in Bulldogs,[7,8,13] a Collie,[7] and Manx cats.[9] Although a subcutaneous mass may be present in these cases, usually there is no apparent mass (**Fig. 2**). Bulldogs have been reported with L7 or sacral dorsal vertebral arch defects and subcutaneous meningoceles with or without slit-like cavitation of the dorsal terminal spinal cord,[8,13] midline caudal hair streaming,[7] and apparent caudal tethering of the filum by a fibrous cord.[14,15] Although reports of attempted surgical repair are rare, 2 reports of Bulldogs that had surgery included a dorsal surgical approach to the caudal spine, opening of the dura, and transection of a fibrous filum terminale, resulting in release of the caudal tether.[14,15]

Box 2
Classification of spinal dysraphism in dogs and cats

Open spinal dysraphism

- Myelomeningocele (Hemimyelomeningocele)
- Myelocele (Hemimyelocele)

Closed spinal dysraphism

- With subcutaneous mass
  - Meningocele
  - Lipomyelomeningocele
  - Terminal myelocystocele
- Without a subcutaneous mass

Simple dysraphic states

- Dorsal spina bifida
  - Intradural and intramedullary lipoma
  - Filum terminale lipoma
  - Dermal sinus tract, dermoid and epidermoid cysts

Complex dysraphic states

- Split cord malformations (diastematomelia and diplomyelia)
- Segmental spinal dysgenesis/agenesis
- Hydromyelia

Data from Rossi A, Gandolfo C, Morana G, et al. Current classification and imaging of congenital spinal anomalies. Semin Roentgenol 2006;41(4):250–73.

Sacrocaudal dysgenesis in the Manx cat

Sacrocaudal dysgenesis is a complex CSD consisting of dysgenesis or agenesis of the coccygeal and sacral vertebrae and the associated sacral and caudal spinal cord segments, and occasionally caudal lumbar spinal cord segments. Associated abnormalities include subcutaneous cysts with or without fistulas opening to the dorsal skin with constant cerebrospinal fluid (CSF) leakage, meningoceles, shortening/absence of the spinal cord and cauda equina, central canal defects, syringomyelia, diastematomyelia, abnormal gray matter differentiation/disorganization, and intradural or filum terminal lipomas with or without tethered spinal cord.[9,11,16]

The macroscopic lesions in Manx cats were first described by Kerruisch[17] in 1964 and microscopically by James and colleagues[9] in 1969. Autosomal dominant inheritance occurs with incomplete penetrance.[16,18] Kittens are variably affected including (a) normal tails and no neurologic deficits, (b) short tails with minimal neurologic signs (stumpies), and (c) no visible tail with few or absent coccygeal vertebrae and more severe neurologic dysfunction (rumpies). Clinical signs include a palpable dorsal vertebral defect caudally over the sacral area or an apparent subcutaneous mass (lipoma or meningocele), bunny hopping pelvic limb gait, plantigrade stance, paraparesis, pelvic limb ataxia, urinary or fecal incontinence, megacolon, atonic bladder, hyporeflexia of the pelvic limbs, anal sphincter, urinary bladder and sphincter, and alterations in nociception to perineal area and possibly to the pelvic limbs.[16,18] Occasionally fistulation of a cyst or meningocele occurs, leading to a caudal pinpoint midline patency that constantly leaks CSF, wetting the fur. This condition can be a cause of ascending meningitis and provoke rapid decline in function.

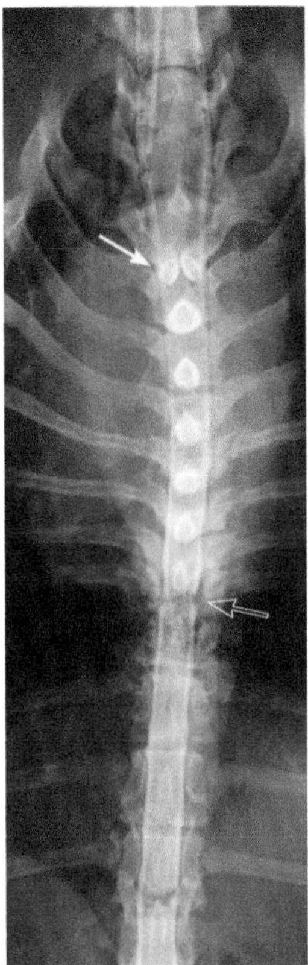

Fig. 1. Ventrodorsal projection radiograph of the thoracic vertebral column. Dorsal spina bifida can be seen in this dog that presented with signs of a T3 to L3 myelopathy. Note the 2 spinous processes seen at T2 (*solid white arrow*). The restrictive band of fibrous tissue seen at T8 to T9 was the source of the clinical signs in this case (*arrow*).

Diagnostic modalities include survey spinal radiographs and computed tomography (CT) for assessment of bony anomalies and/or magnetic resonance imaging (MRI) for assessment of neural structures within and around the spinal canal, especially if surgical treatment is considered. CSF analysis is indicated with a patent fistula and when secondary infection is apparent or likely. Urinary tract infections and constipation are frequent complications, and treatment of severely affected animals is not recommended. Surgical management in one reported case (also with an intradural lipoma and tethered spinal cord) resulted in the cat returning to normal neurologic function.[11] Tailless animals with mild neurologic deficits can lead full lives. The practice of continued breeding of affected cats is unethical and should be stopped.

Dermal sinus tract

A dermal sinus tract is caused by incomplete dysjunction of the neural tube from skin ectoderm during embryonic development.[19] This anomaly is not synonymous with pilonidal cysts (which are acquired) or dermoid cysts, as discussed later. Dermal sinus tracts are (blind) tubular sacs extending ventrally from the dorsal midline into the underlying tissues, occurring most commonly in the cervical, cranial thoracic, and lumbosacral regions.[12] This anomaly was first described by Steyn and colleagues[20]

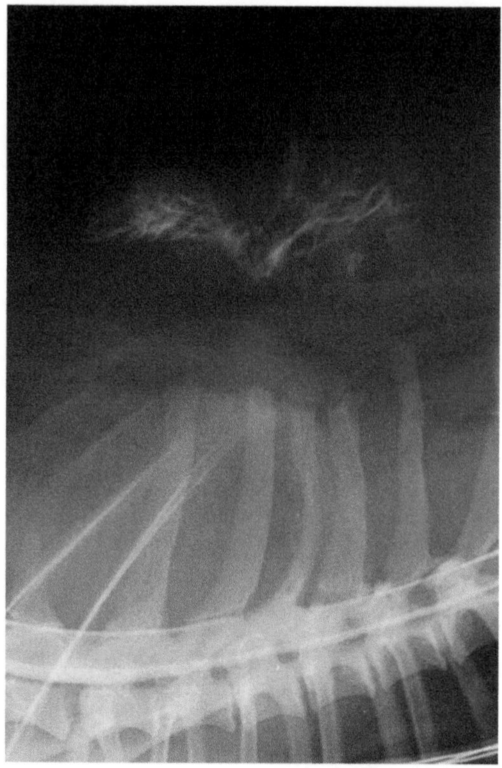

Fig. 2. Lateral projection radiograph of the thoracic vertebral column post myelogram in a 4-year-old Shetland sheepdog that presented for acute paraplegia. A dorsal meningocele can be seen with subcutaneously arborizing tracts and a lipomatous mass was present at surgery extending through a laminal defect associated with T3 dorsal spina bifida.

in South Africa in 1939 and later in North America by Lord and colleagues[21] in 1957. The most common breeds affected are Rhodesian Ridgebacks, Ridgeback-crosses, or related dogs (South African Ridged Hottentot dog and Boerboel). Inheritance in Rhodesian Ridgebacks is a dominant mutation in fibroblast growth factor genes.[22] Other reported breeds include Shih Tzu, Boxer, Siberian Husky, Chow Chow, American Cocker Spaniel, Yorkshire Terrier, English Springer Spaniel, Great Pyrenees, Wire Fox Terrier, and Golden Retriever.[12] It is rarely reported in cats.[23,24]

In Rhodesian Ridgebacks the sinus tract is not found within the region defined by the ridge but instead found cranial or caudal to it, especially in the cervical region where it often extends to the spinous process of C2. In other breeds the most common location is in the cranial or mid-thoracic regions. Four[25] or 5 types[12] have been proposed depending on the depth to which they extend (**Fig. 3**). Types I and II extend to the supraspinous ligament (deeply Type II is a closed fibrous band), whereas Type III is a more superficial sac and Type IV extends to the vertebral canal (with or without an obvious laminal defect) and attaches to the dura mater. Type V has been proposed more recently,[12] but this entity is a true cyst, with no tract or skin opening, and should be referred to as a dermoid cyst.[26]

On the surface of the skin, the sinus tract may appear grossly as a small (1–5 mm) indentation/invagination (**Fig. 4**). On palpation it may feel like a subcutaneous cord or

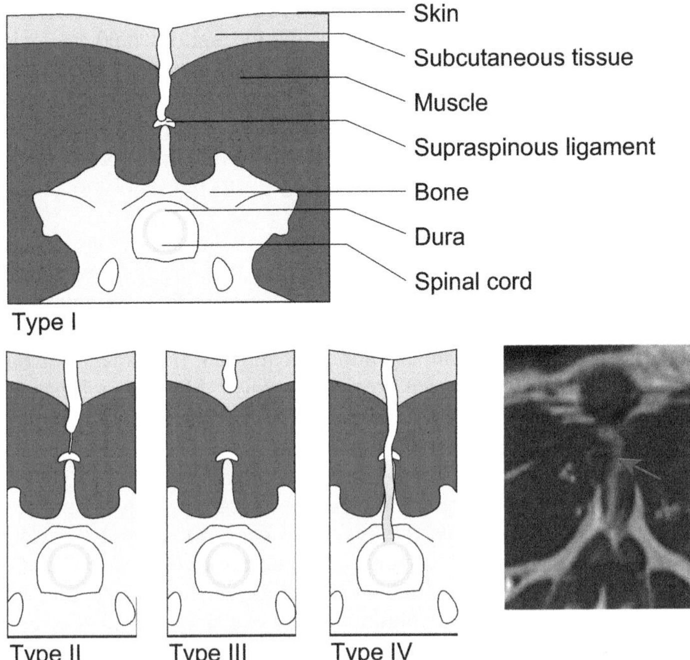

Fig. 3. Diagram of the 4 types of dermal sinus tracts (I–IV), illustrating the extent of tissue depth involved. For comparison, a cervical transverse T2-weighted MRI of a Type IV dermal sinus tract is shown. Note the serpentine appearance of the tract as it courses ventrally (*arrows*) through a laminal defect to the dura mater. (*MRI Courtesy of* Dr Jim Lavely.)

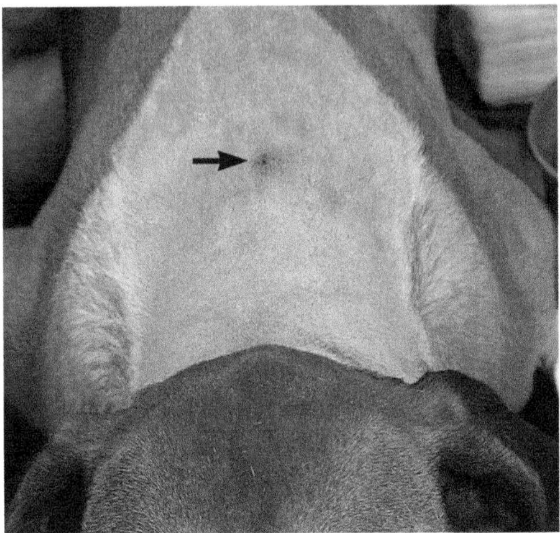

Fig. 4. Photograph of the shaved dorsal cervical region of a 1-year-old Rhodesian ridgeback dog in preparation for surgery and removal of a dorsal sinus tract. Note the pinpoint surface indentation indicating the most superficial extent of the tract (*arrow*). (*Courtesy of* Dr Jim Lavely.)

band of fibrous tissue. Histologically it is lined with squamous epithelium and adenexal structures, and often filled with epithelial debris (keratin, sebum, hair) and/or inflammatory cells and bacteria. When inflamed or infected it will enlarge and become painful. The most common reported infections are *Staphylococcus intermedius* and *Enterococcus* spp.[12] With Type IV dermal sinuses, neural structures may become infected or inflamed causing spinal pain and/or myelopathy due to spinal cord compression, empyema/abscess, and/or osteomyelitis. In dogs with ridges, Type IV cysts more often occur in the sacrococcygeal region.[12]

Clinical diagnosis can be made with palpation, or clipping of the hair and visual inspection. Survey vertebral column radiographs may identify vertebral laminal defects or osteomyelitis. Advanced imaging (MRI and/or CT) is recommended when vertebral canal involvement is suspected and/or prior to surgical exploration to provide adequate presurgical planning and limit the risk of inadvertent damage to the spinal cord (see **Fig. 3**). In recent reports, however, MRI did not clearly indicate the full extent of the tract[27] and was misleading in another case of a single dermoid cyst without a tract.[26]

Myelogram and/or CT may provide similar information in cases demonstrating a myelopathy. Fistulography is contraindicated because infection or dermal elements may be introduced into deeper tissues. Surgical excision without disruption of the sinus is the treatment of choice in clinically affected cases (**Fig. 5**).[12] Good visualization through appropriate exposure, knowledge of regional anatomy, and experience handling neural tissues is needed when surgically excising dermal sinuses involving the meninges and/or spinal cord. Deep culture should be taken and broad-spectrum antibiotics used if there is apparent infection or contamination of surrounding structures.

Dermal sinus tracts may also be seen with other anomalies of the spine.[28] In addition, dermoid and epidermoid cysts without sinus tracts (as noted earlier) are congenital anomalies of misplaced dermal elements that have also been described to cause spinal disease.[29]

Spinal dysraphism in Weimaraner dogs

McGrath[30,31] first reported this malformation in the Weimaraner as syringomyelia in 1956 and later, in 1965, renamed the condition spinal dysraphism. Previous investigators,[32,33] and even McGrath,[31] have questioned whether this condition should be described as spinal dysraphism. Although there is complete closure of the neural tube, anomalies including hydromelia are present, which are seen in other dysraphic anomalies of the spinal cord, and therefore warrant (at least at this time) its inclusion under CSD.

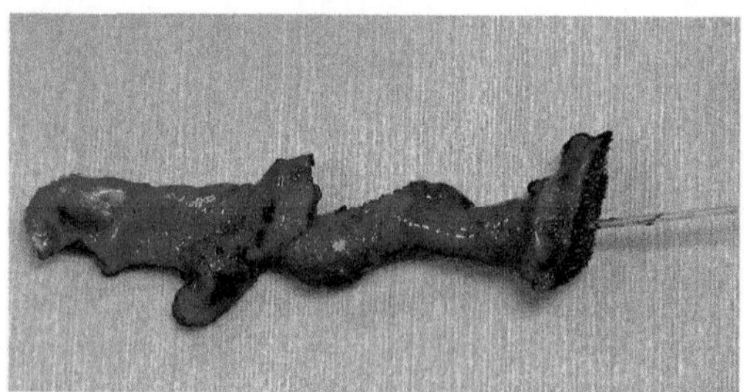

Fig. 5. Photograph of the dorsal sinus tract once removed surgically *en bloc*. (*Courtesy of* Dr Jim Lavely.)

Spinal dysraphism is caused by an inheritance of a codominant lethal gene with reduced penetrance and variable expression: homozygotes die; heterozygotes are variably clinically affected.[32] The primary lesion is caused by abnormal migration of mantle cells following neural tube closure ventral to the central canal in the floor plate of the developing spinal cord (24–28 days' gestation).[32] Various anomalies result including gray matter ectopias and disruption of spinal nuclei, absence of the ventral median fissure with associated fusion and flattening of the ventral horns, ventral diverticuli of the central canal and/or duplication, stenosis or absence of the central canal, disruption of the dorsal median septum, central gray matter loss, failure of separation of dura mater from vertebral arch, and syringohydromyelia and hydromyelia are also seen. The thoracic, lumbar, and sacral spinal cord segments are most commonly affected although the severity, extent, and location vary widely.[31–34]

Clinical signs usually are evident by 4 to 6 weeks of age and include a classic symmetric (bunny) hopping pelvic limb gait, crouched and wide based stance, unilateral pelvic limb abduction, and decreased pelvic limb proprioception. The syndrome is generally nonpainful and nonprogressive in nature, without urinary and fecal incontinence. Other less common anomalies concomitantly seen include scoliosis, koilosternia, and abnormal hair streams in the dorsal neck region.[31] Diagnosis is based on history, signalment, and examination. MRI may demonstrate a syrinx or hydromyelia and in conjunction with CSF analysis, may assist in ruling out other diseases. Although there is no treatment, most affected heterozygote animals can live functional lives.

There are many other case reports of CSD in dogs, with varying degrees of both vertebral column and spinal cord anomalies. The terminology used to describe the anomalies varies considerably, and care should be taken to note the exact description and extent of the pathology. Some examples of breeds reported include a Dalmatian with a C2-T5 extensive dorsal funiculi cavity without vertebral anomaly,[35] a Rottweiler with mid-thoracic so-called hemivertebrae, stenosis, and spinal cord microscopic lesions,[36] and a Samoyed with thoracic scoliosis and dorsal vertebral arch defect as well as syringomyelia.[37]

CONGENITAL ANOMALIES OF THE VERTEBRAL COLUMN

Congenital anomalies of the vertebral column are common in many breeds and are often incidental findings with no clinical significance.[38–40] The anomalies may appear singly or multiply (complex). The cause is generally not apparent; however, certain breeds are overrepresented such as the Bulldog.[38,39,41] Storage diseases, that is, mucolipidosis II, may also result in congenital spinal malformations.[42]

The classification systems used to identify this group of anomalies, both in the human and veterinary literature, are inconsistent, sometimes resulting in confusion and/or overlapping terminology. Most are based on the developmental stage of origin (embryonic vs fetal) with further separation into defects in formation versus defects in segmentation (**Box 3**). In this article the most common small animal vertebral column anomalies are listed, with clear definition of the structural extent of the anomaly, developmental origin (if known), direction of the angular deformity, clinical significance, and reported surgical treatments.

Congenital anomalies of the vertebral column may be associated with anomalies of the spinal cord and/or other systems, particularly those originating in the early (embryonic) developmental period. Reported associated defects in people include cardiac, renal, and gastrointestinal anomalies, and limb deformities as well as spinal cord and cranial malformations including Chiari malformations and various neural tube defects.[43,44]

Box 3
Classification of common congenital vertebral anomalies in dogs and cats

Embryonic period

- Diastematomyelia and centrum median cleft
- Centrum median cleft only (butterfly vertebrae)
- True hemivertebrae
  - with or without segmentation deformity
- Wedge vertebra (mediolateral wedged vertebrae)
  - with or without segmentation deformity
- Transitional vertebra (embryonic or fetal period depending on anomaly)

Fetal period

- Failure of segmentation and or late formation
  - Block vertebrae (partial or complete)
  - Hypoplasia of articular processes
  - Costovertebral joint failure of segmentation
  - Centrum hypoplasia or aplasia (dorsoventral wedged vertebrae)

Complex anomalies are those not readily classifiable or unclassifiable, and may involve any multiple defects of formation and segmentation.

Data from Tsou PM, Yau A, Hodgson AR. Embryogenesis and prenatal development of congenital vertebral anomalies and their classification. Clin Orthop Relat Res 1980;152:211–31.

Diagnosis of many simple vertebral deformities can be readily made with screening survey vertebral column radiographs in orthogonal projections. However, CT myelography or MRI is needed to identify the degree and level of spinal cord involvement. MRI may provide superior parenchymal information with respect to the presence of dysraphism, cyst, syrinx, edema, and alteration in CSF flow. The use of CT, particularly with 3-dimensional reconstruction, can more clearly identify the degree of bony malformation in complex or multiple malformations, and has been recently proposed as the method of classification of these lesions in humans.[45] Presurgical planning with advanced imaging is always advised.

Malformations Originating in the Embryonic Period of Development

Vertebral column anomalies originating in the embryonic period are caused by defects in formation, and may be associated with neural tube defects. Segmentation defects may occur secondarily. Those that involve only the vertebrae include butterfly vertebra and various forms of true or classic hemivertebra.

Butterfly vertebra

Butterfly vertebrae result from incomplete intradiscal migration of notochordal material resulting in bifid centrum formation.[46] The term butterfly vertebra comes from the appearance of a sagittal cleft in the vertebral body on viewing a ventrodorsal radiographic projection (**Fig. 6**). There is partial or complete failure of formation of the ventral and central portions of the vertebral body, leaving 2 dorsolateral fragments of bone attached to the neural arch. If the vertebral body is very diminutive it may result

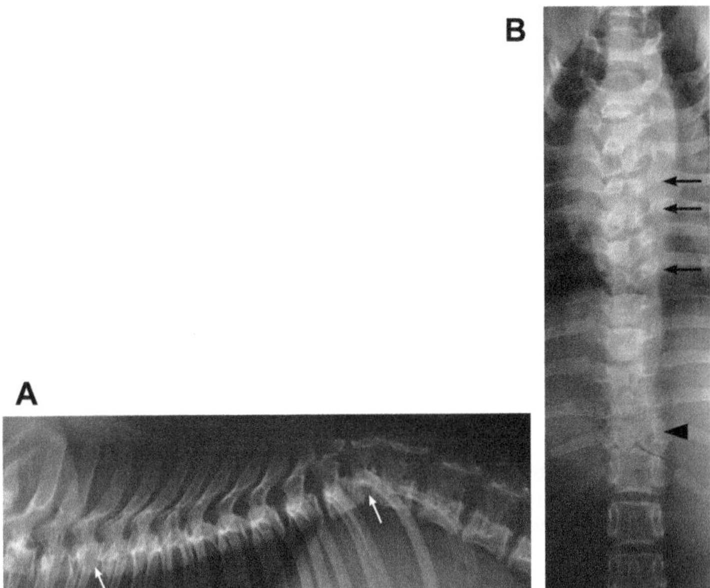

Fig. 6. Radiographs from a French Bulldog puppy. (*A*) The lateral projection shows an obvious vertebral anomaly at T3 and T12 (*white arrow*). (*B*) Ventrodorsal projection shows multiple vertebral anomalies in the cranial thoracic spine (*black arrow*). A butterfly vertebra can be clearly seen at T12 (*arrowhead*).

in kyphotic angulation, especially if associated with centrum hypoplasia. This anomaly is most often seen in brachycephalic, screw-tailed breeds and is often not clinically significant.[38]

Hemivertebra (with or without segmental defects)

Classic hemivertebra results from a failure to form one sagittal half of the vertebrae, including the centrum and neural arch (**Fig. 7**).[46,47] Although the cause is not known it most likely due to congenital absence of vascularization unilaterally,[46] resulting in predominantly scoliotic angulation deformities. An incomplete failure of formation leads to a laterally wedged vertebrae with a variable degree of unilateral hypoplasia; however, there are bilateral pedicles completing the vertebral arch (see **Fig. 7**A).[46,47] Further classification of these anomalies is based on the degree of segmentation failure during the fetal period, resulting in the presence or absence of fusion to vertebral bodies cranially or caudally (see **Fig. 7**B). Defects of segmentation result in a concave angulation on the side of the lateral block with restricted growth, due to loss of growth plates on the affected side.[47] Single or multiple ipsilateral anomalies may result in severe lateral angulation and hence scoliosis. A hemimetameric shift occurs if the angulation is counterbalanced with a contralateral hemivertebrae, with the resulting degree of scoliosis being less pronounced.[46] Mixed malformations may result in complex and not readily classifiable anomalies.

Malformations Originating in the Fetal Period of Development

Vertebral column anomalies originating in the fetal period are associated with defects in formation and particularly segmentation. Such deformities are well differentiated and occur late in the chrondrification and ossification stages, and are much less

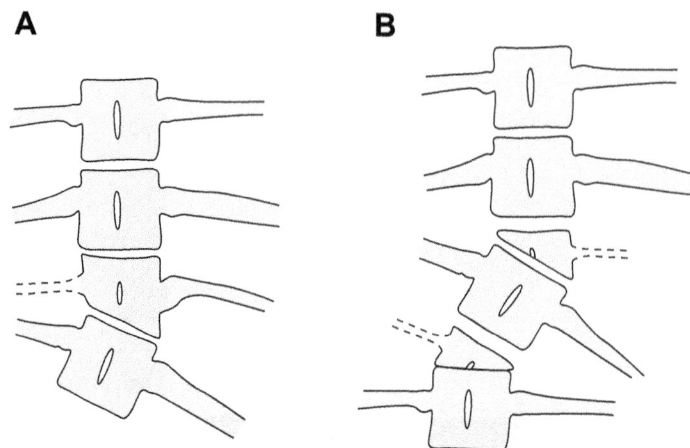

Fig. 7. Vertebral malformations resulting in predominantly scoliotic angulation deformities. (*A*) Wedge-shaped vertebra. (*B*) Hemivertebra unsegmented (*above*) and contralateral partially segmented hemivertebra (*below*). Note that hemivertebra, unlike the wedge vertebra, have an incomplete neural arch. Segmentation may occur partially as shown here, or fully (cranially and caudally).

commonly associated with other defects and spinal cord anomalies because they occur after the formation of those structures.[46] Anomalies originating in this period of development include centrum hypoplasia or aplasia, partial or block vertebra, neural arch apophyseal joint failure, and costovertebral joint failure of segmentation (see **Box 3**).[46]

Vertebral anomalies of the centrum result in predominantly kyphotic angulation deformities caused by diminished vertebral body longitudinal growth. These anomalies affect the vertebral body only (unless a mixed deformity), with normal or near normal neural arch development,[43] and are caused by a defect in formation or segmentation.[46] Centrum hypoplasia or aplasia results in variable loss of the body, and bilateral or unilateral defects may occur (**Fig. 8**). Unilateral centrum defects may result in a degree of scoliosis (kyphoscoliosis) (see **Fig. 8**B). The cause is not known, but in severe forms may be due to congenital absence of vascularization or may be caused by any teratogenic insult to the very active cartilaginous proliferation in the ventral rim. The term hemivertebra is inappropriate for such malformations.[48]

The degree of kyphosis that results is related to the number of vertebrae affected and the severity of the centrum defect. The least deforming is the dorsoventral wedge (see **Fig. 8**C). Other forms have greater propensity for instability, stenosis, and kyphosis with or without scoliosis as evident by their inherent ventral defect (see **Fig. 8**A, B). Dorsal displacement of a severely affected vertebra (centrum aplasia or severe hypoplasia) above the main curvature of the spine may cause severe local angulation and spinal cord compression.

One of the first reports of such anomalies was by Reihart[49] in 1950. The most commonly affected breeds are those with screw tails, namely Bulldog, French Bulldog, Pug, and Boston Terrier.[38,39] Other breeds have been described, including the German short-haired pointer with an autosomal recessively inherited trait.[50] The most common area involved is the coccygeal segments in screwtail breeds and the mid to caudal thoracic region. Such anomalies are described rarely in cats[51] and may be associated with storage disorders such as autosomal recessively acquired

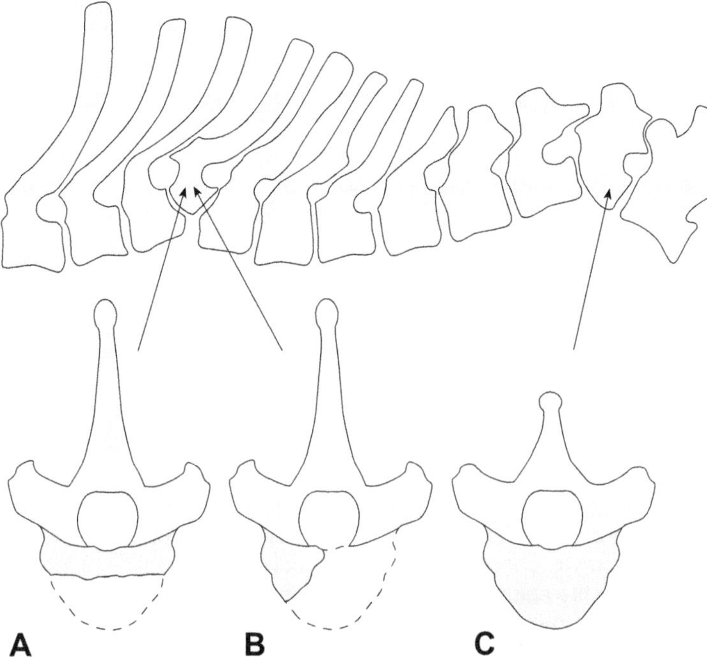

Fig. 8. Vertebral malformations resulting in kyphotic or kyphoscoliotic angulation deformities due to centrum defects. Complex centrum defects may be seen where much of the ventral centrum is missing and severe angulation deformities result (*A*), or (*B*) ventrolateral centrum defect results in kyphoscoliosis. (*C*) A wedge vertebra (ventrodorsal) with the apex ventral.

mucolipidosis II.[42] Although these defects are present at birth, often they are not clinically apparent until 4 to 10 months of age (adolescence) when the most dramatic and rapid curvatures may be seen during periods of accelerated growth.[43,52] Clinical signs are often progressive until skeletal maturity occurs and onset may be acute, chronic, or intermittent. If associated with a degenerative process, for example, intervertebral disc degeneration and subsequent protrusion/extrusion, ligamentous hypertrophy, or articular remodeling, onset of neurologic signs may occur in mature animals.

Lateral projection radiographs may reveal ventrodorsal wedging of the body, with the apex orientated ventrally (**Fig. 9**). Advanced imaging, especially MRI, provides

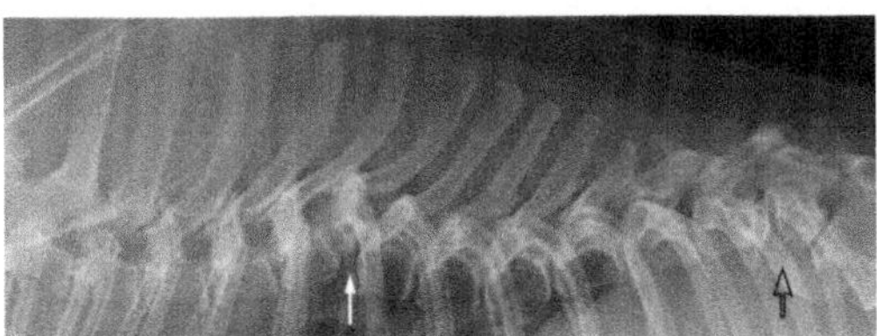

Fig. 9. Lateral projection radiograph of the thoracic vertebral column illustrating centrum defects. Note the 2 kyphotic angulation deformities: severe centrum defect at T6 (*arrow*) and wedge vertebra (ventrodorsal) at T13 (*open arrow*).

necessary information regarding both extrinsic (degree of compression) and intrinsic spinal cord changes (**Fig. 10**).

Surgical decompression or an attempt to realign the vertebral column has been infrequently reported for such vertebral anomalies in animals (**Figs. 11** and **12**). In 2007 Aikawa and colleagues[52] reported 9 dogs and Jeffery and colleagues[53] reported 3 dogs with predominantly thoracic kyphotic deformations. Dorsal laminectomy or hemilaminectomy provided decompression, and most cases were stabilized with pins and polymethylmethacrylate, with some success.[52,53] Recently Havlicek and colleagues[51] reported a cat that underwent dorsal decompression for a kyphotic thoracic anomaly without stabilization, and returned to full ambulation and only mild residual ataxia.

People with kyphotic deformities more frequently suffer neurologic deficits than those with scoliotic deformities. Early intervention is strongly recommended both to prevent progressive neurologic deterioration and to avoid the need for late correction in the mature spine. Dorsal arthrodesis of the facets is often done when the angular deformity is less than 45° as determined by the modified Cobb method.[43] In many cases this can adequately limit the deformity when done early in children younger than 5 years. If greater than 45°, anterior release is required, usually with strut grafting, instrumentation, and posterior arthrodesis to correct and stabilize the deformity.[54] In humans, laminectomy is considered absolutely contraindicated.[54,55] Laminectomy is ineffective because the spinal cord is often not compressed posteriorly and removal of the posterior bony structures destabilizes the spine, resulting in more rapid progression of the kyphosis and greater anterior spinal cord compression. In cases where there are complex anomalies, stenosis of the vertebral canal and/or instability lateral posterior corpectomy and instrumentation with fusion to decompress the anterior surface of the spinal cord at the maximum point of angulation is appropriate, with care to preserve segmental arterial supply to the spinal cord.[55]

Block vertebrae

Block vertebrae are another example of failure of segmentation during embryogenesis, and result from partial or complete fusion of 2 or more vertebrae (**Fig. 13**). In some cases this fusion may occur predominantly in one plane or unilaterally, resulting in a bony bar

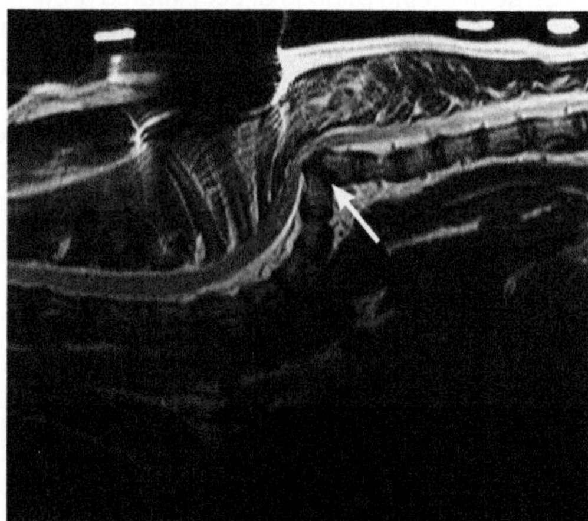

Fig. 10. Sagittal T2-weighted MRI of the thoracic region of a French bulldog. Note the severe kyphotic deformity and ventral compression of the spinal cord (*arrow*). T5 and T7 are wedge-shaped and T6 has a severe centrum defect.

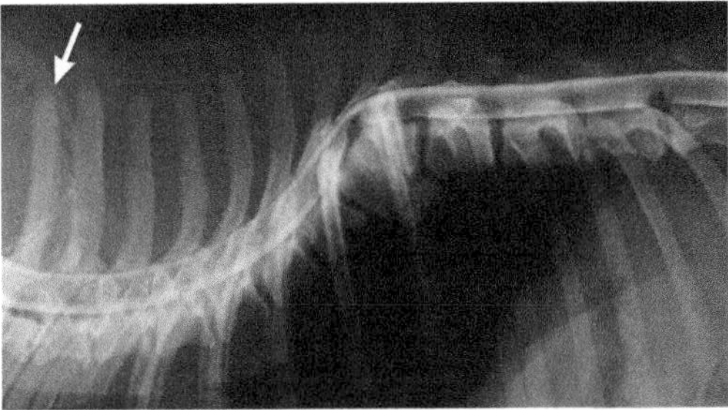

Fig. 11. Lateral projection myelogram from an 8-year-old Pug with acute onset of paraplegia. A centrum anomaly (wedge vertebra) resulting in kyphosis with ventral spondylosis at T9 is apparent. Ventral extradural compression at the T8 to T9 disc space is noted. Note also the bifid spine that is visible at T1 (*arrow*). This dog resumed normal ambulation after surgical decompression was performed.

restricting growth, and may cause an angular deformity in that plane. Any adjoining part(s) of the vertebrae may be involved, that is, vertebral arch with fused nonarticulated processes, or centrum with or without the intervertebral disc formed. The segments may be of normal length or shortened. Often these anomalies are not associated with neurologic deficits, but may occur in cases of angular deformation, stenosis of the vertebral canal, or if there is abnormal loading of adjacent vertebra, leading to intervertebral disc degeneration/protrusion, instability, or ligament hypertrophy.[56]

Articular facet aplasia/dysplasia

Articular facet aplasia/dysplasia is an anomaly relating to reduced formation or absence of the articular processes or facet (zygapophyseal, diarthrodial synovial joints). In dogs such entities are apparently frequent, but poorly reported.[38] The

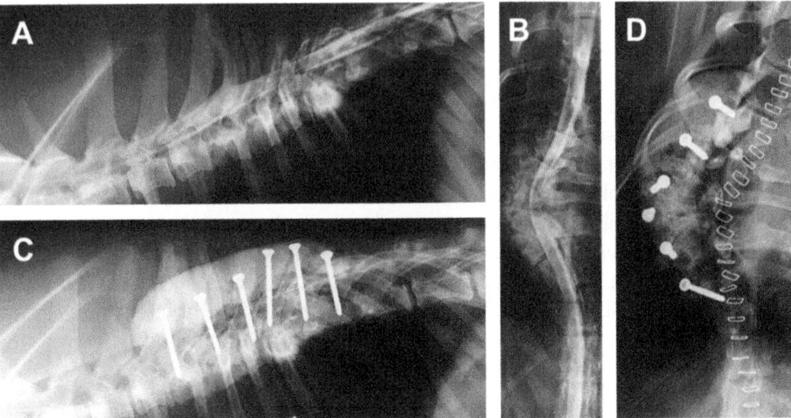

Fig. 12. Radiographic study of a 7-month-old shepherd cross with progressive paraparesis. At the time of presentation she was nonambulatory. (*A*) Lateral projection myelogram showing multiple vertebral anomalies in the cranial and mid-thoracic spine. Note the meningocele at T4. (*B*) Ventrodorsal projection myelogram showing marked scoliosis secondary to complex vertebral anomalies. (*C, D*) Lateral ventrodorsal projection postoperative radiographs. Surgical decompression from T4 to T10 with stabilization using screws and bone cement was performed. The puppy was ambulatory again 2 weeks later.

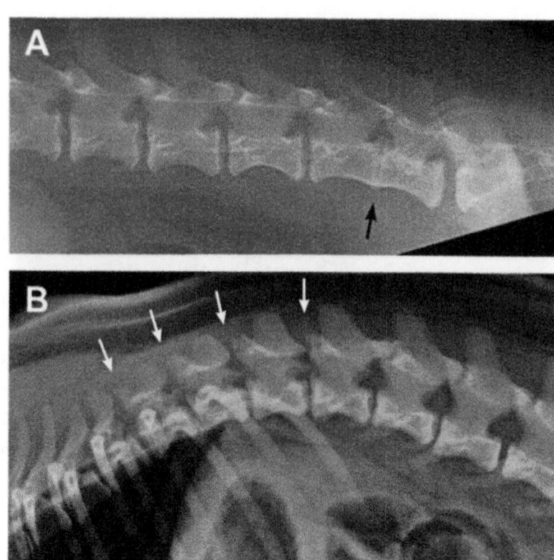

Fig. 13. Lateral projection radiograph of the lumbar spine. (*A*) Note the partially fused L6 to L7 vertebrae (*arrow*). Ten-month-old Pug dog with articular facet aplasia clearly evident from T10-11 caudally to L1-2 (*arrows*) (*B*). This dog had 7 lumbar vertebrae but only 12 thoracic vertebrae (with bilateral costa) counting from T1. The anticlinal vertebra was T10. The dog had no pain or neurological deficits referable to this area.

pathogenesis has not been fully determined, but is postulated to result from either dysgenesis of the 2 neural arch centers of ossification or abnormal development of secondary ossification centers.[57]

In 1968 Morgan[38] observed in a series of 145 dogs that almost every case had some degree of anomalous change to the articular facet(s). In general, this involved just mild changes to shape and size. More severe changes were noted to include uni- or bilateral absence of the articular process, and most commonly the anomalies were found cranial to T10 in the thoracic region.[38] More recently, 3 other articles have also demonstrated such anomalies and have attempted to review the clinical significance. In 2002 Breit[58] examined 140 spines in neurologically normal large, chondrodystrophic, and small breed dogs, and found T1-T9 segments to be exclusively affected and in small breed dogs only. There was no apparent association of such anomalies and intervertebral disc disease or deformative spondylosis. A case of bilateral aplasia of the caudal T12, both cranial and caudal T13 and cranial L1 articular processes without apparent gross instability, has been reported in a small breed dog, showing possible association with intervertebral disc extrusion.[57] Another series of 4 dogs of varying size had either aplasia (3) or hypoplasia (1) of the caudal facets joints at the thoracolumbar junction (T12–L1) or L5. Associated with this was cranial articular process degeneration and proliferation of the joint capsule and ligamentum flavum, causing stenotic myelopathy in the 3 cases with aplasia.[59]

Transitional vertebrae

Transitional vertebrae are congenital anomalies usually found at the junction between 2 divisions of the vertebral column, that is, cervicothoracic, thoracolumbar, lumbosacral, or sacrocaudal, and may result in variations in the number of vertebrae found within a division. Characteristics of adjacent divisions are exhibited in a single vertebra, unilaterally or bilaterally. This condition most commonly involves the presence or absence of a costa or transverse process.[38] Examples are elongated C7 transverse process resembling a costa, absence of a rib at T13 and/or short misshapen transverse process, L7 attached to sacrum by fused transverse process and/or body (sacralization of L7), or partially divided S1-S2 segment (lumbarization of S1) and variation in the level of the anticlinal vertebra (T10 or T11). The cause of these anomalies is not known, but involves border shifts of somites and is a defect of segmentation (**Fig. 14**).

Transitional vertebrae are one of the most common anomalies, and have been well described in most breeds of dogs[38] and cats.[40] In general, animals remain asymptomatic. As described for block vertebrae, changes in force dynamics to adjacent vertebrae can result in instability or intervertebral disc herniation. The German Shepherd dog and relatives are well described in the literature regarding lumbosacral involvement and associated stenosis (see article on degenerative lumbosacral stenosis in this issue). Recognition of a transitional segment is especially important during surgery of the spine because failure to do this may result in performing a procedure at a level cranial or caudal to that expected, particularly in the thoracolumbar spine.

Spinal stenosis

Spinal stenosis is a narrowing or stricture of the vertebral canal or intervertebral foramen, in any plane or level. It can occur focally, segmentally, or generalized throughout the spine. Several classification systems have been applied to spinal stenosis in humans, including a classification based on primary elements producing the stenosis,[60] presumed etiology,[61] location of the anatomic narrowing,[62] and others. In this article the spinal stenoses recognized in domestic animals are classified by presumed etiology into congenital/developmental and acquired causes.

Congenital spinal stenoses are malformations that are present at the time of birth but for which there is no active underlying cause. This type of stenosis

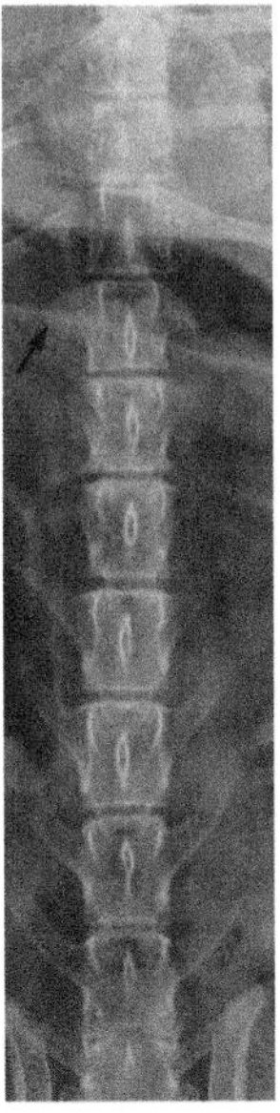

Fig. 14. Ventrodorsal projection radiograph of the thoracolumbar vertebral column with a transitional vertebra. Note the missing costa and small perpendicular deformed transverse process on the right side of T13 (*arrow*).

may occur alone or in association with other congenital anomalies of the spine or spinal cord, including spinal dysraphism, hemivertebrae, and block vertebrae (**Figs. 15** and **16**).[60] A mid-sagittal vertebral canal diameter that is small enough to result in compression of neural elements directly is referred to as absolute stenosis, whereas a diameter that is less than normal (for the breed), but not causing neural compression or clinical signs, is termed relative stenosis. This type of stenosis may become symptomatic if another space-occupying pathological condition is superimposed, such as disc protrusion or ligamentous hypertrophy.[60]

Doberman Pinschers have been described with cranial thoracic (T3–T6) dorsoventral diameter of the canal, often with impingement of the spinal cord without overt compression.[41] The malformation is apparent on routine spinal radiographs most commonly affect the T3 to T6 vertebrae associated with mild spinal curvature (kyphosis). On myelography or MRI the vertebrae show a decrease in the dorsoventral diameter of the vertebral canal as compared with adjacent vertebrae, but spinal cord compression is not usually present. Two unrelated 5-month-old Dogues de Bordeaux were reported with dorsolateral cranial thoracic stenosis (T2–4 and T4–6) and thickening of the pedicle, causing spinal cord compression. Decompressive dorsal laminectomy and medial pediculectomy without stabilization was done, with slow recovery to reasonable function.[63] The authors also have seen several giant breed puppies, usually Bull Mastiffs or Great Danes between 8 and 15 months of age, that have segmental spinal stenosis commonly seen in the T2 to T4 region. These dogs generally have spinal cord compression on imaging studies. Additional similar case reports include a 3-month-old Basset Hound with progressive paraparesis due to T12 to T13 stenosis and malformation of the lamina causing spinal cord compression,[64] and a bulldog with T3 to T4 bony dorsolateral stenosis.[65] This dog also had wedged-shaped vertebrae most likely due to ventral centrum hypoplasia at T9 and T10, without spinal cord compression at that level. Thoracic congenital spinal stenosis was also reported in 2 English Bulldogs.[66] In addition, transitional vertebrae may frequently be stenotic or may predispose to acquired stenosis, especially in the lumbosacral location (see on degenerative lumbosacral stenosis in this issue).

Developmental stenoses are malformations that are present at the time of birth with an active underlying cause that remains present throughout the growth period until the

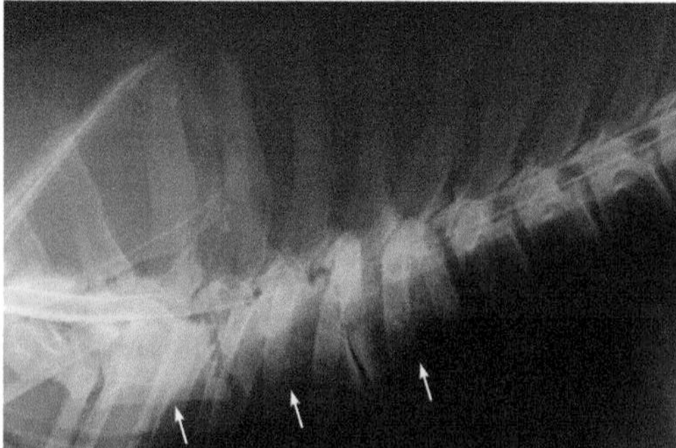

Fig. 15. Lateral projection myelogram of the cervicothoracic spine in a 16-month-old Labrador retriever with progressive paraparesis. There are multiple complex block vertebra at C7-T1, T2-T3, and T4-T5 (*arrows*), and associated segmental spinal stenosis (T1-T5).

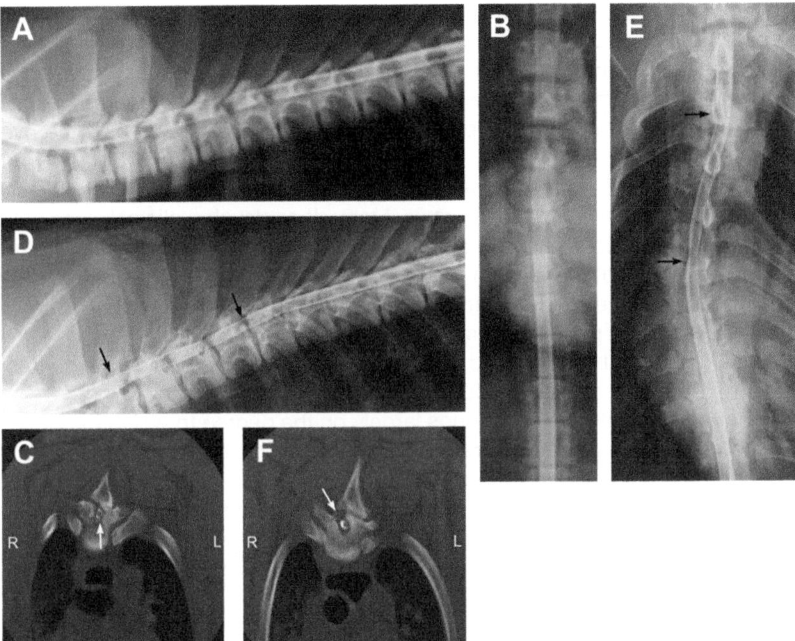

Fig. 16. Myelogram images from a Doberman Rottweiler cross puppy with a progressive T3-L3 myelopathy. (*A, B*) Lateral and ventrodorsal radiographs obtained at 6 months of age when the puppy first presented for nonambulatory paraparesis. A segmental stenosis can be seen from T2 to T5. (*C*) Axial CT image at the level to T3. Note the profound osseous thickening of the vertebral arch compressing the spinal cord (*arrow*). Decompressive surgery was performed over the length of this region via hemidorsal laminectomy on the right side, and the puppy became ambulatory shortly thereafter. (*D*) Four months later the puppy again developed progressive paraparesis and diagnostic CT myelography was repeated. On this lateral radiograph the stenosis is again evident over the same region (*arrows*), only more pronounced this time. (*E*) Ventrodorsal images obtained showed that scoliosis was occurring as well, possibly secondary to the "destabilizing" effects of previous surgical procedure. (*F*) Regrowth of bone over previous laminectomy site and ongoing stenosis on the unoperated side can be seen. A second decompressive surgery was done once the dog reached skeletal maturity, and the dog regained the ability to walk. Ten years later the dog remained ambulatory without clinical reoccurrence of stenosis.

vertebrae have reached maturity. Developmental stenosis in humans may be caused by genetic mutations leading to inborn errors in the metabolism of cells involved in ossification and/or bone growth.[60] Generalized spinal stenosis usually results, although it may be more clinically significant in one region of the spine over another. This type of stenosis is relatively common in people, and has been associated with hypochondroplasia and achondroplasia. In this condition a disproportion between a narrowed vertebral canal and the volume of neural elements within the canal often leads to clinical signs, especially affecting the lower lumbar region.[60] This condition is also present in chondrodysplastic dogs[67] and may be part of the reason that clinically significant disc disease is so common in these breeds.

Cats have also been described with stenosis of the thoracolumbar spine caused by bony proliferation associated with mucopolysaccharidosis VI.[68,69]

Acquired spinal stenoses may be associated with conditions such as hypertrophied ligaments, intervertebral disc protrusion, degenerative articular changes, synovial cysts, and malarticulation-malformation syndromes with or without associated vertebral anomalies[60]; this may be caused by a multifactorial etiology whereby superimposed acquired stenosis causes a previously subclinical disease to become overtly significant.

As with all spinal malformations, the clinical signs of spinal stenosis reflect the site(s) of the lesion localization along the neuraxis. Many dogs develop clinical signs associated with congenital stenosis in adult life. The signs may have an acute or chronic onset, and be symmetric or asymmetric in nature. The course of the disease may be that of steady decline or a more stepwise progression. Diagnosis of spinal stenosis can often be made by plain radiography; however, if surgical treatment is contemplated, advanced imaging is needed. CT and/or MRI allow more accurate characterization of the bony and soft tissue components of the spinal stenoses.

Treatment of spinal stenoses depends largely on the degree to which the patient is affected neurologically, whether there is ongoing neurologic deterioration and/or pain, and the age of the animal. In the authors' experience, most dogs respond well to surgical decompression with or without spinal stabilization. However, in dogs that have surgery before bony development is complete, reoccurrence secondary to regrowth is possible. In this situation, reoperation of the stenosis after skeletal maturity is reached is generally successful.

Atlantoaxial Instability

Instability of the atlantoaxial (AA) region allows excessive flexion of the joint that may result in subluxation, traumatic spinal cord injury, and compression. This condition usually occurs secondary to congenital or developmental abnormalities of the bones or ligaments of the AA joint, traumatic injury to the joint, or a combination of both.[70–72] In many instances, the abnormalities present are associated with the dens and include agenesis/hypoplasia of the dens, dorsal angulation of the dens, and fracture or avulsion of the dens with the axis. Absence or rupture of associated AA ligaments often contributes to the instability caused by congenital anomalies in the region.[70–72] Dorsal displacement of the cranial portion of the body of the axis into the vertebral canal, acutely or chronically, causes compression, edema, and inflammation of the spinal cord that may extend cranially into the caudal brainstem (**Fig. 17**).

The atlas (C1) and axis (C2) normally form a pivotal joint that allows free movement of the head about the longitudinal axis of the spine. During development, part of the atlas centrum fuses with that of the axis so that at birth the axis has 7 ossification centers, with the dens or odontoid process morphologically derived from the atlas and lying within the vertebral foramen of the atlas.[70] On the apical tip of the dens there is a transient ossification seen in many animals called the proatlas, which is most likely a remnant vertebra interposed between the skull and the atlas. The proatlas centrum forms as a nodule or cap on the cranial end of the dens and eventually fuses with it by about 3 months of age.[70] An un-united proatlas centrum may mistakenly be interpreted as fracture of the dens. There are several reports of fractures of the dens and the apparent absence of the dens causing AA instability in dogs.[72–74] It is not clear whether the absence of the odontoid process is always due to a congenital absence of an ossification center or whether it may be caused by traumatically induced ischemic necrosis in some breeds of dogs.[75]

Most of the rotational movement of the AA joint centers around the dens, which projects cranially from the rostral aspect of the body of the axis and is held in position relative to the atlas by the apical, alar, and transverse ligaments. The atlas articulates

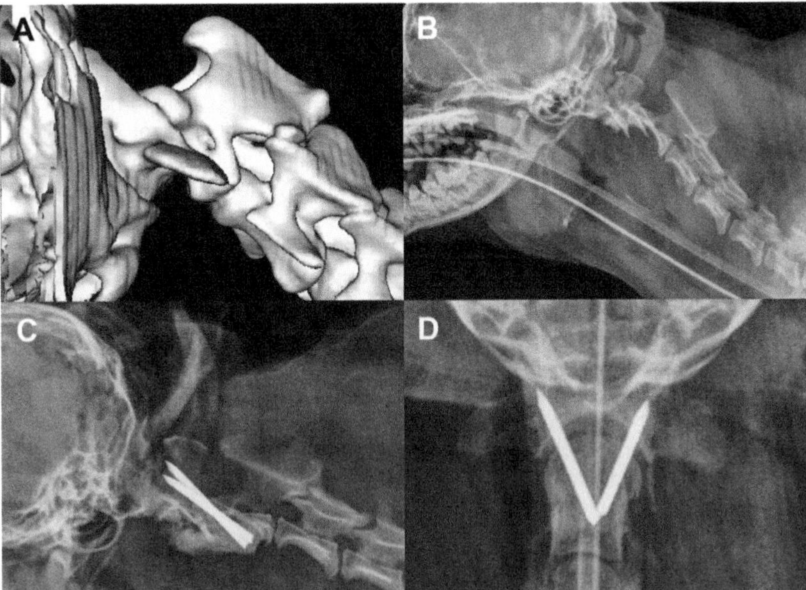

Fig. 17. Atlantoaxial instability and ventral surgical repair of a 10-month-old Yorkshire terrier. (*A*) Three-dimensional CT reconstruction and (*B*) lateral projection radiograph of the cervical vertebral column. Note the dorsal displacement of C2 relative to C1, and the separation of the dorsal aspects of C1 and C2 lamina. (*C*) Postoperative lateral radiograph, (*D*) postoperative ventrodorsal radiograph.

rostrally with the occipital condyles of the skull and forms a joint of which the main movements are flexion and extension of the head. Caudally, the atlas articulates with the axis allowing lateral (and rotational) movement of the head. Working together, these 2 joints allow free motion of the head in all directions. The large nuchal ligament, which attaches the spinous process of C2 with those of T1 and T2, functions in suspension of the head by forming a fulcrum at the AA joint.

AA instability with subluxation of C2 relative to C1 is a frequent cause of cervical pain and/or myelopathy in toy and miniature breeds of dogs, occurring most frequently in Chihuahuas, Yorkshire terriers, Toy and Miniature poodles, Pomeranians, Japanese Chin, Maltese dogs, and others. On rare occasions, large breeds of dogs, and cats, may also be affected.[71,72,76,77] Clinical signs of a C1-C5 myelopathy and/or cervical pain occur and may be acute or chronic in onset, and progressive, nonprogressive, or intermittent in nature. Often the signs occur secondary to mild "trauma" such as jumping off the bed or roughhousing with other dogs. Onset of signs commonly occurs within the first year of life, although they may occur in dogs older than a year, including middle- to older-aged animals. Severity in clinical signs varies from mild cervical pain to profound cervical pain to tetraparesis, respiratory paralysis, and caudal brainstem signs (eg, hypoventilation, vestibular signs). Because AA subluxation is a potentially life-threatening problem, it is important to recognize when AA instability *may* be present so that the patient is handled appropriately; this will prevent exacerbation of the clinical signs until a definitive diagnosis is made and appropriate treatment is instituted. Occasionally dogs with AA instability may present with a history of seizure-like signs occurring intermittently, with or without transient apnea and paresis.[41] Often these episodes can be related to a mild trauma such as jumping off furniture, and usually occur with malformations of the dens, specifically agenesis of the dens or dorsal angulation of the dens.

Differential diagnoses for dogs with this clinical presentation should include intervertebral disc disease, cervical trauma/spinal fracture, infectious/inflammatory disease (eg, granulomatous meningoencephalitis [GME]), other craniospinal anomalies (eg, syringomyelia, Chiari-like malformation), and neoplasia (cervical spine or brain). A diagnosis of instability at the AA joint should be considered a clinically significant finding and treated promptly.

Plain cervical radiography usually provides the diagnosis in most instances.[78] Because it is essential that positioning be accurate when evaluating the AA region of the cervical spine, general anesthesia is necessary. Radiographically the body of the axis is displaced dorsally and cranially into the vertebral canal, and the distance between the dorsal arch of the atlas and spinous process of the axis is increased (see **Fig. 17**B) If lateral views are not diagnostic, slight flexion of the head may be necessary to demonstrate subluxation or instability of the AA joint. Abnormalities of the dens may be seen clearly on oblique lateral views, in which the wings of the atlas are not superimposed on the dens, and/or ventrodorsal views. Myelography (via lumbar injection) and/or CT imaging may be required to confirm that subluxation is present, to further delineate regional problems when multiple congenital anomalies are present and/or to rule out other differential diagnoses in the same region of localization (eg, disc disease) (see **Fig. 17**).

MRI may be very useful in the diagnosis of AA subluxation, especially in patients with clinical signs of brain or brainstem disease as well as cervical pain and myelopathy (**Fig. 18**). The extent of the parenchymal injury to the cervical cord and/or caudal brainstem is best visualized on MRI. A region of hyperintensity on T2-weighted images typically is visible in the cranial cervical spinal cord and/or caudal brainstem on MR images. In addition, MR imaging is useful for ruling out the presence of concurrent diseases with clinical signs localizing to the same region and for identifying underlying disease that may influence long-term prognosis. Collection of CSF is recommended in cases where the diagnosis is not straightforward on imaging, especially in breeds of dogs typically prone to inflammatory disease (eg, GME) of the brain.

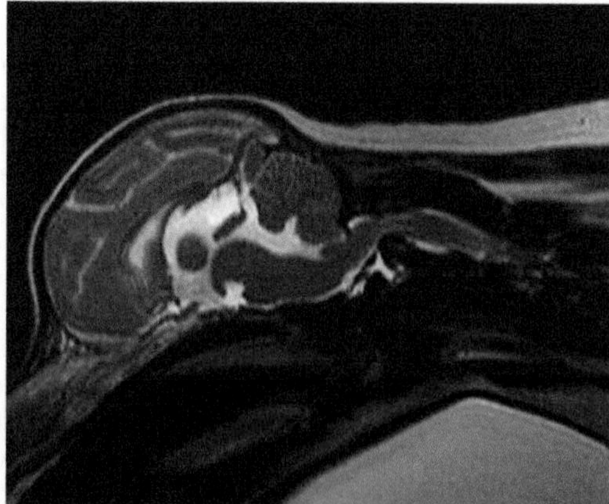

Fig. 18. Sagittal T2-weighted MRI of the brain and C1 to C2 region. The dens (C2) is causing ventral compression of the cervical spinal cord secondary to dorsal displacement of C2, and there is hyperintensity in the spinal cord consistent with edema/inflammation.

Animals with cervical pain only or minimal neurologic deficits may respond well to splinting of the head and neck in mild extension and strict cage rest for at least 6 weeks. However, clinical signs often recur when the animal returns to normal activity. Surgical decompression and stabilization is indicated in animals with moderate to severe neurologic deficits, intense pain, or those that are unresponsive to nonsurgical treatment.[78–80] Surgery is also recommended in animals in which angulation of the dens results in spinal cord injury. Animals younger than 6 months are best treated conservatively, if possible, to allow for more complete mineralization of bone and closure of vertebral physes before attempting surgical stabilization. Conservative treatment certainly should be attempted in situations where financial constraints do not allow surgical repair to be done. The reader is referred to standard medical and surgical texts for details on current surgical and nonsurgical treatment options.

The prognosis for animals with AA subluxation varies depending on the chronicity and severity of the spinal cord injury that occurs. Generally speaking, long-term outcome is very good to excellent for animals treated surgically that have clinical signs of pain and/or mild to moderate neurologic deficits. Animals presenting with severe tetraparesis/plegia and respiratory distress, especially with a chronic history, have a guarded prognosis for good recovery of neurologic function.[79,81] Recently reported success rates of ventral surgical techniques vary from 79% to 92% for a good to excellent outcome[79,81–84] with no one method proving to be superior to the others with respect to long-term survival. The experience and comfort level of the surgeon in performing surgery in the AA region is likely one of most important influences on the overall outcome of patients with AA disease.

A recent study looking at the long-term outcome of dogs treated nonsurgically found that dogs with an acute onset of clinical signs and no prior history of signs of AA instability had a good outcome about 60% of the time, regardless of the severity of the presenting neurologic status.[80] Dogs treated nonsurgically that had clinical signs for longer than 30 days were significantly more likely to have a poor final outcome.

VASCULAR MALFORMATIONS

Vascular malformations of the spine are rare in dogs. There are 8 case reports of vascular malformations resulting in myelopathy in dogs: cavernous angioma,[85] intramedullary hamartoma,[86] arteriovenous malformation in the cervical[87] and thoracolumbar region,[88] lumbosacral angioectatic malformation,[89] ectatic radicular arteries due to aplasia of the right subclavian artery[90] (**Fig. 19**), intramedullary cavernous malformation,[91] and intramedullary vascular cyst–like anomaly.[92] Treatment has been accomplished using endovascular occlusion via arteriography[90] and open surgical excision and decompression in dogs.[86,92]

In cats, the reported vascular malformation of the spine is vertebral angiomatosis, and was first reported in 1987.[93] All cats had thoracic spine involvement, most often between T10 and T12 or cranially (T2, T4).[93–95] All cats were younger than 2 years with a slowly, apparently painful, progressive myelopathy. Myelography and CT showed extradural compression with proliferative or lytic changes to the vertebra (mottled appearance). Pathology consisted of bony and vascular benign proliferations (angiomas). In 2 cats hemilaminectomy was done, decompression afforded, with good outcome,[93,94] and another died during anesthetic recovery from a hemilaminectomy, cause not determined.[95]

In humans vascular malformations of the spine are well described and arteriovenous malformations are the most common.[96,97] Treatment of such entities is well reported

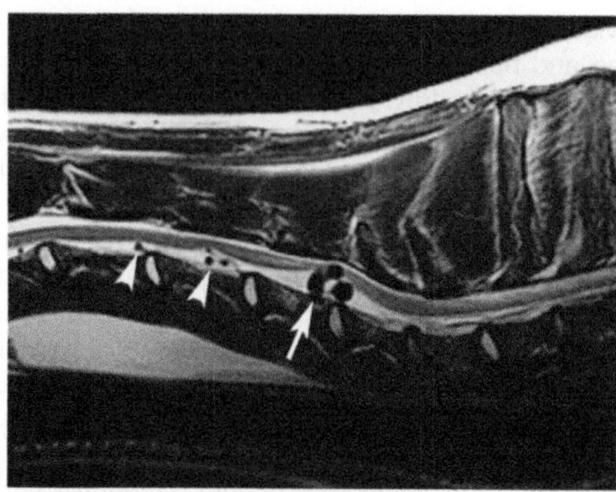

Fig. 19. Sagittal T2-weighted MRI of the cervical spinal cord with a vascular anomaly. Large flow voids consistent with abnormally dilated vascular structures are evident at C5 to C6 (*arrow*) causing marked spinal cord compression. Additional smaller flow voids are present at the level of the body of C3 and C4 (*arrowheads*).

with endovascular management using prothrombotic devices such as coils, or surgical excision and/or bypass techniques.[96,97]

ARACHNOID DIVERTICULA

Previously commonly called arachnoid cysts (a misnomer), arachnoid diverticula are an accumulation of CSF and dilation of a focal area of the meninges, and may be apparently congenital or acquired.[98] These relatively uncommon structures have also been called intra-arachnoid or subarachnoid cysts, meningeal cysts, leptomeningeal cysts, and pseudocysts. In humans, cyst-like structures of the meninges have been classified into 3 types,[98] with Type III (intradural forms) best fitting those that are described in dogs.[99–102] Further classification in humans relating to continuity versus isolation of the cyst-like structure to the subarachnoid space has also been reported.[103] In dogs, as in people, these entities are not true cysts, having no epithelial cell lining; nor are they typically closed, in fact usually there is an obvious connection to the subarachnoid space.

Histopathologically the structures are lined by meningothelial cells and are separated from the spinal cord by intact pia mater. The histopathologic descriptions vary from no apparent change, to fibrosis and/or hyperplasia of the meninges and/or arachnoid trabeculae, with/or without mild inflammatory infiltrate.

The etiology of these entities is unknown, and most are idiopathic.[100] In young dogs and children they are considered congenital. Anomalous structures occurring dorsally may be caused by diverticulae in the septum posticum.[104] Congenital forms may be associated with a neural tube defects and syringohydromyelia[100] and vertebral column spinal deformities.[104,105] Arachnoid diverticulae are also recognized in mature dogs, where they may be acquired versus late onset, with expansion of a congenital anomaly due to alterations in local CSF flow dynamics and arachnoid trabeculae structure. Acquired forms may occur at a site of previous trauma, arachnoiditis, intervertebral disc disease, previous surgery, hematomas, or meningitis.

Since first described by Gage and colleagues[106] in 1968, there have been numerous case reports and case series with more than 54 cases represented.[102] Although most commonly reported to occur in the Rottweiler, many breeds have been reported.

Almost any segment of the spine may be affected. The cervical region, specifically C2 to C4, is most commonly affected in larger breeds, whereas that of the caudal thoracic or thoracolumbar region occurs in any breed, but particularly smaller breeds. Extent is variable from less than 1 to multiple vertebral lengths. Multiple and ventrally situated diverticulae have also been reported, and may occur in propinquity or remotely.[99] Congenital arachnoid diverticulae are occasionally reported in cats.[107]

Presentation usually is of a slowly progressive myelopathy, with or without apparent pain. Fecal and urinary incontinence are commonly reported. Age of onset is very variable but congenital forms may show onset within the first few months of life. Diagnosis can be made using myelography or MRI. Myelographic appearance is of focal accumulation of contrast, usually dorsally or dorsolaterally. It is often tapered caudally and ends more abruptly cranially as a "teardrop" shape on the lateral projection, although orientation may be vice versa. MRI appearance is as described for myelography on sagittal images with focal accumulation of CSF at the level of the dilation (**Figs. 20** and **21**). There may also be, particularly cranially to point of greatest compression, T2-weighted hyperintensity within the spinal cord parenchyma, consistent with edema, malacia, and/or syringohydromyelia. Neural tube defects may also be apparent. Occasionally MRI has been used to document CSF flow into and within the dilation.[101,103]

CSF analysis has been variably reported. Often there is a normal cell count and albuminocytological disassociation with mild to markedly elevated protein (up to 200 mg/dL) versus very mild mononuclear pleocytosis, that is, less than 10 cells/μL.[99]

Conservative therapy with prednisone may be considered and in some cases can stabilize the myelopathy, with even low doses achieving good effect. No analysis in the literature of such treatment and long-term outcome has been performed, however, thus there are no specific recommendations.

Surgery is often indicated and in progressive cases should be recommended. Care should be taken to review for any other underlying disease as outlined earlier that may otherwise contribute to reformation of the diverticulae or result in lack of resolution of signs. Routine approach and exposure of the spinal cord with hemilaminectomy

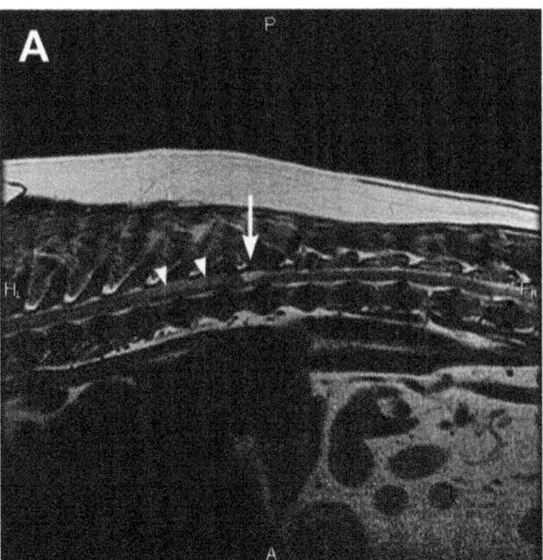

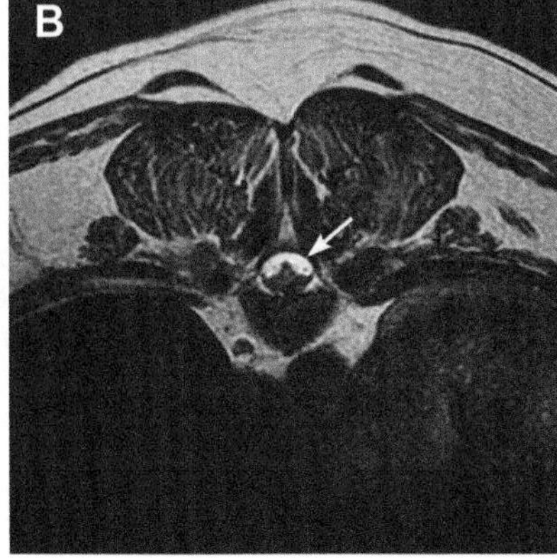

Fig. 20. (*A*) Sagittal T2-weighted MRI at the level of T10 with arachnoid diverticula. There is a teardrop-shaped diverticulum dorsolaterally at T10 (*arrow*) and hyperintensity within the spinal cord cranial to this, consistent with intramedullary edema (*arrowheads*). (*B*) Transverse T2-weighted MRI at T10 with bilobed arachnoid diverticula compressing the spinal cord dorsally (*arrow*).

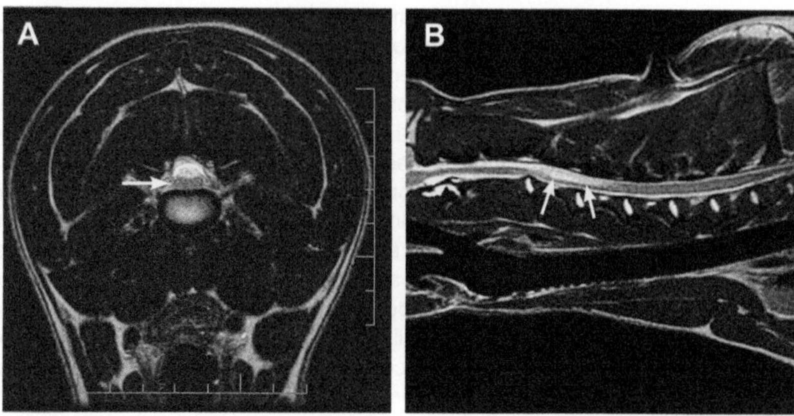

Fig. 21. (*A*) Transverse T2-weighted MRI at C2. A fluid-filled arachnoid diverticulum can be seen dorsal to the spinal cord (*arrow*) with slightly different MR intensity than the overlying subarachnoid space. (*B*) Sagittal T2-weighted MRI at the level of C2 with arachnoid diverticulum dorsal to the spinal cord. Edema within the spinal cord can be seen caudal to the diverticulum in the C3 and C4 spinal cord segments.

versus laminectomy is done. Occasionally even a ventral slot approach may be indicated.[99] In general at least fenestration, and if possible excision, of the affected tissue should be attempted if small and accessible; however, often the diverticula is more extensive and full excision is not possible. Marsupialization has also been reported with success. It is also important to gently break down any adhesions, open up the full extent of the lesion, and ensure there are no adhesions tethering the spinal cord.[100,101] Immediate postoperative complications include hemorrhage and hypoventilation that may require use of a ventilator.[99] Long-term outcomes are inconsistently reported, but 60% to 85% of cases appear to have good functional outcomes; however, at least 10% to 20% may have recurrence of signs.[100]

SUMMARY

Congenital malformations of the spine occur frequently in dogs and cats. Many spinal anomalies do not produce overt neurologic disease and are detected as incidental findings. In animals with neurologic disease, any spinal malformation that is seen within the region of neuroanatomic localization must be investigated carefully to establish its clinical significance. Although severe malformations may result in poor quality of life and euthanasia, there are a large number of conditions that remain surgically treatable. Recent advances in imaging and surgical techniques have improved our understanding and treatment of these diseases.

ACKNOWLEDGMENTS

The authors would like to acknowledge the invaluable assistance of John Doval with the provided figures.

REFERENCES

1. Summers BA, Cummings JF, de Lahunta A. Malformations of the central nervous system. Veterinary neuropathology. St. Louis (MO): Mosby; 1995. p. 86–90.

2. Dias MS, McLone DG, Partington M. Normal embryology of the spinal cord and spine. Youmans neurological surgery. 5th edition. Philadelphia: WB Saunders; 2004. p. 4239–88.
3. Rossi A, Gandolfo C, Morana G, et al. Current classification and imaging of congenital spinal anomalies. Semin Roentgenol 2006;41(4):250–73.
4. Chesney CJ. A case of spina bifida in a Chihuahua. Vet Rec 1973;93:120–1.
5. Clayton HM, Boyd JS. Spina bifida in a German shepherd puppy. Vet Rec 1983; 112:13–5.
6. Frye FL, McFarland LZ. Spina bifida with rachischisis in a kitten. J Am Vet Med Assoc 1965;146(5):481–2.
7. Wilson JW, Kurtz HJ, Leipold HW, et al. Spina bifida in the dog. Vet Pathol 1979; 16:165–79.
8. Parker AJ, Park RD, Byerly CS, et al. Spina bifida with protrusion of spinal cord issue in a dog. J Am Vet Med Assoc 1973;163(2):158–60.
9. James CC, Lassman LP, Tomlinson BE. Congenital anomalies of the lower spine and spinal cord in Manx cats. J Pathol 1969;97(2):269–76.
10. Umphlet RC, Vicini DS, Godshalk CP. Intradural-extramedullary lipoma in a dog. Compend Contin Educ Vet 1989;11(10):1192–6.
11. Plummer SB, Bunch SE, Khoo LH, et al. Tethered spinal cord and an intradural lipoma associated with a meningocele in an Manx-type cat. J Am Vet Med Assoc 1993;203(8):1159–61.
12. Miller L, Tobias K. Dermoid sinuses: description, diagnosis and treatment. Compend Contin Educ Vet 2003;25(4):295–9.
13. Brunetti A, Fatone G, Cuomo A, et al. Meningomyelocele and hydrocephalus in a bulldog. Prog Vet Neurol 1993;4(2):54–8.
14. Fingeroth JM, Johnson GC, Burt JK, et al. Neuroradiographic diagnosis and surgical repair of tethered cord syndrome in an English bulldog with spina bifida and myeloschisis. J Am Vet Med Assoc 1989;194(9):1300–2.
15. Shamir M, Rochkind S, Johnston D. Surgical treatment of tethered spinal cord syndrome in a dog with myelomeningocele. Vet Rec 2001;48:755–6.
16. Leipold HW, Huston K, Baluch B, et al. Congenital defects of the caudal vertebral column and spinal cord in Manx cats. J Am Vet Med Assoc 1974;164(5): 520–3.
17. Kerruisch DW. The Manx cat and spina bifida. J Cat Genet 1964;1:16–7.
18. Deforest ME, Basrur PK. Malformations and the Manx syndrome in cats. Can Vet J 1979;20:304–14.
19. Oskouian JR Jr, Sansur CA, Shaffrey CI. Congenital abnormalities of the thoracic and lumbar spine. Neurosurg Clin N Am 2007;18:479–98.
20. Steyn HP, Quinlan J, Jackson C. A skin condition seen in Rhodesian ridgeback dogs: report on two cases. J S Afr Vet Med Assoc 1939;10(4):170–4.
21. Lord LH, Cawley AJ, Gilray J. Mid-dorsal Dermoid sinuses in Rhodesian Ridgeback dogs—a case report. J Am Vet Med Assoc 1957;131(11):515–8.
22. Salmon Hillbertz NH, Isaksson M, Karlsson EK. Duplication of FGF3, FGF4, FGF19 and ORAOV1 causes hair ridge and predisposition to dermoid sinus in ridgeback dogs. Nat Genet 2007;19(11):1318–20.
23. Henderson JP, Pearson GR, Smerdon TN. Dermoid cyst of the spinal cord associated with ataxia in a cat. J Small Anim Pract 1993;34:402–4.
24. Rochat MC, Campbell GA, Panciera RJ. Dermoid cysts in cats: two cases and a review of the literature. J Vet Diagn Invest 1996;8:505–7.
25. Mann GE, Stratton J. Dermoid sinus in the Rhodesian ridgeback. J Small Anim Pract 1966;7:631–42.

26. Davies ES, Transson BA, Gavin PR. A confusing magnetic resonance imaging observation complicating for a dermoid cyst in a Rhodesian ridgeback. Vet Radiol Ultrasound 2004;45:307–9.
27. Rahal S, Mortari AC, Yamashita S. Magnetic resonance imaging in the diagnosis of type 1 dermoid sinus in two Rhodesian ridgeback dogs. Can Vet J 2008;49:871–6.
28. Fatone G, Brunetti A, Lamagna F, et al. Dermoid sinus and spinal malformations in a Yorkshire terrier: diagnosis and follow-up. J Small Anim Pract 1995;36: 178–80.
29. Capello R, Lamb CR, Rest JR. Vertebral epidermoid cyst causing hemiparesis in a dg. Vet Rec 2006;158:865–7.
30. McGrath JT. Neurologic examination in the dog. Philadelphia: Lea and Febiger; 1956. p. 136.
31. McGrath JT. Spinal dysraphism in the dog. With comments on syringomyelia. Pathol Vet 1965;2(Suppl):1–36.
32. Engel HN, Draper DD. Comparative prenatal development of the spinal cord in normal and dysraphic dogs: fetal stage. Am J Vet Res 1982;43(10):1735–43.
33. Engel HN, Draper DD. Comparative prenatal development of the spinal cord in normal and dysraphic dogs: embryonic stage. Am J Vet Res 1982;43(10): 1729–34.
34. Confer AW, Ward BC. Spinal dysraphism: a congenital myelodysplasia in the Weimaraner. J Am Vet Med Assoc 1972;160(10):1423–6.
35. Neufeld JL, Little PB. Spinal dysraphism in a Dalmatian dog. Can Vet J 1974; 15(11):335–6.
36. Shell LG, Carrig CB, Sponberg DP, et al. Spinal dysraphism, hemivertebra and stenosis of the spinal canal in a Rottweiler puppy. J Am Anim Hosp Assoc 1987; 24:341–4.
37. Furneaux RW, Doige CE, Kaye MM. Syringomyelia and spina bifida occulta in a Samoyed dog. Can Vet J 1973;14(12):317–21.
38. Morgan JP. Congenital anomalies of the vertebral column of the dog: a study of the incidence and significance based on a radiographic and morphologic study. J Am Vet Rad Soc 1968;IX:21–9.
39. Done SH, Drew RA, Robins GM, et al. Hemivertebrae in the dog: clinical and pathological observations. Vet Rec 1975;96:313–7.
40. Newitt A, German AJ, Barr FJ. Congenital abnormalities of the feline vertebral column. Vet Radiol Ultrasound 2008;49(1):35–41.
41. Bailey CS, Morgan JP. Congenital spinal malformations. Vet Clin North Am 1992; 22:985–1015.
42. Mazrier H, Van Hoeven M, Wang P, et al. Inheritance, biochemical abnormalities, and clinical features of feline mucolipidosis II: the first animal model of human I-cell disease. J Hered 2003;94:363–673.
43. McMaster MJ, Singh H. Natural history of congenital kyphosis and kyphoscoliosis. J Bone Joint Surg Am 1999;81(10):1367–83.
44. Kaplan KM, Spivak JM, Bendo JA. Embryology of the spine and associated congenital abnormalities. Spine J 2005;5(5):564–76.
45. Kawakami N, Tsuji T, Imagama S. Classification of congenital scoliosis and kyphosis: a new approach to the three-dimensional classification for progressive vertebral anomalies requiring operative treatment. Spine 2009;41(17): 1756–65.
46. Tsou PM, Yau A, Hodgson AR. Embryogenesis and prenatal development of congenital vertebral anomalies and their classification. Clin Orthop Relat Res 1980;152:211–31.

47. Hedequist D, Emans J. Congenital scoliosis. J Pediatr Orthop 2007;27(1): 106–16.
48. Tsou PM. Embryology of congenital kyphosis. Clin Orthop Relat Res 1977;128: 18–25.
49. Reihart OF. Congenital scoliosis of the anterior dorsal spine. North Am Vet 1950; 21:464.
50. Kramer JW, Schiffer WP, Sande RD, et al. Characterization of heritable thoracic hemivertebra of the German Shorthaired pointer. J Am Vet Med Assoc 1982;15: 814–5.
51. Havlicek M, Mathis KR, Beck JA. Surgical management of vertebral malformation in a Manx cat. J Feline Med Surg 2009;11(6):514–7.
52. Aikawa T, Kanazono S, Yoshigae Y, et al. Vertebral stabilization using positively threaded profile pins and polymethylmethacrylate, with or without laminectomy, for spinal canal stenosis and vertebral instability caused by congenital thoracic vertebral anomalies. Vet Surg 2007;36:432–41.
53. Jeffery ND, Smith PM, Talbot CE. Imaging findings and surgical treatment of hemivertebrae in 3 dogs. J Am Vet Med Assoc 2007;230(4):532–6.
54. McMaster MJ, Singh H. The surgical management of congenital kyphosis and kyphoscoliosis. Spine 2001;26(9):2146–54.
55. Winter RB. Congenital kyphosis. Clin Orthop Relat Res 1977;128:26–32.
56. Malik Y, Konar M, Wernick M, et al. Chronic intervertebral disk herniation associated with fused vertebrae treated by lateral corpectomy in a cat. Vet Comp Orthop Traumatol 2009;22:170–3.
57. Werner T, McNicholas TW, Kim J, et al. Aplastic articular facets in a dog with intervertebral disc rupture of the 12th to 13th thoracic vertebral space. J Am Anim Hosp Assoc 2004;40:490–4.
58. Breit S. Osteological and morphometric observations on intervertebral joints in the canine pre-diaphragmatic thoracic spine (Th1-Th9). Vet J 2002;164:216–23.
59. Penderis J, Schwarz T, McConnell JF, et al. Dysplasia of the caudal articular facets in four dogs: results of radiographic, myelographic and magnetic resonance investigations. Vet Rec 2005;156:601–5.
60. Verbiest H. Lumbar spinal stenosis. In: Youmans JR, editor. Neurological surgery, vol. 4. 3rd edition. Philadelphia: WB Saunders; 1990. p. 2805–55.
61. Arnoldi CC, Brodsky AE, Caichois J, et al. Lumbar spinal stenosis and nerve root entrapment syndromes. Clin Orthop 1976;115:4–5.
62. Manzanec DJ, Vinod PR, Augusto H. Lumbar canal stenosis: start with nonsurgical therapy. Cleve Clin J Med 2002;69(11):909–17.
63. Stalin CE, Pratt JN, Smith PM, et al. Thoracic stenosis causing lateral compression of the spinal cord in two immature Dogues de Bordeaux. Vet Comp Orthop Traumatol 2009;22(1):59–62.
64. Stigen O, Hagen G, Kolbjornsen O. Stenosis of the thoraco-lumbar vertebral canal in a basset hound. J Small Anim Pract 1990;31:621–3.
65. Wheeler SJ. Vertebral abnormalities in dogs. J Small Anim Pract 1991;32: 149–50.
66. Knecht CD, Blevins WE, Raffe MR. Stenosis of the thoracic spinal canal in English bulldogs. J Am Anim Hosp Assoc 1979;15:181–3.
67. Morgan JP, Atilola M, Bailey CS. Vertebral canal and spinal cord mensuration: a comparative study of its effect on lumbosacral myelography in the Dachshund and German shepherd dog. J Am Vet Med Assoc 1987;191:951–7.
68. Haskins ME. Animal models for mucopolysaccharidosis disorders and their clinical relevance. Acta Paediatr Suppl 2007;96(455):56–62.

69. Marioni-Henry K, Vite CH, Newton AL, et al. Prevalence of diseases of the spinal cord of cats. J Vet Intern Med 2004;18(6):851–8.
70. Evans HE. Arthrology. In: Evans HE, editor. Miller's anatomy of the dog. Philadelphia (PA): SB Saunders Co; 1993. p. 223–8.
71. McCarthy RJ, Lewis DD, Hosgood G. Atlantoaxial subluxation in dogs. Compend Contin Educ Pract Vet 1995;17:215–27.
72. Oliver JE, Lewis RE. Lesions of the atlas and axis in dogs. J Am Anim Hosp Assoc 1973;9:304–13.
73. Gage ED, Smallwood JE. Surgical repair of atlanto-axial subluxation in a dog. Vet Med Small Anim Clin 1970;65:583–92.
74. Ladds P, Guffy M, Blauch B, et al. Congenital odontoid process separation in two dogs. J Small Anim Pract 1970;12:463–71.
75. Watson AG, Stewart JS. Postnatal ossification centers of the atlas and axis in Miniature Schnausers. Am J Vet Res 1990;51:264–8.
76. Jaggy A, Hutto VL, Roberts RE, et al. Occipitoatlantoaxial malformation with atlantoaxial subluxation in a cat. J Small Anim Pract 1991;32(7):366–72.
77. Wheeler SJ. Atlantoaxial subluxation with absence of the dens in a rottweiler. J Small Anim Pract 1992;33(2):90–3.
78. Sharp NJH. Atlantoaxial subluxation. In: Sharp NJH, Wheeler SJ, editors. Diagnosis and surgery of small animal spinal disorders. 2nd edition. Philadelphia (PA): Elsevier; 2005. p. 161–80.
79. Beaver DP, Ellison GW, Lewis DD, et al. Risk factors affecting the outcome of surgery for atlantoaxial subluxation in dogs: 46 cases (1978-1998). J Am Vet Med Assoc 2000;216(7).
80. Havig ME, Cornell KK, Hawthorne JC, et al. Evaluation of nonsurgical treatment of atlantoaxial subluxation in dogs: 19 cases (1992-2001). J Am Vet Med Assoc 2005;227(2):257–62.
81. Knipe MF, Sturges BK, Vernau KM, et al. Atlantoaxial instability in 17 dogs. 20th Annual ACVIM Forum Proceedings. Dallas (TX): J Vet Intern Med; 2002.
82. Schulz KS, Waldron DR, Fahie M. Application of ventral pins and polymethylmethacrylate for the management of atlantoaxial instability: results in nine dogs. Vet Surg 2004;33:349–54.
83. Sanders SG, Bagley RS, Silver GM, et al. Outcomes and complications associated with ventral screws, pins, and polymethyl methacrylate for atlantoaxial instability in 12 dogs. J Am Anim Hosp Assoc 2004;40:204–10.
84. Platt SR, Chambers JN, Cross A. A modified ventral fixation for surgical management of atlantoaxial subluxation. Vet Surg 2004;33:349–54.
85. Zaki FA. Vascular malformation (cavernous angioma) of the spinal cord in a dog. J Small Anim Pract 1979;20(7):417–22.
86. Sanders SG, Bagley RS, Gavin PR, et al. Surgical treatment of an intramedullary spinal cord hamartoma in a dog. J Am Vet Med Assoc 2002;221:659–61.
87. Hayashida E, Ochiai K, Kadosawa T, et al. Arteriovenous malformation of the cervical spinal cord in a dog. J Comp Pathol 1999;121:71–6.
88. Cordy DR. Vascular malformations and hemangiomas of the canine spinal cord. Vet Pathol 1979;6:275–82.
89. Vandevelde M, Frankenhauser R. Zur Pathologie der Ruckenmarksblutungen beim Hund. Schweiz Arch Tierheilkd 1972;114:463–75.
90. Westworth DR, Vernau KM, Cullen SP. Vascular anomaly causing subclavian steal and cervical myelopathy in a dog: diagnosis and endovascular management. Vet Radiol Ultrasound 2006;47(3):265–9.

91. MacKillop E, Olby NJ, Linder KE, et al. Intramedullary cavernous malformation of the spinal cord in two dogs. Vet Pathol 2007;44(4):528–32.
92. Alexander K, Huneault L, Foster R, et al. Magnetic resonance imaging and marsupialization of a hemorrhagic intramedullary vascular anomaly in the cervical portion of the spinal cord of a dog. J Am Vet Med Assoc 2008;232(3):399–404.
93. Wells MY, Weisbrode SE. Vascular malformations in the thoracic vertebrae of three cats. Vet Pathol 1987;24:360–1.
94. Kloc PA II, Scrivani PV, Barr SC, et al. Vertebral angiomatosis in a cat. Vet Radiol Ultrasound 2001;42(1):42–5.
95. Schur D, Rademacher N, Vasanjee S, et al. Spinal cord compression in a cat due to vertebral angiomatosis. J Feline Med Surg 2010;12(2):179–82.
96. Spetzler RF, Detweiler PW, Riina HA, et al. Modified classification of spinal cord vascular lesions. J Neurosurg 2002;96:145–56.
97. da Costa L, dehdashti AR, terBrugge KG. Spinal cord vascular shunts: spinal cord vascular malformations and dural arteriovenous fistulas. Neurosurg Focus 2009;26(1):E6 1–9.
98. Nabors MW, Pait TG, Byrd EB, et al. Updated assessment and current classification of spinal meningeal cysts. J Neurosurg 1988;68:366–77.
99. Rylander H, Lipsitz D, Berry WL, et al. Retrospective analysis of spinal arachnoid cysts in 14 dogs. J Vet Intern Med 2002;16:690–6.
100. Skeen TM, Olby NJ, Munana KR, et al. Spinal arachnoid cysts in 17 dogs. J Am Anim Hosp Assoc 2003;39:271–82.
101. Gnirs K, Ruel Y, Blot S, et al. Spinal subarachnoid cysts in 13 dogs. Vet Radiol Ultrasound 2003;44(4):402–8.
102. Jurina K, Grevel V. Spinal arachnoid pseudocysts in 10 rottweilers. J Small Anim Pract 2004;45:9–15.
103. Lee Brooks M, Jolesz FA, Patz S. MRI pulsatile CSF motion within arachnoid cysts. Magn Reson Imaging 1988;6:575–84.
104. Petridis AK, Doukas A, Barth H, et al. Spinal cord compression caused by idiopathic intradural arachnoid cysts of the spine: review of the literature and illustrated case. Eur Spine J 2010;19(Suppl 2):124–9.
105. Parker AJ, Adams WM, Zachary JF. Spinal arachnoid cysts in a dog. J Am Anim Hosp Assoc 1983;19:1001–8.
106. Gage ED, Hoerlein BF, Bartels JE. Spinal cord compression resulting from a leptomeningeal cyst in the dog. J Am Vet Med Assoc 1968;152:1664–70.
107. Vignoli M, Rossi F, Sarli G. Spinal subarachnoid cyst in a cat. Vet Radiol Ultrasound 1999;40(2):116–9.

Degenerative Lumbosacral Stenosis in Dogs

Björn P. Meij, DVM, PhD[a,*], Niklas Bergknut, DVM, MS[a,b]

KEYWORDS

- Degenerative lumbosacral stenosis • Cauda equina syndrome
- Lumbosacral disease • Lumbosacral instability
- Intervertebral disc degeneration • Dogs

Degenerative lumbosacral stenosis (DLSS) is a common disorder seen mainly in large breed dogs.[1–4] DLSS has been attributed many names over the past 40 years: cauda equina syndrome, cauda equina compression, lumbosacral stenosis or disease, lumbosacral instability, and DLSS.[2,4–8] All these terms refer to a degenerative disorder that is of multifactorial origin in which intervertebral disc (IVD) degeneration plays a major role. IVD degeneration, and bony and soft-tissue proliferations contribute to spinal stenosis and cauda equina compression leading to pain, lameness, and neurologic signs. This article describes current knowledge on the pathogenesis of IVD degeneration and recent advances in the management of DLSS. The biomechanics, pathogenesis, clinical manifestation, and treatments of lumbar disc herniation are very similar between dogs and humans. Hence many studies in humans with lumbar disc herniation can contribute to a better understanding of DLSS in dogs, and dogs may in turn be used as a spontaneous animal model for lumbar disc herniation in humans.

CLINICAL ANATOMY

Development

During embryonic development, the spinal cord (derived from the ectoderm) and the vertebral column (derived from the mesoderm) grow at a different rate, leading in the newborn animal to the spinal column being longer than the spinal cord. In most dogs the conus medullaris (end point of the spinal cord) is located in the caudal half of L6

There are no conflicts of interest to report and no external funding has been received.
[a] Department of Clinical Sciences of Companion Animals, Faculty of Veterinary Medicine, Utrecht University, PO Box 80.154, Yalelaan 108, NL-3508 TD, Utrecht, The Netherlands
[b] Division of Small Animals, Department of Clinical Sciences, Faculty of Veterinary Medicine and Animal Sciences, Swedish University of Agricultural Sciences, Box 7054, Ulls väg 12, 750 07 Uppsala, Sweden
* Corresponding author.
E-mail address: B.P.Meij@uu.nl

Vet Clin Small Anim 40 (2010) 983–1009
doi:10.1016/j.cvsm.2010.05.006 vetsmall.theclinics.com
0195-5616/10/$ – see front matter

and the cranial part of L7 (**Fig. 1**).[9] In smaller breed dogs this is further caudally.[9] The dural sac extends into the sacrum in more than 80% of the dogs[10] but varies considerably in its caudal extension (**Fig. 2**).

The cauda equina originates from the conus medullaris and is composed of the spinal nerves L6, L7, S1-S3, and Cd1-Cd5 (see **Fig. 1**; **Table 1**) and stretches from vertebra L6 to Cd5. The structures surrounding the cauda equina are (1) ventral: the dorsal longitudinal ligament, the L7-S1 IVD, and neighboring vertebral bodies; (2) lateral: the pedicles of L7 and S1 and intervertebral foramina; and (3) dorsal: the interarcuate ligament and the lamina of L7 and S1.

The IVD and 2 synovial facet joints connect L7 and S1, which is further stabilized by the ventral and dorsal longitudinal ligaments, the interarcuate ligament, the interspinous ligament, and the surrounding fascia and muscular tissues.

The Intervertebral Disc

The lumbosacral IVD has a triangular appearance on a lateral view, being thicker on the ventral side than on the dorsal side, and is entirely dependent on osmosis and

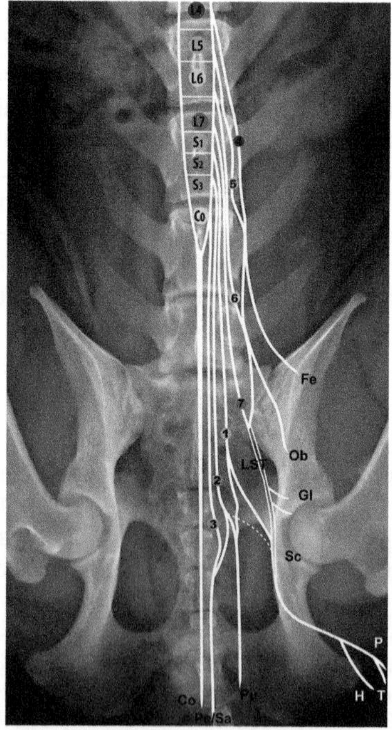

Fig. 1. Ventrodorsal radiograph of the lumbosacral area of a dog. The overlay outlines the approximate location of the spinal segments, the caudal extent of the spinal cord, and the origin of the spinal nerves comprising the cauda equina. Each individual spinal segment (lumbar 4–7 and sacral 1–3) and its corresponding spinal nerve have been marked with the same number and color. Co, coccygeal spinal segment and nerve; Fe, femoral nerve; Gl, gluteal nerve; LST, lumbosacral trunc; Ob, obturator nerve; Pe/Sa, pelvic and sacral nerves; Pu, pudendal nerve; Sc, sciatic nerve. (*Modified from* Wheeler SJ. Lumbosacral disease. Vet Clin North Am Small Anim Pract 1992;22:937–50; with permission.)

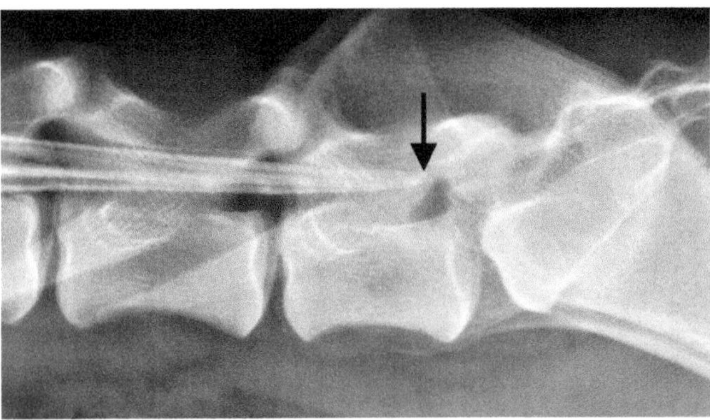

Fig. 2. Lateral radiograph of the lumbosacral spine of a dog after myelography, illustrating the extension of the dural sac (*arrow*).

diffusion for nutrients to reach its cells.[11,12] The IVD is made up of 3 different parts (**Figs. 3** and **4**):

1. The annulus fibrosus (AF) provides tensile strength and connects the 2 adjoining vertebrae rigidly together. The AF is comprised of well-organized lamellar layers of type I collagen.
2. The nucleus pulposus (NP) evenly distributes the load over the vertebral end plates and acts as a shock absorber when the spine is subjected to compressive forces. The gelatinous NP contains 80% to 88% water.[13–15] The remaining 18% to 20% is made up of disorganized type II collagen and negatively charged proteoglycans attracting water and nutrients into the NP through osmosis.[16,17] Therefore, positively

Table 1
Peripheral nerves with clinical significance originating from the cauda equina: normal function and dysfunction in dogs with degenerative lumbosacral stenosis (DLSS)

Nerve	Segment	Reflex	Function	Neurologic Findings in DLSS
N. femoralis (Femoral nerve)	L4–L6	Patellar	Flexion hip Extension stifle	Normal or pseudo-hyperreflexia
N. ischiadicus (Sciatic nerve)	L6–S1	Cranial tibial Gastrocnemius Withdrawal	Extension hip Flexion stifle Flexion and extension of tarsus Proprioception	Muscle atrophy Normal or decreased reflexes Normal or decreased conscious proprioception
N. pelvicus and sacrales (Pelvic and sacral nerves)	S1–S3		Urinary bladder	None or urinary incontinence
N. pudendus (Pudendal nerve)	S1–S3	Perineal Anal	Anal and urinary bladder sphincters	None or decreased perineal reflex None or urinary or fecal incontinence
N. caudales (Tail nerves)	Cd1–Cd5		Tail tone	Normal or hypotonia

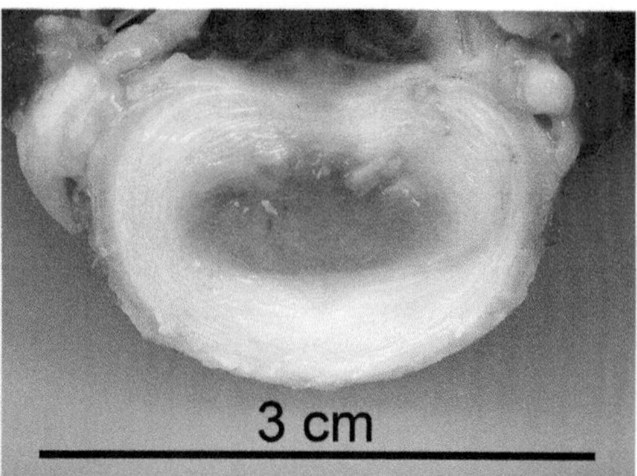

Fig. 3. Transverse view of a healthy canine intervertebral disc showing a clear demarcation between the lamellar structure of the annulus fibrosus and the gelatinous nucleus pulposus.

charged antibiotics such as aminoglycosides (eg, gentamicin) penetrate more easily into the NP than negatively charged ones such as cefuroxime or penicillin.[18]

3. The cartilaginous end plate is a thin structure of hyaline cartilage covering the vertebral end plates. It functions as a semipermeable membrane so that nutrients can enter the disc by diffusion or osmosis.[12,19]

PATHOPHYSIOLOGY

General

DLSS is a multifactorial degenerative disorder resulting in stenosis of the spinal canal and compression of the cauda equina or its blood supply. Several pathologies contribute to DLSS such as:

- Hansen type II (or less commonly type I) IVD herniation.[2,3] IVD herniation is preceded by degeneration of the disc[20,21]
- Ventral subluxation of S1 (lumbosacral instability),[20,22–25] and misalignment of the facet joints[26–28]
- Congenital vertebral anomalies such as symmetric or asymmetric transitional or extra vertebrae[29–34]
- Proliferation of the soft tissues surrounding the cauda equina such as hypertrophy of the interarcuate ligament, the joint capsule, and epidural fibrosis[35]
- Sacral osteochondrosis[36–38]
- Vascular compromise of the blood supply to the spinal nerves.[8,35,39]

Pathogenesis

The following pathogenesis is proposed for DLSS in dogs:

1. An abnormal motion pattern of the lumbosacral junction (commonly caused by repetitive stress, genetic or congenital abnormalities) predisposes for degeneration of the L7-S1 disc.[20,22–25]
2. IVD degeneration is initiated by degradation of the proteoglycans; subsequently less nutrients and water are being drawn into the disc leading to dehydration, further degeneration, and loss of disc width.[40,41]
3. The load bearing of the unstable spinal segment is then shifted from the central axis of the IVD to the peripheral parts of the spine (facet joints and ventral aspect of the vertebral bodies). Due to the angulation of the facet joints, there can also be

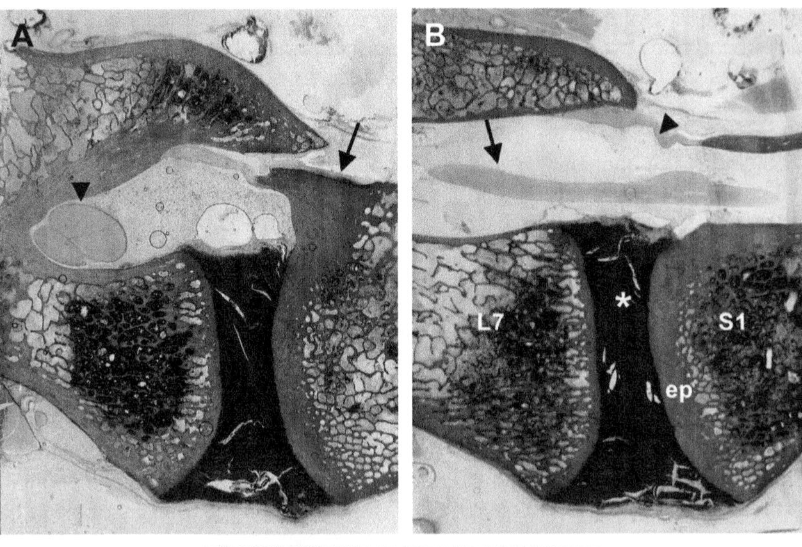

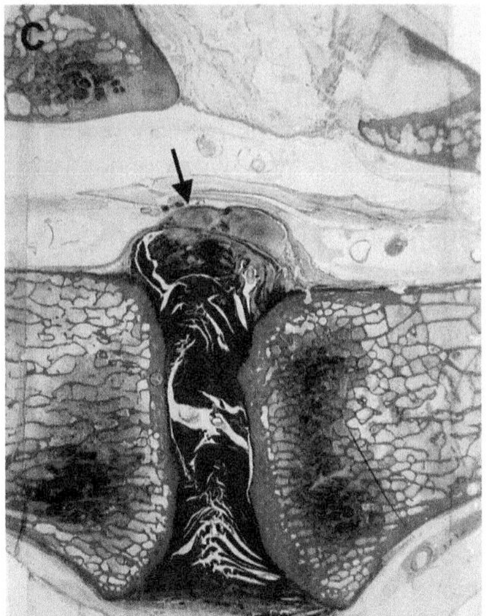

Fig. 4. Histologic sections of the lumbosacral region of the dog. (*A*) A parasagittal section showing the L7 spinal root ganglion in the dorsal radix (*arrowhead*) of the intervertebral foramen and the articular cartilage (*arrow*) of the facet joint. (*B*) A midsagittal section illustrating the dural sac (*arrow*), the interarcuate ligament (*arrowhead*), and the spinal unit consisting of the end plates (ep) and the intervertebral disc (*asterisk*). (*C*) Midsagittal section in a dog with degenerative lumbosacral stenosis demonstrating intervertebral disc degeneration, with type 2 disc protrusion (*arrow*) and dorsal displacement of the dural sac.

a ventral subluxation of the sacrum at this point causing dynamic impingement of the cauda equina.

4. To compensate for the increasing instability, there is a proliferation of the surrounding soft-tissue structures causing hypertrophy of the interarcuate ligament, epidural fibrosis, and thickening of the capsules of the articular processes.

To compensate for the loss of load-bearing properties, the cartilaginous end plates thicken and bony proliferations develop, such as osteophytes and ventral spondylosis. This process further impairs the nutritional supply to the disc, triggering a negative spiral leading to structural failure of the disc.[16,42]

5. Narrowing of the IVD width and loss of AF compliance to compressive forces lead to bulging of the annulus fibrosus and type II disc herniation.[20,43]
6. Cell-mediated inflammatory responses lead to ingrowth of blood vessels and nerves into the damaged disc, which contributes to the lumbosacral pain.[20,44]

Biomechanics of the Lumbosacral Area

Axial compressive forces in humans are similar to those in dogs.[45,46] The IVD is the most important structure for maintaining stability between adjoining vertebrae.[20,23,25] The healthy L7-S1 segment has a greater mobility in flexion-extension (FE) than the other lumbar segments in dogs.[47–49] The most prominent motion direction is FE, although lateral bending and torsion are also possible.[49,50] Torsional stiffness is smaller in the LS segment than in the other caudal lumbar segments.[51] The angulation of the facet joints is reported to have a significant effect on the mobility of the lumbosacral junction.[28] Dogs with DLSS have been shown to have a reduced range of motion in FE of the lumbosacral segment compared with healthy dogs.[52] A kinematic study of the spinal movement of healthy malinois dogs found significant differences in the motion patterns between dogs with normal lumbosacral junctions compared with dogs with radiographic changes of degeneration or transitional vertebrae in the lumbosacral region.[53] Dorsal laminectomy with concomitant facetectomy has been demonstrated to increase instability in healthy cadaveric lumbosacral spines[54] whereas dorsal laminectomy and nucleotomy alone did not increase instability in flexion and extension.[55] However, a later, extended, and more detailed study by the same investigators showed that stability was negatively affected in all 3 motion directions in the healthy lumbosacral spine after dorsal laminectomy and nucleotomy.[56]

EPIDEMIOLOGY

Several studies have reported on the common occurrence of DLSS in large breed dogs, with a predisposition for the German Shepherd dog and working dogs.[1–3,57] The average age at presentation is 7 years, and DLSS is more common in males than females.[1–3] It is not directly possible to relate case-based measures (proportional measures) from larger referral hospitals to the occurrence in the base population. However, basing the estimations on a canine population insured for veterinary care in Sweden (in general dogs $\leq$12 years of age), the incidence in the Swedish dog population was further explored. Data of 200,000 dogs from the insurance company Agria (Agria pet insurance, Stockholm, Sweden) were used spanning a 12-year period (1995–2006), previously reported as representative for the whole Swedish dog population of more than 800,000 dogs.[58–60] Incidence rates were calculated based on dog years at risk (**Table 2**). The main differences from previous studies is that the occurrence of DLSS increases with age and is not most common around the age of 7, as previously stated. The most likely reason for this discrepancy is that older dogs diagnosed with DLSS are more seldom referred for surgery. It must be emphasized that the epidemiologic data of the Swedish population may not apply to canine populations from other countries.

Table 2
Breed-specific incidence rates for the 15 most common dog breeds presented with DLSS per 10,000 dog years at risk (DAR) in the Swedish canine insurance population (data from 1995 to 2006)

Dog Breed	Incidence Rate (No. of Cases/ 10,000 DAR)
German Shepherd dog	33.7
Boxer	21.7
Rottweiler	18.0
Doberman Pinscher	17.5
Briard	17.4
Rhodesian Ridgeback	15.7
Bernese Mountain dog	14.9
Dalmatian dog	13.6
Hovawart	10.5
Greyhound	10.0
Riesenschnauzer	9.1
Great Dane	8.9
Labrador Retriever	8.8
Nova Scotia Duck Tolling Retriever	8.2
Standard Poodle	7.8

CLINICAL SIGNS

History, Clinical Signs, and Clinical Examination

The majority of dogs with DLSS are presented with a history of caudal lumbar or lumbosacral pain. Owners may report pelvic limb lameness, hyperesthesia or self-mutilation of the lumbosacral area or pelvic limbs, difficulty with rising, sitting, or lying down, reluctance to jump or climb, dragging of toes, a low carriage of the tail, and urinary or fecal incontinence.[1–3,61] Working dogs may refuse to perform certain exercises like jumping. In companion animals the clinical signs may only be evident after heavy exercise or play, after which the dog may show muscle tremors or pacing before lying down. In these situations it may help to ask the owner to record a home video.

The clinical signs of DLSS in dogs have been well documented.[61–66] In general, findings during clinical examination are related to the compression of the cauda equina, for example, lumbosacral pain, hyperesthesia of the lumbosacral region, difficulty rising, jumping, and/or getting into the car, unilateral or bilateral pelvic limb lameness, and posterior paresis (**Fig. 5**). The most consistent finding during clinical examination in dogs with DLSS is pain evoked by pressure applied over the lumbosacral region.[61] Specific tests in the standing or recumbent animal can be performed to evoke this pain response. Hyperextension of the caudal lumbar spine with lumbosacral pressure (lordosis test), tail hyperextension, and the lumbosacral pressure test may evoke resistance or a pain response. An experienced clinician is able to differentiate between pain evoked by hyperextension of the hip joints and pain on hyperextension of the lumbosacral region. Lumbosacral pain can further be examined by individual hyperextension of each pelvic limb and simultaneous lumbosacral pressure to confirm lateralization (left or right) of the lumbosacral pain.

In some dogs with DLSS, nonweight-bearing pelvic limb lameness is the most evident clinical sign (see **Fig. 5**). This unilateral lameness may be the result of unilateral

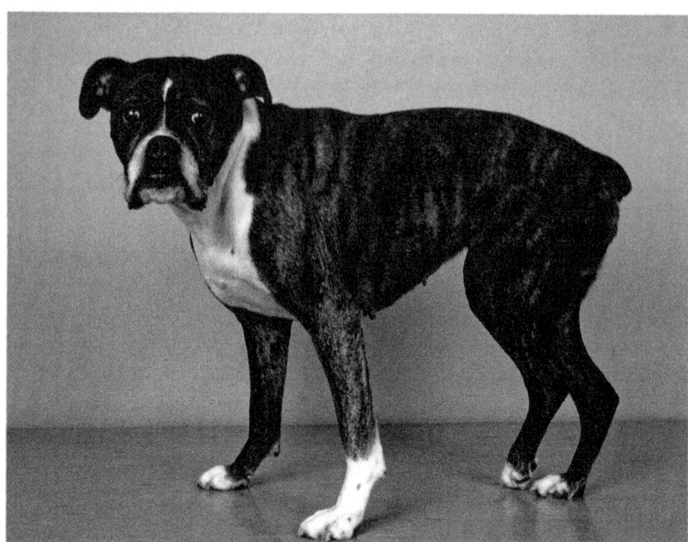

Fig. 5. Typical posture of an 8-year-old Boxer with degenerative lumbosacral stenosis. The clinical signs resemble other orthopedic conditions, but in this case the dog shows the so-called nerve root signature due to left nerve root entrapment at L7-S1.

entrapment of the L7 and/or S1 nerves with radiating nerve root pain, resulting in the so-called nerve root signature. Typical in these dogs is that the lameness can be evoked by hyperextension of the affected limb together with lumbosacral pressure.

Frequently, the dog with DLSS is more an orthopedic patient than a neurologic patient. Profound neurologic deficits in dogs with DLSS are rare, simply because the stenosis affects the cauda equina (and not the spinal cord), which is resistant to compressive forces.[67] In dogs with DLSS showing proprioceptive ataxia and proprioceptive deficits, other conditions, such as degenerative myelopathy, thoracolumbar IVD herniation, or neoplasia must also be considered. Neurologic deficits in DLSS include lower motor neuron signs of the pelvic limbs such as paresis, atrophy of muscles innervated by the sciatic nerve (L6, L7, S1), hyporeflexia of the withdrawal reflex or cranial tibial reflex, or pseudo-hyperreflexia of the patellar reflex ("patellar override"). The patellar reflex is not affected by lumbosacral disease so the muscle tone of the stifle extensors (femoral nerve, L4-L6) will override that of the flexors (sciatic nerve) (see **Table 1**). In severely affected dogs, urinary and/or fecal incontinence is often reported,[61] but other causes than DLSS should also be considered.

DIAGNOSIS

The preliminary diagnosis of DLSS in dogs is based on history and clinical signs, combined with the results of orthopedic and neurologic examinations. Imaging techniques are needed to confirm DLSS.

Imaging Techniques

Conventional radiography, stress radiography, myelography, epidurography, and discography have been used to diagnose DLSS.[68] Computed tomography (CT) and magnetic resonance imaging (MRI) have become increasingly available and are now standard diagnostic tools for DLSS,[68–70] eliminating the need for standard radiographic studies. Moreover, normal radiographs do not exclude DLSS.[71,72] However, because many veterinarians rely on routine radiographic techniques for the diagnosis of DLSS, the most important aspects are reported here.

Conventional radiography

The lateral radiographic view is the most informative for DLSS.[69,73–75] Common findings in dogs with DLSS include collapse of the IVD space, sclerosis of the vertebral end plates, elongation of the sacral lamina ("telescoping") in the caudal aperture of L7, lumbosacral step formation with ventral subluxation of S1, the vacuum phenomenon, and ventral spondylosis (**Figs. 6** and **7**).[2] Sacral osteochondrosis, symmetric or asymmetric transitional vertebrae, an additional eighth lumbar vertebra, or congenital sacral anomalies may also play a role in DLSS.[29–33,36–38] Survey radiographs help to exclude neoplasia with bone involvement (eg, metastatic disease from prostate carcinoma), traumatic luxation, and discospondylitis. Stress radiography of the lumbosacral region, such as dynamic flexion/extension studies, may enhance the lumbosacral step formation.[76]

Myelography

The usefulness of myelography in DLSS is debated because it depends on the extension of the dural sac over the lumbosacral junction. In large dogs the spinal cord ends at L6 and the dural sac extends further caudally (see **Fig. 2**). In myelography, nonionic contrast medium is injected into the subarachnoid space at the cerebellomedullary

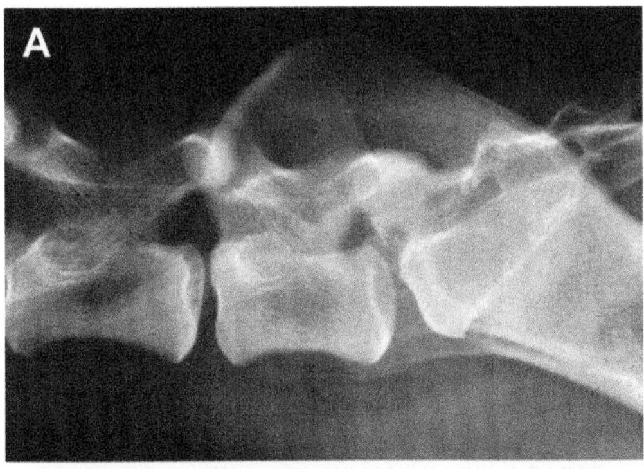

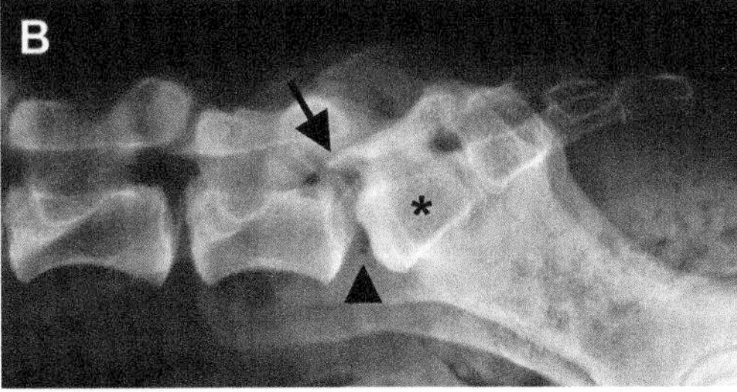

Fig. 6. Lateral radiograph of the lumbosacral region. (*A*) Normal dog. (*B*) Dog with degenerative lumbosacral stenosis and a transitional vertebra (*asterisk*), telescoping of the lamina of S1 into the caudal aperture of L7 (*arrow*), and vacuum phenomenon between L7 and S1 (*arrowhead*).

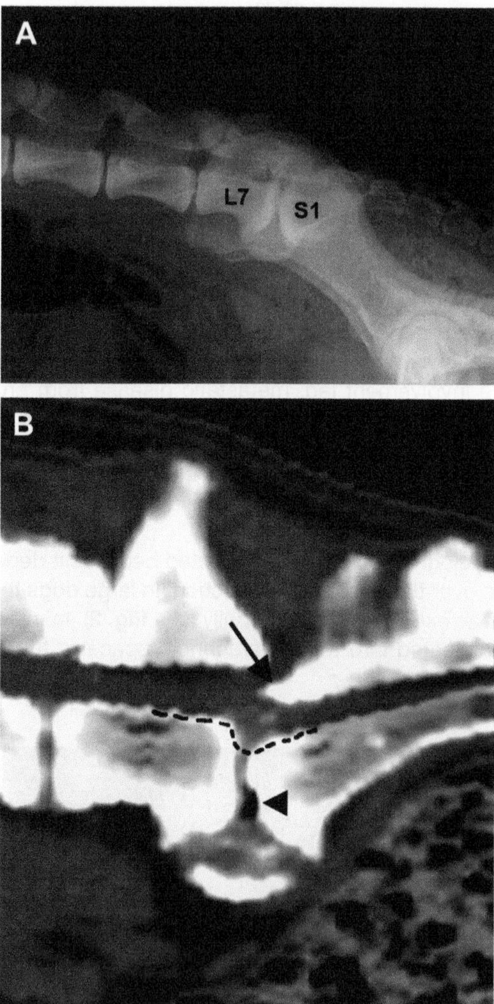

Fig. 7. Lateral radiograph (*A*) and sagittal CT reconstruction (*B*) of the lumbosacral region in a dog with degenerative lumbosacral stenosis. Typical findings are: collapse of the intervertebral disc space, end plate sclerosis, vacuum phenomenon (*arrowhead*), ventral spondylosis, ventral subluxation of S1 (*dotted line*), and elongation of the sacral lamina in the caudal aperture of L7 (*arrow*).

cistern or at a caudal lumbar site (L5-L6),[69,77] so only the dural sac is visualized at the lumbosacral level. Myelography has been reported to be successful in the diagnosis of DLSS.[10] However, lumbosacral stenosis may be present although no abnormalities are seen on myelography.[78] Myelography is more sensitive than routine radiography, and its sensitivity can be increased by dynamic flexion/extension studies.[79,80]

Epidurography

In epidurography, the contrast medium is injected into the epidural space at the lumbosacral or sacrococcygeal junction. Epidurography is technically easier than myelography and has a low morbidity.[68] An epidurogram in dogs with DLSS may show narrowing, elevation, deviation, or obstruction of the epidural contrast-medium lines, especially when combined with dynamic flexion/extension studies[81] (**Fig. 8**). Superimposition of structures, adipose tissue, incomplete filling, and leakage through the intervertebral foramina make interpretation of the epidurogram difficult.[68] Usually the lateral view is the most informative view. Epidurography gives minimal information on lateralization of compressive lesions.[68]

Discography

In discography, contrast medium is injected through the dorsal AF into the NP and leaks into the degenerated disc (more than 0.3 mL is abnormal).[77,82,83] The technique is controversial because disc puncture itself can initiate disc degeneration.[84,85] Both discography and epidurography are rarely used nowadays because of the availability of CT and MRI.

Computed tomography

CT provides better soft-tissue contrast resolution than conventional radiography.[68,86–88] Transverse CT images can be reconstructed to view structures in the sagittal, dorsal, or oblique planes and computer processing techniques also allow for 3-dimensional reconstructions. The CT findings in DLSS are the same as for radiography, but in addition CT shows Hansen type II disc herniation, hypertrophy of the interarcuate ligament, and joint capsules (see **Fig. 7; Fig. 9**). Transverse views are helpful to identify entrapment of thickened nerve roots and pre- and poststenotic dilatation of the dural sac. Parasagittal, dorsoplanar, and transverse views give detailed information on the L7-S1 intervertebral foramina.[89] Disc protrusion can be central or eccentric, and may vary between moderate (<50% of the spinal canal diameter) or severe (>50%) protrusion. In the case of disc protrusion and hypertrophy of the interarcuate ligament, the dural sac and nerves may no longer be protected by epidural fat.

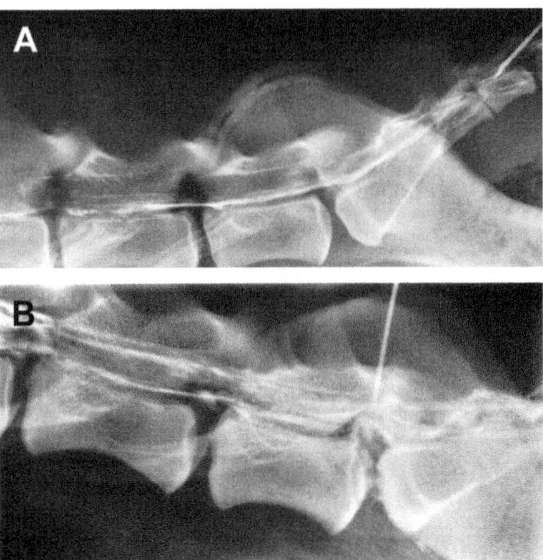

Fig. 8. (*A*) Normal epidurogram. (*B*) Epidurogram in a dog with degenerative lumbosacral stenosis showing dorsal elevation of the ventral contrast line indicating cauda equina compression.

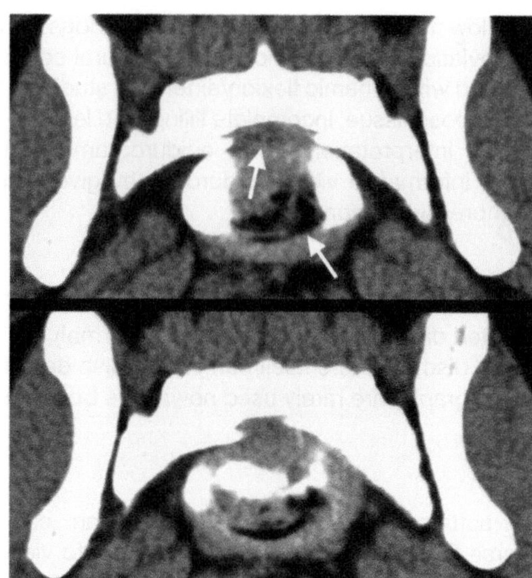

Fig. 9. Transverse CT images of the lumbosacral intervertebral disc space in a dog with degenerative lumbosacral stenosis: severe disc protrusion (*top arrow*), dorsal displacement of the dural sac and nerves, and accumulation of nitrogen gas, the so-called vacuum phenomenon (*bottom arrow*).

The vacuum phenomenon is formed when nitrogen gas accumulates in a ruptured degenerated disc. CT is often less sensitive than MRI for discriminating soft tissues within the spinal canal[69] but is more sensitive for soft-tissue calcifications, cortical bone spurs, and degenerative changes in the facet joints.

Magnetic resonance imaging

MR findings in dogs with DLSS are the same as for CT,[90] but MRI provides more detailed information on IVD degeneration, dural sac, and/or nerve root displacement as well as loss of epidural fat (**Fig. 10**). On T1-weighted images, the IVD is of uniform medium signal intensity, slightly greater than that of the spinal cord, nerve roots, and bone marrow. Epidural fat has a very high signal intensity and appears bright white (see **Fig. 10**). On sagittal T2-weighted images, normal IVDs have a high NP signal surrounded by a medium AF signal. The signal intensity is related to the concentrations of matrix hyaluronic acid and glycosaminoglycans (GAG), which in turn attract and hold water.[91,92] The NP normally possesses the highest GAG concentration, and therefore has a prominent T2 signal. IVD degeneration is characterized by a decreased T2 signal intensity within the NP (see **Fig. 10**).[93–95] Parasagittal and transverse MR images provide valuable information on stenosis of the L7-S1 intervertebral foramina.[96] There is a high degree of agreement between CT and MRI findings in dogs with DLSS but less so between imaging findings and surgical findings.[90,97]

Electrodiagnostic techniques

Electromyography (EMG) is a diagnostic tool that can be used to support the diagnosis of DLSS,[98,99] but it does not provide information regarding the source and direction of compression. Somatosensory evoked potentials (SEPs) provide information about lesion location and sensory nerve root involvement. SEP abnormalities (delay

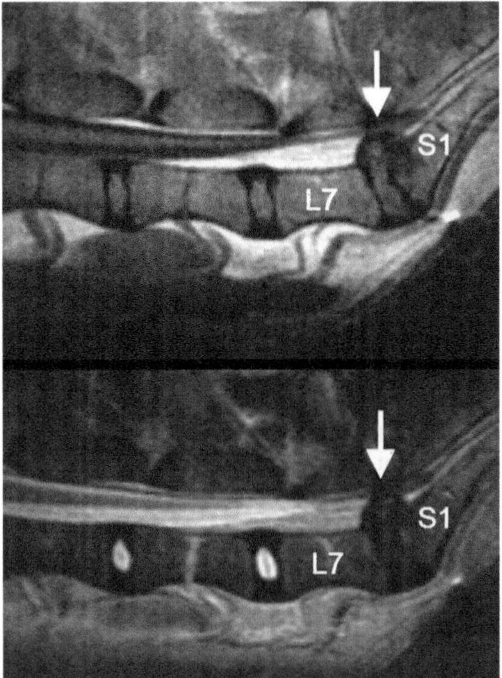

Fig. 10. Sagittal MR images of a dog with degenerative lumbosacral stenosis. The T1-weighted (*top*) and T2-weighted (*bottom*) midsagittal images demonstrate severe disc bulging at L7-S1 (*arrow*), attenuation of epidural fat on T1, and loss of the nucleus pulposus water signal on T2 indicating disc degeneration.

in latency and reduction in amplitude) occurred before deficits in an experimental canine model of lumbosacral stenosis.[67] In a study comparing tibial nerve SEPs in dogs with DLSS with those in healthy dogs, SEPs recorded over the lumbosacral spine were delayed by 1 to 2 milliseconds.[100] Measurement of SEPs in dogs is technically demanding and time consuming, and therefore remains largely a research tool.

Force plate analysis

Measurement of ground reaction forces (GRFs) using force plate analysis (FPA) enables noninvasive, objective measurement of the locomotion in dogs. The propulsive forces of the pelvic limbs in dogs with DLSS were significantly lower than those of healthy dogs,[2,101] reflecting impaired use of the pelvic limbs due to cauda equina compression. FPA has been used to evaluate short- and long-term outcome after dorsal laminectomy in dogs with DLSS.[2,101]

DIFFERENTIAL DIAGNOSIS

Other orthopedic conditions resemble DLSS in clinical signs, age, and breed predisposition. For the German Shepherd dog the differential diagnosis of DLSS may include cranial cruciate ligament rupture, hip dysplasia, psoas muscle injury, and gracilis and semitendinosus contracture. When neurologic deficits are evident, the differential diagnosis of DLSS may be extended with degenerative myelopathy (also often seen in the German Shepherd dog), thoracolumbar IVD disease, neoplasia (eg, peripheral nerve sheath tumor), and severe discospondylitis.[35,66]

TREATMENT

Conservative Treatment

The conservative treatment of DLSS consists of the use of nonsteroidal anti-inflammatory drugs (NSAIDs), a change in exercise pattern, and body weight reduction, the same as for degenerative osteoarthritis. The use of systemic corticosteroid treatment is controversial because the analgesic effect provided through their anti-inflammatory actions can be achieved using NSAIDs, which has significantly fewer side effects.

Lumbosacral epidural injections of corticosteroids have recently been reported as a treatment method in dogs, showing improvement in 79% of the patients.[102] For treatment of epidural injections of corticosteroids to be successful, the patients must not have any proprioceptive deficits in the hind limbs nor display urinary or fecal incontinence.[102] The treatment regime proposed constituted of 3 injections of 1 mg/kg of methylprednisolone acetate, injected at day 1, day 14 and finally at day 42. Local epidural injections of steroids may cause adverse effects and lower the immune response, and result in a flare-up of an unrecognized discospondylitis.

The exercise pattern in dogs with DLSS should include regular short leash walks to maintain muscle mass. Also, regular walking on an underwater treadmill may help recovery. Working dogs with recurrent episodes of lumbosacral pain may improve when work demands are decreased. Conservative treatment does not cure the underlying problem (ie, IVD disease) but may result in sufficient pain management. No studies evaluating conservative treatment of DLSS in dogs can be found in the literature.

Surgical Treatment

Surgical treatment of DLSS is indicated in dogs with moderate to severe lumbosacral pain unresponsive to conservative treatment and in dogs with neurologic deficits. The aim of the surgery is to decompress the cauda equina and free the entrapped nerve roots. The primary surgical procedure comprises dorsal laminectomy, which is extended with additional procedures when further decompression is required: (1) partial discectomy consisting of dorsal fenestration (or dorsal annulectomy) and nuclear pulpectomy (or nucleotomy); (2) foraminotomy[1,103–105]; and rarely, (3) facetectomy. Stabilization by fixation and fusion is indicated when ventral subluxation of S1 is present, or to prevent further development of lumbosacral instability. In some patients foraminotomy on its own, without concurrent dorsal laminectomy, has been reported.[96]

Dorsal laminectomy

Dorsal laminectomy is performed with a motorized burr. The caudal two-thirds of the L7 laminar bone is removed, leaving a cranial laminar bridge; however, the slot may be extended up to L6 when necessary (**Fig. 11**). Bone is removed as far lateral as possible, including sublaminar extensions of the interarcuate ligament extending under the caudal facet of L7, thereby freeing entrapped L7 and S1 nerve roots in the lateral recesses (**Fig. 12**). The cauda equina nerve roots and dural sac are identified and inspected for swelling and adhesions. In the case of adhesions, the nerve tissue is gently freed from the disc protrusion, taking care not to damage the venous sinuses (**Fig. 13**). Partial discectomy is performed to further relieve compression. This procedure is started with a dorsal fenestration (or annulectomy) (**Fig. 14**) and is continued

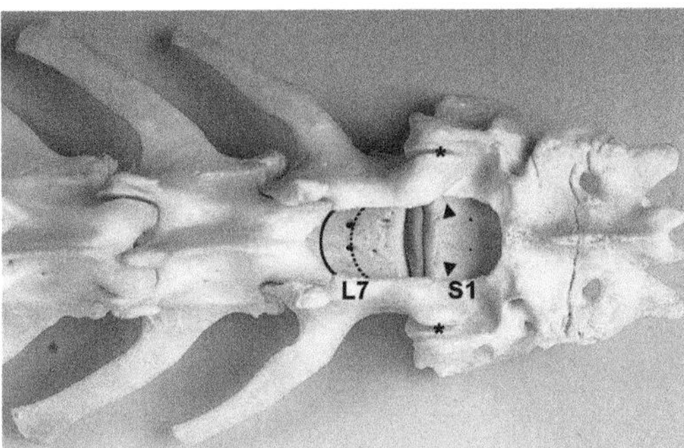

Fig. 11. Bony specimen of the canine lumbosacral spine showing the extension of dorsal laminectomy. The facet joints (*asterisk*) are left intact. The laminectomy usually includes the caudal two-thirds of L7 (*dashed line*) but may be extended cranially (*uninterrupted line*). The lamina of S1 should be removed as far lateral as possible (*arrowheads*) to free the L7 and S1 nerves in the lateral recesses.

with a nuclear pulpectomy (or nucleotomy) (**Fig. 15**). A small bone spoon or curette is used to remove degenerated disc material. The IVD space is routinely swabbed for bacterial culture.

Further decompression may be achieved by facetectomy and/or foraminotomy. Facetectomy should be avoided whenever possible because this will increase lumbosacral instability.[54]

Following decompression a free subcutaneous fat graft is harvested, a small piece (1 cm $\times$ 0.5 cm) is used as a ventral sling under the cauda equina (**Fig. 16**), and a large piece is transplanted dorsally to the laminectomy site to prevent dural adhesions and new bone formation.[106,107] Inadequate closure techniques and poor hemostasis may result in seroma formation and a high risk of postoperative infection.[4,63,104,108]

Over the last decade, several studies have reported on short- and long-term results after decompressive surgery (**Table 3**). Outcome assessed by veterinary surgeons or owners is good to excellent for treatment of caudal lumbar pain, but results may be

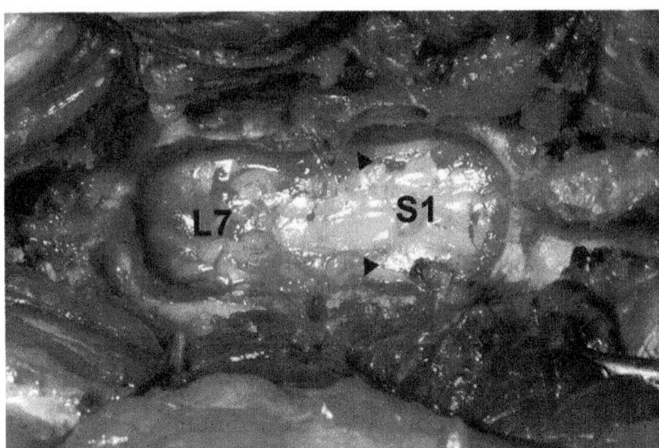

Fig. 12. Dorsal laminectomy includes the caudal two-thirds of the L7 lamina and the complete S1 lamina. The S1 lamina should be removed as far lateral (*arrowheads*) as possible, extending under the caudal L7 facet and giving the laminectomy a keyhole appearance.

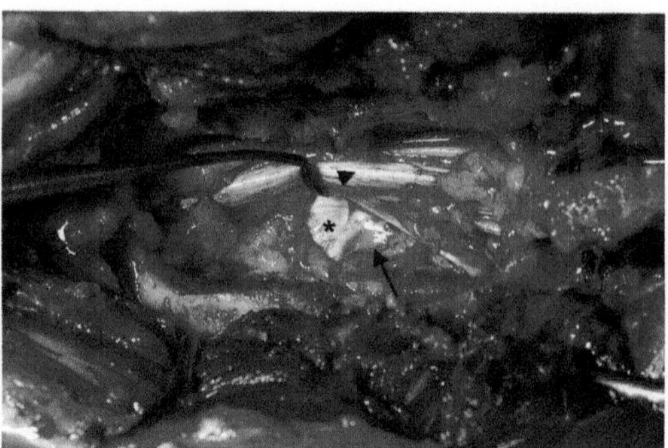

Fig. 13. The cauda equina and dural sac (*arrowhead*) are gently retracted, exposing the disc protrusion (*asterisk*). Care should be taken not to damage the venous sinuses (*arrow*).

biased. In studies that involved working dogs, results were less favorable because of higher demands on performance. Objective assessment of gait using FPA showed that propulsive forces were not restored after decompressive surgery in dogs with DLSS, although owners were very satisfied with the outcome of surgical treatment.[101] Resolution of urinary and/or fecal incontinence after surgery is poor.[2,3,109] Recurrence of clinical signs has been reported in 18% of dogs after dorsal laminectomy.[1]

Foraminotomy

In some patients, if clinical signs and diagnostic imaging combined suggests that nerve root compression is the core problem and no spinal canal stenosis is seen on CT or MRI, surgical treatment consisting of only lateral foraminotomy via a lateral approach has proved sufficient to achieve a good to excellent outcome in 8 of 8 dogs.[96] Lateral foraminotomy can also be combined with a standard dorsal laminectomy as described, or via a mini-dorsal laminectomy assisted by endoscope.[89] A cadaveric study has demonstrated the accessibility to the lumbosacral foramina via a transiliac approach,[110] and suggests that this could be a less invasive approach

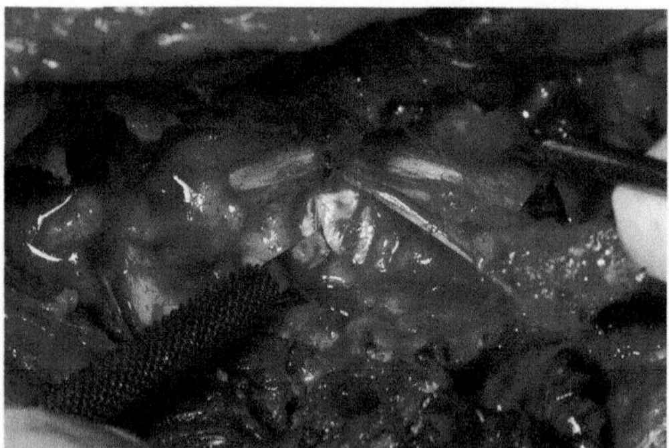

Fig. 14. The dorsal annulus fibrosus is excised in a 2-step procedure with a Beaver knife, always pointing the cutting edge away from the nerves: first, incision of the ipsilateral side while retracting the cauda equina (like a curtain) to the contralateral side, followed by incision of the contralateral side while retracting the cauda equina to the ipsilateral side.

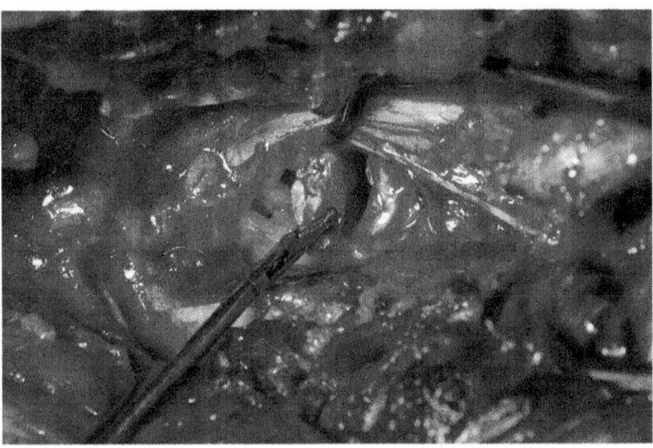

Fig. 15. Following dorsal annulectomy and nucleotomy with a grasping forceps, an empty intervertebral disc remains.

to surgically treat DLSS. The clinical usefulness of this method, however, is yet to be proven in vivo.

Fixation

Dorsal distraction fixation-fusion The goal is to restore disc width and the foraminae, to relieve the pressure on neural tissues, and to stabilize the lumbosacral joint with pins or screws. Fusion is promoted by placing a cancellous bone graft over the dorsal lamina. After distraction, fixation is achieved by embedding pin ends or screw heads in polymethylmethacrylate, which functions as an internal fixator along the dorsal aspect of the lumbosacral spine.[111,112] This procedure may be combined with dorsal laminectomy.[112,113] In the dorsal cross-pinning technique pins are driven in a cross-directive fashion through the base of the L7 spinous process, across the L7-S1 facet joints into the ilial wings.[114] This technique is dependent on the integrity of the spinous process of L7, so dorsal laminectomy can only be focused on S1. A complications of fixation techniques is implant failure.[111,113]

Pedicle screw and rod fixation Lumbosacral fixation with pedicle screw and rod fixation aims at alignment and fusion of the vertebral bodies. In dogs with DLSS, ventral subluxation of S1 is common (see **Figs. 6** and **7**), whereas in humans with

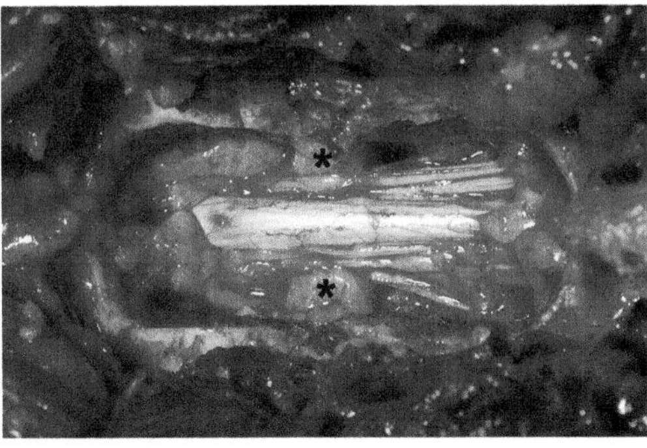

Fig. 16. To protect the cauda equina on the ventral side, a free fat graft sling (*asterisk*) is positioned under the cauda equina.

Table 3
Studies from 1999 to 2009 including results of decompressive surgery in dogs with degenerative lumbosacral stenosis

	Danielsson and Sjöstrom, 1999[1]	Janssens et al, 2000[118]	Jones et al, 2000[97]	De Risio et al, 2001[3]	Linn et al, 2003[109]	Kinzel et al, 2004[119]	Van Klaveren et al, 2005[120]	Suwankong et al, 2007[101]	Gödde and Steffen, 2007[96]	Suwankong et al, 2008[2]
Retrospective/ Prospective study	Retrospective	Retrospective	Prospective	Retrospective	Retrospective	Retrospective	Prospective	Prospective	Retrospective	Retrospective
Number of dogs	131	35	12 military	69	29 military	86	12	31	20	156
German Shepherd dogs	56.5%	23%	25%	27.5%	31%	83.7%	25%	29%	40%	25.6%
Male:female ratio	2:1	2.5:1	Males	2.6:1	4.8:1	2.9:1	1.4:1	2.4:1	0.7:1	1.7:1
Age (years); Mean ± SD or median (ranges)	5.5 ± 2.0	7.2 (2–12)	6.7 (4–9)	6.8 ± 2.8 (2–13)	7.4	5.2 (0.6–11)	4.7 ± 2.5	5.4 ± 2.3	5.7 (2–11)	5.8 ± 2.5
Lumbosacral pain	84.7%	90%	100%	76.8%	72.4%	100%	100%	100%	100%	68.6%
Proprioceptive deficits	9.2%	0%	0%	39.1%	55.2%	39.5%	0%	0%	45%	NA
Lameness	54.2%	55%	100%	37.7%	72.4%	29.1%	58.3%	64.5%	100%	41%
Urinary incontinence	9.2%	0%	0%	14.5%	6.9%	0%	0%	0%	0%	5.8%
Disc protrusion	85.5%	100%	91.7%	75% or 98%	50%	?	75%	93.6%	35%	95.2%

Follow up method[a]	MR & T	Q	SPT & MR	MR & T & Q	MR	?	FPA	FPA & MR & Q	MR & T	MR & Q
Follow-up period (years) Mean ± SD/ median (ranges)	2.2 ± 1.5	2.5	0.5	3.1 ± 1.9	2.7 ± 3.5 (0.6–5.2)	2	0.5	2.2 ± 0.5	1.3 (0.5–3.5)	MR: 1.6 (0.2–3.5) Q: 2.1 (0.3–5)
Postoperative improvement	93.2%	85% Short term 69% Long term	66.7%	78%	79.3%	96.5%	GRF improved	GRF not improved Q: 91%	95%	MR: 79% Q: 76%
Urinary incontinence improved	11 of 12 dogs	—	—	5 of 10 dogs	1 of 2 dogs	—	—	—	—	MR: 4 of 8 dogs Q: 3 of 8 dogs

[a] *Abbreviations:* FPA, force plate analysis; GRF, ground reaction forces; MR, medical record; NA, not available; Q, written questionnaires; SPT, standardized performance test; T, telephone interview.

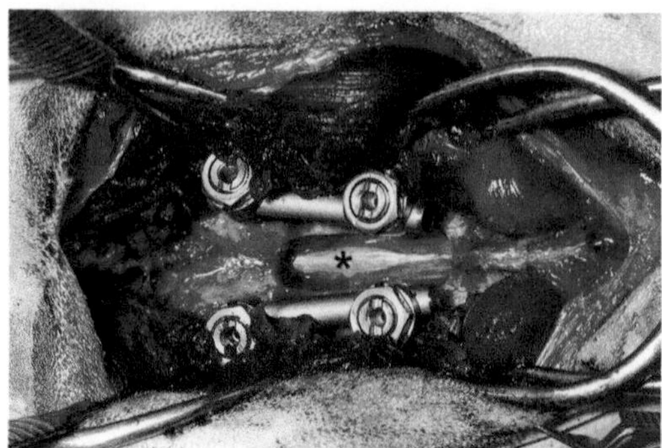

Fig. 17. After dorsal laminectomy (*asterisk* indicates dural sac) the lumbosacral junction can be stabilized using pedicle screw-rod fixation. The pedicle screws are inserted into the L7 and S1 pedicles and connected with 2 titanium rods.

spondylolisthesis L5 is displaced anteriorly. Pedicle screw and rod fixation treats preexistent lumbosacral instability. The technique can be combined with dorsal laminectomy (**Fig. 17**). Distraction of vertebral bodies widens the intervertebral foramina. Spinal fusion is promoted by packing a cancellous bone graft (from the spinous processes and the laminar bone) in the IVD space after nucleotomy and careful removal of the cartilaginous end plates by curettage. The titanium screws are inserted under fluoroscopic control and are connected with contoured titanium rods.[115] The implants may be visualized postoperatively with radiographs (**Fig. 18**), CT, and/or MRI. The surgical technique and biomechanical characteristics of pedicle screw and rod fixation for the canine lumbosacral spine have been described.[55] In humans, adjacent segment disease is a major problem after spinal fusion.[116,117]

POSTOPERATIVE MANAGEMENT AND REHABILITATION

Postoperative treatment consists of analgesic medication and limited, controlled exercise. Antibiotic treatment is only indicated when needed. One study showed that in dogs operated for DLSS, 23% of bacterial cultures of disc material were positive.[2] Because the clinical signs and deficits caused by DLSS can vary considerably between patients, it is important to tailor rehabilitation programs to the needs of the individual patient. Close cooperation between veterinary surgeons and qualified

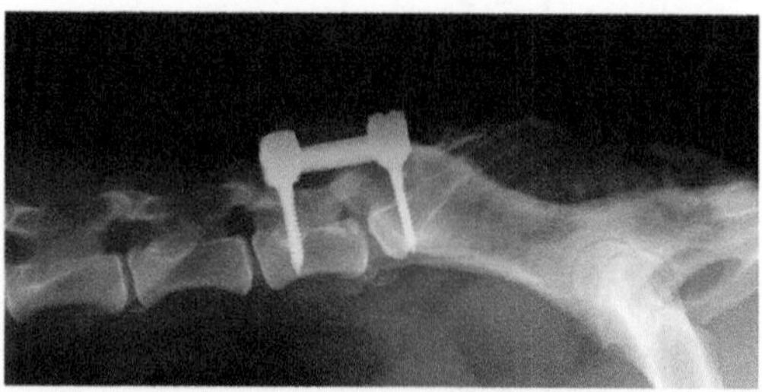

Fig. 18. Lateral radiograph of the lumbosacral region after pedicle screw-rod fixation of L7 and S1.

animal physiotherapists during the rehabilitation program, including the use of underwater treadmills, can improve long-term functional outcome.

SUMMARY

- DLSS is the most common cause of lumbosacral pain in dogs.
- IVD degeneration plays an important role in DLSS.
- Advanced diagnostic imaging techniques such as CT and MRI have greatly contributed to our knowledge on DLSS and enable treatments tailored to the individual patient.
- The most common surgical treatment is dorsal decompressive laminectomy.
- Well-designed clinically controlled studies are needed to assess the value of lumbosacral spinal fusion in the management of dogs with DLSS.

ACKNOWLEDGMENTS

The support of Joop Fama (photography), Agneta Egenvall (epidemiology), and Niyada Suwankong and Luc Smolders (manuscript) is highly appreciated.

REFERENCES

1. Danielsson F, Sjöstrom L. Surgical treatment of degenerative lumbosacral stenosis in dogs. Vet Surg 1999;28:91–8.
2. Suwankong N, Meij BP, Voorhout G, et al. Review and retrospective analysis of degenerative lumbosacral stenosis in 156 dogs treated by dorsal laminectomy. Vet Comp Orthop Traumatol 2008;21:285–93.
3. De Risio L, Sharp NJ, Olby NJ, et al. Predictors of outcome after dorsal decompressive laminectomy for degenerative lumbosacral stenosis in dogs: 69 cases (1987–1997). J Am Vet Med Assoc 2001;219:624–8.
4. Oliver JE Jr, Selcer RR, Simpson S. Cauda equina compression from lumbosacral malarticulation and malformation in the dog. J Am Vet Med Assoc 1978;173:207–14.
5. Wheeler SJ. Lumbosacral disease. Vet Clin North Am Small Anim Pract 1992;22:937–50.
6. Koppel E, Rein D. [Lumbosacral instability. The cauda equina compression syndrome in dogs]. Tierarztl Prax 1992;20:637–45 [in German].
7. Orendacova J, Cizkova D, Kafka J, et al. Cauda equina syndrome. Prog Neurobiol 2001;64:613–37.
8. Tarvin G, Prata RG. Lumbosacral stenosis in dogs. J Am Vet Med Assoc 1980;177:154–9.
9. Fletcher TF, Kitchell RL. Anatomical studies on the spinal cord segments of the dog. Am J Vet Res 1966;27:1759–67.
10. Lang J. Flexion-extension myelography of the canine cauda equina. Vet Radiol 1988;29:242–57.
11. Maroudas A, Stockwell RA, Nachemson A, et al. Factors involved in the nutrition of the human lumbar intervertebral disc: cellularity and diffusion of glucose in vitro. J Anat 1975;120:113–30.
12. Urban JP, Smith S, Fairbank JC. Nutrition of the intervertebral disc. Spine 2004;29:2700–9.
13. Hendry NG. The hydration of the nucleus pulposus and its relation to intervertebral disc derangement. J Bone Joint Surg Br 1958;40:132–44.

14. Hansen HJ. A pathologic–anatomical study on disc degeneration in dog, with special reference to the so-called enchondrosis intervertebralis. Acta Orthop Scand Suppl 1952;11:1–117.
15. Bray JP, Burbidge HM. The canine intervertebral disk: part one: structure and function. J Am Anim Hosp Assoc 1998;34:55–63.
16. Raj PP. Intervertebral disc: anatomy–physiology–pathophysiology-treatment. Pain Pract 2008;8:18–44.
17. Roughley PJ. Biology of intervertebral disc aging and degeneration: involvement of the extracellular matrix. Spine 2004;29:2691–9.
18. Tai CC, Want S, Quraishi NA, et al. Antibiotic prophylaxis in surgery of the intervertebral disc. A comparison between gentamicin and cefuroxime. J Bone Joint Surg Br 2002;84:1036–9.
19. Humzah MD, Soames RW. Human intervertebral disc: structure and function. Anat Rec 1988;220:337–56.
20. Adams MA, Roughley PJ. What is intervertebral disc degeneration, and what causes it? Spine 2006;31:2151–61.
21. Gordon SJ, Yang KH, Mayer PJ, et al. Mechanism of disc rupture. A preliminary report. Spine (Phila Pa 1976) 1991;16:450–6.
22. Tanaka N, An HS, Lim TH, et al. The relationship between disc degeneration and flexibility of the lumbar spine. Spine J 2001;1:47–56.
23. Zhao F, Pollintine P, Hole BD, et al. Discogenic origins of spinal instability. Spine (Phila Pa 1976) 2005;30:2621–30.
24. Kaigle AM, Holm SH, Hansson TH. Experimental instability in the lumbar spine. Spine (Phila Pa 1976) 1995;20:421–30.
25. Krismer M, Haid C, Ogon M, et al. [Biomechanics of lumbar instability]. Orthopade 1997;26:516–20 [in German].
26. Seiler GS, Hani H, Busato AR, et al. Facet joint geometry and intervertebral disk degeneration in the L5-S1 region of the vertebral column in German Shepherd dogs. Am J Vet Res 2002;63:86–90.
27. Rossi F, Seiler G, Busato A, et al. Magnetic resonance imaging of articular process joint geometry and intervertebral disk degeneration in the caudal lumbar spine (L5-S1) of dogs with clinical signs of cauda equina compression. Vet Radiol Ultrasound 2004;45:381–7.
28. Benninger MI, Seiler GS, Robinson LE, et al. Effects of anatomic conformation on three-dimensional motion of the caudal lumbar and lumbosacral portions of the vertebral column of dogs. Am J Vet Res 2006;67:43–50.
29. Aihara T, Takahashi K, Ogasawara A, et al. Intervertebral disc degeneration associated with lumbosacral transitional vertebrae: a clinical and anatomical study. J Bone Joint Surg Br 2005;87:687–91.
30. Damur-Djuric N, Steffen F, Hassig M, et al. Lumbosacral transitional vertebrae in dogs: classification, prevalence, and association with sacroiliac morphology. Vet Radiol Ultrasound 2006;47:32–8.
31. Fluckiger MA, Damur-Djuric N, Hassig M, et al. A lumbosacral transitional vertebra in the dog predisposes to cauda equina syndrome. Vet Radiol Ultrasound 2006;47:39–44.
32. Morgan JP. Transitional lumbosacral vertebral anomaly in the dog: a radiographic study. J Small Anim Pract 1999;40:167–72.
33. Meij BP, Voorhout G, Wolvekamp WT. Epidural lipomatosis in a six-year-old dachshund. Vet Rec 1996;138:492–5.

34. Steffen F, Berger M, Morgan JP. Asymmetrical, transitional, lumbosacral vertebral segments in six dogs: a characteristic spinal syndrome. J Am Anim Hosp Assoc 2004;40:338–44.
35. Sharp N, Wheeler S. Small animal spinal disorders. 2nd edition. Philadelphia: Elsevier; 2005. p. 181–3.
36. Mathis KR, Havlicek M, Beck JB, et al. Sacral osteochondrosis in two German Shepherd dogs. Aust Vet J 2009;87:249–52.
37. Lang J, Häni H, Schawalder P. A sacral lesion resembling osteochondrosis in the German Shepherd dog. Vet Radiol Ultrasound 1992;33:69–76.
38. Hanna FY. Lumbosacral osteochondrosis: radiological features and surgical management in 34 dogs. J Small Anim Pract 2001;42:272–8.
39. Sugawara O, Atsuta Y, Iwahara T, et al. The effects of mechanical compression and hypoxia on nerve root and dorsal root ganglia. An analysis of ectopic firing using an in vitro model. Spine 1996;21:2089–94.
40. Roughley PJ, Alini M, Antoniou J. The role of proteoglycans in aging, degeneration and repair of the intervertebral disc. Biochem Soc Trans 2002;30:869–74.
41. Bray JP, Burbidge HM. The canine intervertebral disk. Part two: degenerative changes—nonchondrodystrophoid versus chondrodystrophoid disks. J Am Anim Hosp Assoc 1998;34:135–44.
42. Colombini A, Lombardi G, Corsi MM, et al. Pathophysiology of the human intervertebral disc. Int J Biochem Cell Biol 2008;40:837–42.
43. Brinckmann P, Grootenboer H. Change of disc height, radial disc bulge, and intradiscal pressure from discectomy. An in vitro investigation on human lumbar discs. Spine (Phila Pa 1976) 1991;16:641–6.
44. Freemont AJ, Peacock TE, Goupille P, et al. Nerve ingrowth into diseased intervertebral disc in chronic back pain. Lancet 1997;350:178–81.
45. Zimmerman MC, Vuono-Hawkins M, Parsons JR, et al. The mechanical properties of the canine lumbar disc and motion segment. Spine 1992;17:213–20.
46. Smit TH. The use of a quadruped as an in vivo model for the study of the spine—biomechanical considerations. Eur Spine J 2002;11:137–44.
47. Braund KG, Taylor TK, Ghosh P, et al. Spinal mobility in the dog. A study in chondrodystrophoid and non-chondrodystrophoid animals. Res Vet Sci 1977;22:78–82.
48. Benninger MI, Seiler GS, Robinson LE, et al. Three-dimensional motion pattern of the caudal lumbar and lumbosacral portions of the vertebral column of dogs. Am J Vet Res 2004;65:544–51.
49. Burger R, Lang J. [Kinetic studies of the lumbar vertebrae and the lumbosacral transition in the German shepherd dog. 2. Our personal investigations]. Schweiz Arch Tierheilkd 1993;135:35–43 [in German].
50. Burger R, Lang J. [Kinetic study of the lumbar vertebrae and the lumbosacral passage in German shepherd dogs. 1. Functional anatomy and kinetic foundation]. Schweiz Arch Tierheilkd 1992;134:411–6 [in German].
51. Hediger KU, Ferguson SJ, Gedet P, et al. Biomechanical analysis of torsion and shear forces in lumbar and lumbosacral spine segments of nonchondrodystrophic dogs. Vet Surg 2009;38:874–80.
52. Schmid V, Lang J. Measurements on the lumbosacral junction in normal dogs and those with cauda-equina compression. J Small Anim Pract 1993;34:437–42.
53. Gradner G, Bockstahler B, Peham C, et al. Kinematic study of back movement in clinically sound malinois dogs with consideration of the effect of radiographic changes in the lumbosacral junction. Vet Surg 2007;36:472–81.

54. Smith M, Bebchuk T, Shmon C. An in vitro biomechanical study of the effects of surgical modification upon the canine lumbosacral spine. Vet Comp Orthop Traumatol 2004;17:17–24.
55. Meij BP, Suwankong N, Van der Veen AJ, et al. Biomechanical flexion–extension forces in normal canine lumbosacral cadaver specimens before and after dorsal laminectomy–discectomy and pedicle screw-rod fixation. Vet Surg 2007;36: 742–51.
56. Smolders LA, Bergknut N, van der Veen AJ, et al. Biomechanical testing of a lumbosacral nucleus pulposus prosthesis: a canine cadaver study. In: European Veterinary Conference, 2009;24.
57. Moore GE, Burkman KD, Carter MN, et al. Causes of death or reasons for euthanasia in military working dogs: 927 cases (1993–1996). J Am Vet Med Assoc 2001;219:209–14.
58. Egenvall A, Bonnett BN, Olson P, et al. Gender, age, breed and distribution of morbidity and mortality in insured dogs in Sweden during 1995 and 1996. Vet Rec 2000;146:519–25.
59. Egenvall A, Bonnett BN, Olson P, et al. Validation of computerized Swedish dog and cat insurance data against veterinary practice records. Prev Vet Med 1998; 36:51–65.
60. Egenvall A, Hedhammar A, Bonnett BN, et al. Survey of the Swedish dog population: age, gender, breed, location and enrollment in animal insurance. Acta Vet Scand 1999;40:231–40.
61. Indrieri RJ. Lumbosacral stenosis and injury of the cauda equina. Vet Clin North Am Small Anim Pract 1988;18:697–710.
62. Mayhew PD, Kapatkin AS, Wortman JA, et al. Association of cauda equina compression on magnetic resonance images and clinical signs in dogs with degenerative lumbosacral stenosis. J Am Anim Hosp Assoc 2002;38: 555–62.
63. Ness M. Degenerative lumbosacral stenosis in the dog: a review of 30 cases. J Small Anim Pract 1994;35:185–90.
64. Morgan JP, Wind A, Davidson AP. Lumbosacral disease. Hannover: Schlutersche GmbH & Co. KG; 2000.
65. Palmer RH, Chambers JN. Canine lumbosacral diseases. Part I. Anatomy, pathophysiology, and clinical presentation. Compend Contin Educ Pract Vet 1991; 13:61–8.
66. De Risio L, Thomas WB, Sharp NJ. Degenerative lumbosacral stenosis. Vet Clin North Am Small Anim Pract 2000;30:111–32.
67. Delamarter RB, Bohlman HH, Dodge LD, et al. Experimental lumbar spinal stenosis. Analysis of the cortical evoked potentials, microvasculature, and histopathology. J Bone Joint Surg Am 1990;72:110–20.
68. Ramirez O 3rd, Thrall DE. A review of imaging techniques for canine cauda equina syndrome. Vet Radiol Ultrasound 1998;39:283–96.
69. Sande RD. Radiography, myelography, computed tomography, and magnetic resonance imaging of the spine. Vet Clin North Am Small Anim Pract 1992;22: 811–31.
70. Brawner W. Neuroradiology. In: Slatter D, editor. Textbook of small animal surgery. Philadelphia: W.B. Saunders; 1993. p. 1008–22.
71. Steffen F, Hunold K, Scharf G, et al. A follow-up study of neurologic and radiographic findings in working German Shepherd dogs with and without degenerative lumbosacral stenosis. J Am Vet Med Assoc 2007;231:1529–33.

72. Scharf G, Steffen F, Grunenfelder F, et al. The lumbosacral junction in working German shepherd dogs—neurological and radiological evaluation. J Vet Med A Physiol Pathol Clin Med 2004;51:27–32.
73. Morgan J. Techniques of veterinary radiography. 5th edition. Ames (IA): Iowa State University Press; 1993.
74. Middleton DL. Radiographic positioning for the spine and skull. Vet Clin North Am Small Anim Pract 1993;23:253–68.
75. Dennis R. Radiographic examination of the canine spine. Vet Rec 1987;121: 31–5.
76. Lang J, Jaggy A. [X-ray studies of the cauda equina of dogs]. Schweiz Arch Tierheilkd 1989;131:299–309 [in German].
77. Morgan J, Bailey C. Cauda equina syndrome in the dog: radiographic evaluation. J Small Anim Pract 1990;31:69–76.
78. Hachcock JT, Pechmanm RD, Dillon AR, et al. Comparison of three radiographic contrast procedures in the evaluation of the canine lumbosacral spinal canal. Vet Radiol 1988;29:4–15.
79. Kirberger R, Roos C, Lubbe A. The radiological diagnosis of thoracolumbar disc disease in the Dachsund. Vet Radiol 1992;33:255–61.
80. Olby N, Dyce J, Houlton J. Correlation of plain radiographic and lumbar myelographic findings in thoracolumbar disc disease. J Small Anim Pract 1994;35: 345.
81. Robert RE, Selcer BA. Diagnostic imaging: myelography and epidurography. Vet Clin North Am Small Anim Pract 1993;23:307–29.
82. Barthez PY, Morgan JP, Lipsitz D. Discography and epidurography for evaluation of the lumbosacral junction in dogs with cauda equina syndrome. Vet Radiol Ultrasound 1994;35:152–7.
83. Park RD. Diagnostic imaging of the spine. Prog Vet Neurol 1990;1:371–86.
84. Masuda K, Aota Y, Muehleman C, et al. A novel rabbit model of mild, reproducible disc degeneration by an annulus needle puncture: correlation between the degree of disc injury and radiological and histological appearances of disc degeneration. Spine (Phila Pa 1976) 2005;30:5–14.
85. Sobajima S, Kompel JF, Kim JS, et al. A slowly progressive and reproducible animal model of intervertebral disc degeneration characterized by MRI, X-ray, and histology. Spine (Phila Pa 1976) 2005;30:15–24.
86. Jones JC, Wilson ME, Bartels JE. A review of high resolution computed tomography and a proposed technique for regional examination of the canine lumbosacral spine. Vet Radiol Ultrasound 1994;35:339–46.
87. Jones JC, Sorjonen DC, Simpson ST, et al. Comparison between computed tomographic and surgical findings in nine large-breed dogs with lumbosacral stenosis. Vet Radiol Ultrasound 1996;37:247–56.
88. Jones JC, Inzana KD. Subclinical CT abnormalities in the lumbosacral spine of older large-breed dogs. Vet Radiol Ultrasound 2000;41:19–26.
89. Wood BC, Lanz OI, Jones JC, et al. Endoscopic-assisted lumbosacral foraminotomy in the dog. Vet Surg 2004;33:221–31.
90. Suwankong N, Voorhout G, Hazewinkel HA, et al. Agreement between computed tomography, magnetic resonance imaging, and surgical findings in dogs with degenerative lumbosacral stenosis. J Am Vet Med Assoc 2006;229:1924–9.
91. Pearce RH, Thompson JP, Bebault GM, et al. Magnetic resonance imaging reflects the chemical changes of aging degeneration in the human intervertebral disk. J Rheumatol Suppl 1991;27:42–3.

92. Benneker LM, Heini PF, Anderson SE, et al. Correlation of radiographic and MRI parameters to morphological and biochemical assessment of intervertebral disc degeneration. Eur Spine J 2005;14:27–35.
93. Adams WH, Daniel GB, Pardo AD, et al. Magnetic resonance imaging of the caudal lumbar and lumbosacral spine in 13 dogs (1990–1993). Vet Radiol Ultrasound 1995;36:3–13.
94. de Haan JJ, Shelton SB, Ackerman N. Magnetic resonance imaging in the diagnosis of degenerative lumbosacral stenosis in four dogs. Vet Surg 1993;22:1–4.
95. Karkkainen M, Punto LU, Tulamo RM. Magnetic resonance imaging of canine degenerative lumbar spine diseases. Vet Radiol Ultrasound 1993;34:399–404.
96. Gödde T, Steffen F. Surgical treatment of lumbosacral foraminal stenosis using a lateral approach in twenty dogs with degenerative lumbosacral stenosis. Vet Surg 2007;36:705–13.
97. Jones JC, Banfield CM, Ward DL. Association between postoperative outcome and results of magnetic resonance imaging and computed tomography in working dogs with degenerative lumbosacral stenosis. J Am Vet Med Assoc 2000;216:1769–74.
98. Sisson AF, LeCouteur RA, Ingram JT, et al. Diagnosis of cauda equina abnormalities by using electromyography, discography, and epidurography in dogs. J Vet Intern Med 1992;6:253–63.
99. Kornberg M, Bichsel P, Lang J. [Electromyography and spinal evoked potentials in cauda equina syndrome of dogs]. Schweiz Arch Tierheilkd 1989;131:287–98 [in German].
100. Meij BP, Suwankong N, van den Brom WE, et al. Tibial nerve somatosensory evoked potentials in dogs with degenerative lumbosacral stenosis. Vet Surg 2006;35:168–75.
101. Suwankong N, Meij BP, Van Klaveren NJ, et al. Assessment of decompressive surgery in dogs with degenerative lumbosacral stenosis using force plate analysis and questionnaires. Vet Surg 2007;36:423–31.
102. Janssens L, Beosier Y, Daems R. Lumbosacral degenerative stenosis in the dog. The results of epidural infiltration with methylprednisolone acetate: a retrospective study. Vet Comp Orthop Traumatol 2009;22:486–91.
103. Denny HR, Gibbs C, Holt PE. The diagnosis and treatment of cauda equina lesions in the dog. J Small Anim Pract 1982;23:425–43.
104. Chambers J, Selcer B, Oliver J. Results of treatment of degenerative lumbosacral stenosis in dogs by exploration and excision. Vet Comp Orthop Traumatol 1988;3:130–3.
105. Lenehan T, Tarvin G. Surgical treatment of cauda equina compression syndrome by laminectomy. In: Bojrab M, editor. Current techniques in small animal surgery. 5th edition. Philadelphia: Lea & Febiger; 1998. p. 859–61.
106. Quist JJ, Dhert WJA, Meij BP, et al. The prevention of peridural adhesions, a comparative long-term histomorphometric study using a biodegradable barrier and a fat graft. J Bone Joint Surg Br 1998;80:520–6.
107. Trevor PB, Martin RA, Saunders GK, et al. Healing characteristics of free and pedicle fat grafts after dorsal laminectomy and durotomy in dogs. Vet Surg 1991;20:282–90.
108. Watt PR. Degenerative lumbosacral stenosis in 18 dogs. J Small Anim Pract 1991;32:125–34.
109. Linn LL, Bartels KE, Rochat MC, et al. Lumbosacral stenosis in 29 military working dogs: epidemiologic findings and outcome after surgical intervention (1990–1999). Vet Surg 2003;32:21–9.

110. Carozzo C, Cachon T, Genevois JP, et al. Transiliac approach for exposure of lumbosacral intervertebral disk and foramen: technique description. Vet Surg 2008;37:27–31.
111. Slocum B, Devine T. L7-S1 fixation-fusion for treatment of cauda equina compression in the dog. J Am Vet Med Assoc 1986;188:31–5.
112. Slocum B. L7-S1 fixation-fusion technique for cauda equina syndrome. In: Bojrab M, editor. Current techniques in small animal surgery. 5th edition. Philadelphia: Lea&Febiger; 1998. p. 861–4.
113. Bagley R. Surgical stabilization of the lumbosacral joint. In: Slatter D, editor. Textbook of small animal surgery. 3rd edition. Philadelphia: Elsevier Science; 2003. p. 1238–43.
114. Jeffery N. Treatment of cauda equina syndrome. ESVOT – Eur Soc Vet Orthop Traumatol. 1998. p. 74.
115. van der Veen AJ, Bergknut N, Voorhout G, et al. Assessment of safe corridors for pedicle screw insertion in canine lumbosacral vertebras. In: European Veterinary Conference, Voorjaarsdagen. 2009. Chapter 5, p. 27.
116. Hoogendoorn RJ, Helder MN, Wuisman PI, et al. Adjacent segment degeneration: observations in a goat spinal fusion study. Spine 2008;33:1337–43.
117. Yang JY, Lee JK, Song HS. The impact of adjacent segment degeneration on the clinical outcome after lumbar spinal fusion. Spine 2008;33:503–7.
118. Janssens L, Moens Y, Coppens P, et al. Lumbosacral degenerative stenosis in the dog. Vet Comp Orthop Traumatol 2000;13:97–103.
119. Kinzel S, Koch J, Stopinski T, et al. [Cauda equina compression syndrome (CECS): retrospective study of surgical treatment with partial dorsal laminectomy in 86 dogs with lumbosacral stenosis]. Berl Munch Tierarztl Wochenschr 2004;117:334–40 [in German].
120. van Klaveren NJ, Suwankong N, De Boer S, et al. Force plate analysis before and after dorsal decompression for treatment of degenerative lumbosacral stenosis in dogs. Vet Surg 2005;34:450–6.

Feline Spinal Cord Diseases

Katia Marioni-Henry, DVM, MRCVS, PhD

KEYWORDS

- Spinal cord • Cat • Feline infectious peritonitis
- Lymphosarcoma • Tumor • Intervertebral disc

Our knowledge on feline spinal cord diseases has increased in recent years thanks to studies on their prevalence, and histologic and magnetic resonance imaging (MRI) characteristics[1–4]; however, the diagnosis and treatment of some spinal cord diseases, such as feline infectious peritonitis (FIP) and spinal lymphosarcoma, are still a challenge. The objective of this article is to review the recent literature that reports on the most common diseases affecting the spinal cord of cats and to draw some general conclusions that will be useful to formulate the diagnosis and prognosis for feline spinal patients. In particular, the results of a postmortem study[1] from the University of Pennsylvania that consisted of 205 cats with spinal cord diseases are compared with other retrospective studies of spinal cord disease that considered different populations of cats and different criteria for disease evaluation. In a population of 205 cats with histologic confirmation of spinal cord disease, inflammatory/infectious diseases were the most common (affecting 32% of the cats), followed by neoplastic diseases (27%), trauma (14%), congenital or inherited diseases (11%), vascular diseases (9%), degenerative diseases (6%), and metabolic/nutritional diseases (1%).[1] Each of these categories of disease is discussed herein.

INFLAMMATORY/INFECTIOUS DISEASES

Inflammatory/infectious diseases were the most common type of spinal cord disease in cats in 2 recent retrospective studies.[1,3] FIP was the most common inflammatory/infectious disease (51%) in 205 North American cats with histologic confirmation of spinal cord disease.[1] This finding was consistent with a population of 286 English cats with central nervous system (CNS) disease confirmed on postmortem in which more than 50% of cats with inflammatory disease had FIP.[3] The other inflammatory/infectious diseases reported in decreasing order of frequency were bacterial myelitis (16%), cryptococcosis (9%), unknown infectious/inflammatory diseases (8%), toxoplasmosis (6%), eosinophilic meningomyelitis (5%), and idiopathic poliomyelitis (5%).[1]

Southern Counties Veterinary Specialists, 6 Forest Corner Farm, Ringwood, Hampshire, BH24 3JW, England, UK
E-mail address: kmhvetneurology@yahoo.co.uk

Vet Clin Small Anim 40 (2010) 1011–1028
doi:10.1016/j.cvsm.2010.05.005 **vetsmall.theclinics.com**
0195-5616/10/$ – see front matter

Feline Infectious Peritonitis

FIP is a fatal disease caused by the FIP virus, a highly virulent feline coronavirus strain that induces an immune-mediated progressive polyserositis (wet form) and pyogranulomatosis (dry form).[5] Neurologic signs are usually associated with the dry or pyogranulomatous form of FIP, with ocular and/or CNS involvement reported in less than 9% of cats with the wet form and in 60% of cats with the dry form.[6] The neurologic signs are often multifocal, and common clinical signs are ataxia, depressed mental status, pathologic nystagmus, tetraparesis/tetraplegia, head tilt, and seizures.[6–8] Most deaths from FIP occur in cats between the ages of 3 and 16 months.[9] Other spinal cord diseases that cause death in cats younger than 2 years include storage diseases, bacterial myelitis, and trauma; however, these occur less frequently than FIP in young cats.[1]

On histopathology, CNS lesions are centered in the meninges, choroid plexus, and ependyma, with submeningeal and parenchymal extension.[10] Lesions are common in the posterior and ventral parts of the brain.[9] Within the spinal cord the cervical region is most commonly affected, and lesions associated with FIP were present in the cervical segments in 93% of cats with spinal FIP (**Fig. 1**).[1]

Obtaining an antemortem diagnosis of neurologic FIP is difficult. In presence of effusion, positive immunofluorescent staining of macrophages is conclusive; however, for the dry form of FIP the definitive diagnosis (based on immunohistochemistry) is not practical if the clinical signs are limited to the CNS.[10,11] Cats with FIP may present some nonspecific hematological abnormalities such as leukocytosis, lymphopenia, nonregenerative anemia, and increased total serum protein caused by hyperglobulinemia (present in about 70% of the cats with the dry form).[11] An albumin/globulin ratio of less than 0.6 is diagnostic for an inflammatory process,[12] and the most common inflammatory processes are FIP. MRI and computed tomography (CT) of the brain of cats with the neurologic form of FIP often show hydrocephalus, and on MRI, periventricular enhancement and cervical syringohydromyelia have also been reported in cases of suspected CNS FIP (see **Fig. 1**).[13–15] Spinal fluid analysis often shows high protein content and pleocytosis with a predominance of neutrophils or lymphocytes, but these findings are not pathognomonic for neurologic FIP, and in some cases cerebrospinal fluid (CSF) analysis may be normal.[6,7] Serum antibody detection is of limited

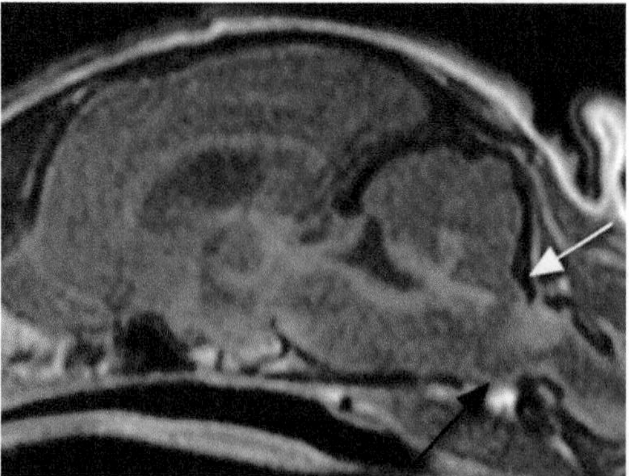

Fig. 1. Sagittal T1-weighted postcontrast image of an 11-month-old Sphynx cat with presumptive diagnosis of FIP. There is ventricular dilation and contrast enhancement associated ventricular lining, consistent with ependymitis, a focal intramedullary contrast-enhancing area at the junction between medulla and first cervical spinal cord segment (*black arrow*), and subtentorial brain herniation (*white arrow*).

help because a high percentage of healthy cats have antibodies against feline coronavirus and will never develop FIP; however, very high titers (≥1:1600) are suggestive of FIP.[10] Detection of feline coronavirus in blood by polymerase chain reaction (PCR) has a high sensitivity, but low specificity, for clinical disease.[10] PCR has accurately differentiated FIP effusions from other types of effusions and can be performed on spinal fluid to diagnose the neurologic form of FIP[10]; however, the author is not aware of any study reporting the sensitivity and specificity of detection of feline coronavirus in spinal fluid by PCR.

There is no treatment with documented efficacy for FIP. Treatment with corticosteroid, cyclophosphamide, ozagrel hydrochloride, ribavirin, melphalan, tylosin, promodulin, human interferon α, feline interferon β or ω, *Propionibacterium acnes*, pentoxifylline, and polyprenyl immunostimulant, as monotherapy or in combination, have been reported, with some cats achieving a remission of the clinical signs.[16,17] In some cases, spontaneous remissions or misdiagnoses may have accounted for responses to treatment; results of some of these studies must be interpreted with caution.[16]

NEOPLASTIC DISEASES

Neoplasms are a common cause of spinal cord disease and were documented in approximately 25% of cases.[1,4] Lymphosarcoma is the most common tumor affecting the spinal cord of cats, with reported prevalence between 28% and 40%.[1,2,4] The second most common tumor was osteosarcoma, representing 27% (14/52) of nonlymphoid tumors; in the same study, glial tumors (9%) and meningioma (7%) were the third and fourth most common tumors affecting the feline spinal cord (**Fig. 2**).[2] By contrast, in 2 retrospective studies with a total of 37 cats with nonlymphoid vertebral or spinal cord tumors treated with surgical cytoreduction, meningioma was the

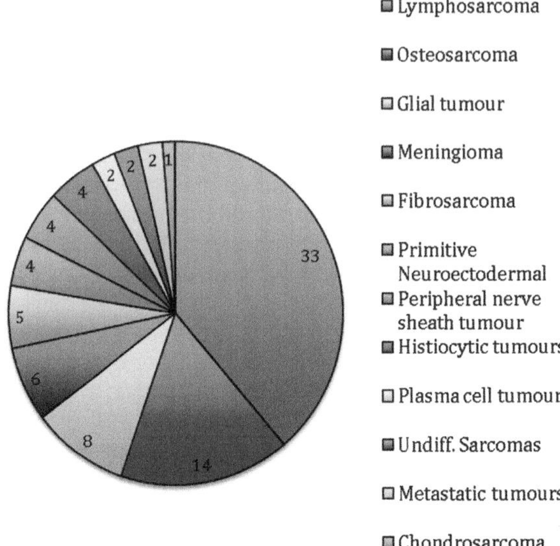

Fig. 2. Prevalence of tumors in a population of 85 cats with histologically confirmed primary or metastatic tumors of the spinal cord or causing spinal cord diseases by local extension from adjacent tissues.

most common tumor representing approximately half (45%–61%) of all the cases.[18,19] In the study by Rossmeisl and colleagues,[19] meningioma was the most common benign tumor (16/18), while osteosarcoma was the most common malignant tumor (3/8). Both the Levy and Rossmeisl studies did not include tumors that were not amenable for surgical cytoreduction, therefore they did not account for intramedullary tumors such as gliomas and primitive neuroectodermal tumors (PNET), and highly invasive and destructive tumors such as advanced osteosarcomas and fibrosarcomas.[18,19]

Lymphosarcoma

Lymphosarcoma was the most common tumor in a retrospective study of 85 cats with definitive diagnosis of spinal cord neoplasms.[2] In this study, cats diagnosed with spinal lymphosarcoma were significantly younger (mean and median age of 6 and 4 years) than cats with other spinal cord tumors (mean and median age of 9 and 10 years).[2] Cats with tumors other than lymphosarcoma had a normal age distribution, with 80% of the cats between the ages of 5 and 14 years; whereas cats with lymphosarcoma presented a bimodal age distribution, with 50% of them younger than 4 years and 25% older than 11 years.[2] The most common clinical signs of spinal lymphosarcoma in cats are progressive asymmetric posterior paresis or paralysis and spinal hyperesthesia,[2,20] as reported for other feline spinal cord tumors; however, cats with lymphosarcoma had a higher prevalence of nonspecific clinical signs such as anorexia, lethargy, weight loss, signs of respiratory tract infection, and abnormal behavior.[2] Presence of nonspecific clinical signs may be explained by immunosuppression associated with positive feline leukemia virus (FeLV) status in 56% of the cats with lymphosarcoma and the postmortem findings of lymphosarcoma involvement of extraneural organs in 85% of the cats.[2] In previous studies the percentage of cats positive for FeLV has been as high as 94%[20] and the percentage of cats with involvement of extraneural sites has been reported as between 43% and 100%.[20,21] A study found that the duration of clinical signs before diagnosis was significantly shorter in cats with lymphosarcoma than in cats with other spinal cord tumors; 93% of the cats with spinal lymphosarcoma were ill for less than 2 months before diagnosis.[2]

Spinal lymphosarcoma represents a challenge for in vivo diagnosis. A definitive diagnosis can be achieved with positive cytology on blood smears in 5% to 13% of the cases,[2,20] bone marrow aspirates in 14% to 67%,[2,22] and spinal fluid analysis in 9% to 35%.[2,20] The variability of positive results in the 3 studies considered is difficult to explain; all 3 studies are retrospective postmortem studies with a similar number of cases,[23–33] and it is possible that the low number of cases is responsible for the different percentages of in vivo tests with a positive result. Combination of multiple diagnostic tests, such as spinal fluid analysis and bone marrow aspirate, may provide a higher diagnostic yield. However, the diagnostic path most likely to provide a definitive in vivo diagnosis of spinal lymphosarcoma appears to be identification of intra- or extraneural masses by physical examination and diagnostic imaging (thoracic radiographs, abdominal ultrasound, spinal radiographs, and MRI or myelography), and fine-needle aspiration (FNA) or biopsy of the mass when possible.[2]

Kidney and bone marrow are the most common extraneural location of spinal lymphosarcoma, based on data from 5 publications, and their investigation may lead to a positive in vivo diagnosis of lymphosarcoma.[2,3,20–22] In cats with spinal lymphosarcoma, lymphosarcoma has been found to affect kidneys in 41% to 100% of cats,[2,20] and bone marrow in 45% to 54% of the cats.[2,22] In the study by Marioni-Henry and colleagues,[2] lymphosarcoma was also found in liver (36%), skeletal muscle (32%), spleen or lymph nodes (27%), and vertebrae or heart (18%). Within the CNS, lymphosarcoma tends to affect multiple regions of the spinal cord, especially thoracic and lumbosacral, and brain; based on 2 postmortem studies, 31% to 43% of cats with spinal lymphosarcoma had also brain involvement.[2,3] Spinal lymphosarcoma may have an exclusively extradural location, which has been reported in 85% to 96% of the cases in publications from the late 1970s and early 1990s[20–22]; however, most recent publications estimate 34% to 38% of feline spinal lymphosarcoma having an exclusive extradural location, with the majority of the cases (61% to 88%) presenting both extradural and intradural components.[2,3]

Prognosis for spinal lymphosarcoma is poor. Spodnick and colleagues[22] reported a complete or partial remission in a series of 6 cats with spinal lymphoma treated with vincristine, cyclophosphamide, and prednisone; the complete remission rate was 50% and the median duration was 14 weeks. Another cat treated with decompressive surgery and chemotherapy had a remission of 62 weeks. Lane and colleagues[20] reported on a series of 4 cats with spinal lymphosarcoma. Three cats were treated with L-asparaginase, vincristine, and prednisone following local spinal radiation, and 1 cat had surgical cytoreduction; 3 of the cats improved, and 1 was alive 13 months following presentation, but the 3 other cats were euthanized or died within 20 weeks of treatment because of systemic relapse. In the Marioni-Henry and colleagues[2] study, one cat with spinal lymphosarcoma was euthanized after recurrence of clinical signs 38 days following a single dose of local radiation therapy and treatment with prednisone, cyclophosphamide, and vincristine; another cat survived 60 days following surgical cytoreduction and treatment with prednisone, asparaginase, and cytarabine.

Osteosarcoma

Feline osteosarcomas affect more often the appendicular than the axial skeleton. In a retrospective study on feline neoplasms, 58% of the 19 cases of osteosarcoma affected the appendicular skeleton and only 2 affected vertebrae.[23] In another retrospective study of 22 feline osteosarcomas, only 32% affected the axial skeleton and none the vertebrae.[24] Nevertheless, vertebral osteosarcoma was the second most common tumor in a postmortem retrospective study on 85 cats with tumors affecting the spinal cord, affecting 14 cats,[2] and information on another 9 cats with histologically confirmed vertebral osteosarcomas has been reported.[18,19,25–28] Taken together, the 14 cats from the study by Marioni-Henry and colleagues[2] and the 9 other cats that all had vertebral osteosarcomas had a mean age of 8.3 years (median age 8 years, range 3–13 years), and included 12 males and 11 females, of which 19 were domestic short-haired (DSH) cats, 1 a Persian, and 1 an Angora cat.[18,19,25–28] The tumors affected the lumbar vertebrae in 9 cases, the thoracic vertebrae in 7 cases, the cervical region in 4 cases, and the sacrum and coccyx in 1 case each.[2,18,19,25–28] Radiographs showed a lytic lesion in 10 of 11 cases, and a pathologic vertebral fracture in 2 cases; CT revealed a pathologic fracture not visible on radiographs in 1 case. Myelography, performed in 5 cases, showed a compressive lesion with deviation or interruption of the flow of contrast in all cases.[2,26–28] MRI revealed presence of a vertebral mass in 2 cases (**Fig. 3**).[2] An FNA was performed in 3 cases; on cytology, the lesion was diagnosed as a neoplasm and an osteosarcoma in 1 case each, and in the last case the neoplasm was misdiagnosed as a lymphosarcoma.[2]

Cytoreductive surgery can prolong survival in cats with vertebral osteosarcoma, but results tend to be highly variable. Following cytoreductive surgery, 5 cats with vertebral osteosarcoma had a mean and median survival time of 145 and 88 days (range 2–518 days)[2,18,19,25–28]; 3 of these cats were part of a retrospective study of

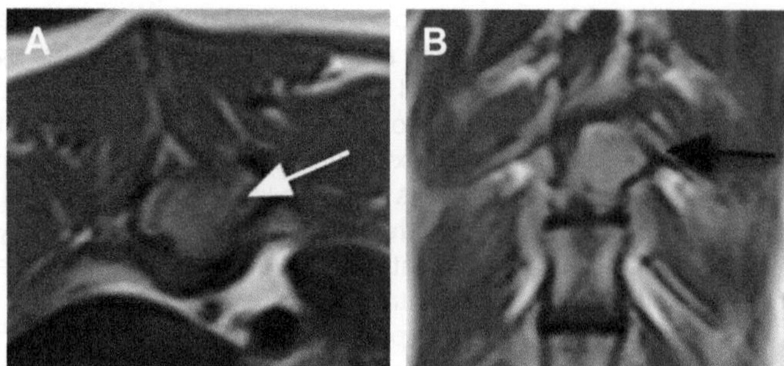

Fig. 3. Vertebral osteosarcoma in a DSH cat. Transverse T1-weighted (*A*) and dorsal T1-weighted postcontrast (*B*) images demonstrate a homogenously contrast-enhancing mass associated with the left pedicle and body of the 10th thoracic vertebra (*arrow*). (*Courtesy of* Sergio Rodenas and Sonia Anor, Neurology Service, Veterinary College, University of Barcelona.)

26 cats with nonlymphoid vertebral or spinal cord neoplasms treated surgically.[19] This study found that cytoreduction is a good palliative treatment, but the prognosis was based on the phenotype of the tumor and the surgeon's impression of a partial or complete excision; in fact, cats with malignant tumors (including the 3 osteosarcomas) were found to have a median survival time of 110.5 days versus 518 days for cats with benign tumors.[19]

Meningioma

Meningioma is the most common feline intracranial tumor, representing 58% of the cases in a recent study[29]; however, spinal meningioma represented only 7% of the cases in a study on histologically confirmed tumors affecting the spinal cord of cats[2] and 8% of the tumors of the feline spinal cord identified by MRI.[4] Based on information on 32 feline spinal meningiomas reported in the literature, the mean and median age of the affected cats is 9.7 and 9 years (range 5–14 years), the majority of cats are DSH (20/27), there is an equal gender distribution with 59% male cats, and the tumors affect more commonly the thoracic spinal cord (19 or 59% of the cases) than the cervical (7 cases) or lumbar (6 cases) spinal cord.[2,18,19,30–34] In all cases in which results of radiographic examination were reported, survey spinal radiographs were normal; myelography revealed an interruption of the normal flow of contrast at the level of the tumor, and in 2 cases where MRI was performed the tumor revealed a strong and homogeneous contrast enhancement (**Fig. 4**).[2,18,19,30–34] Two studies reported the survival time of cats treated with cytoreductive surgery. Levy and colleagues[18] reported a median survival time of 180 days (range 30–600 days) in 4 cats, with a fifth cat alive 1400 days following surgery. Rossmeisl and colleagues[19] reported a median survival time of 426 days (range 211–842 days) in 16 cats; 1 cat in the first study and 5 cats in the second were euthanized due to other conditions, and the reason for euthanasia was unknown in many cases.

TRAUMATIC

Intervertebral Disc Disease

Intervertebral disc disease (IVDD) is uncommon in cats. The incidence of IVDD in cats has been estimated as between 0.02% and 0.12%, whereas in dogs it is estimated at 2%.[35] A postmortem study of IVDD in cats performed in 1958 revealed the presence of

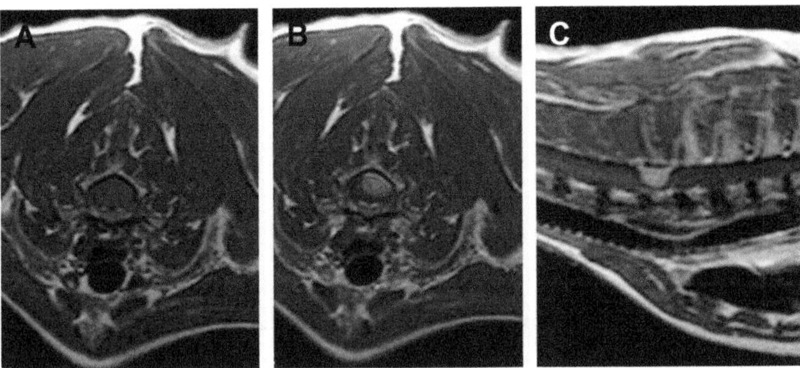

Fig. 4. Meningioma in a 12-year-old male Norwegian Forest cat. Transverse pre- (*A*) and postcontrast (*B*), and sagittal postcontrast (*C*) T1-weighted images at the level of the first thoracic vertebra demonstrate a smoothly marginated, homogenously contrast-enhancing mass displacing the spinal cord to the right. (*Courtesy of* Dr Rodolfo Cappello, North Downs Specialists Referrals, Bletchingley, Surrey, England.)

both Hansen type I (chondroid disc degeneration with annulus fibrosus completely perforated) and type II (fibroid degeneration with bulging annulus fibrosus) disc protrusions.[36] King and colleagues[36] found dorsal disc protrusions in 1 of every 4 cats obtained at random from local general practices, and severe trauma to the spine was the only exclusion criteria. In the same study, Hansen type I protrusions accounted for only 18% (16/91) of all protrusions; the cervical discs had the most protrusions of both types with a peak at C6-7; another peak of incidence was seen at the L4-5 intervertebral disc space.[36] King completed a second postmortem study in 1960, separating type II disc protrusion into small and large. In this study protrusions were more common in the cervical region than in the T10-S1 region; however, if only type I disc protrusions were considered, the cervical and T10-S1 regions had similar incidence (**Fig 5**A).[37] If the small type II protrusions were included, the highest incidence of protrusions was found in the C2-3 disc, and in the T10-S1 region, the incidence peak was not at the thoracolumbar junction as in the dog, but at L4-5.[37] Disc protrusions were found more frequently in older cats, in particular those older than 15 years.[38]

Recently, various investigators have published single case reports or case series of cats with IVDD, and there are 17 reports describing a total of 44 clinically affected cats with 50 intervertebral disc protrusions published between 1981 and November 2009.[1,35,39–53] One case report from 1971 was not considered, because the author later included the same case in a study on spinal lymphosarcoma.[54] Based on the information provided in these publications and including data from 8 cats from Marioni-Henry and colleagues,[1] the median and mean age of cats with clinical signs of IVDD was 8 years (range 1.5–17 years; 28 male cats and 16 female). Twenty-two cats were DSH, 10 domestic long-haired, 2 domestic medium-haired, and 10 (22%) were pure breed cats. The onset of clinical signs was acute in 13 of 43 cats and insidious with a progressive course in 30 of 43 (70%). Spinal hyperesthesia was reported in 22 of 24 (92%) cats. There were Hansen type I disc protrusions in 30 of 45 (67%) and type II in 15 of 45 cats. The most commonly affected intervertebral discs were L4-5 (9 cats), L7-S1, (7 cats), and T13-L1 (6 cats) (**Fig. 5**B). Two case series reports focused on lumbar and lumbosacral intervertebral disc disease in cats, and may have skewed the distribution of IVDD toward those locations, however, also in the study by King and Smith[37] the L4-5 disc space represented the peak of incidence for IVDD of both type I

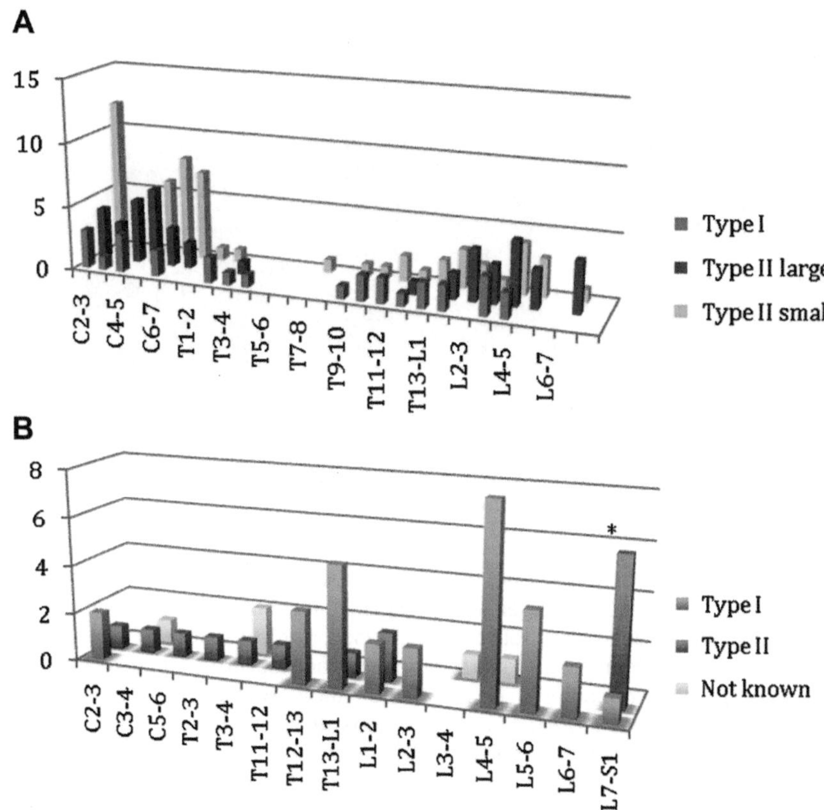

Fig. 5. (*A*) Prevalence of intervertebral disc protrusions in a population of 100 clinically unaffected cats (135 protrusions). (*Modified from* King AS, Smith RN. Disc protrusion in the cat: distribution of dorsal protrusion along the vertebral column. Vet Rec 1960;72:335–7; with permission.) (*B*) Prevalence of intervertebral disc protrusions in a population of 44 clinically affected cats (50 protrusions) published in veterinary literature between 1981 and 2009.[1,35,39–53] *Includes data from a study that only considered L7-S1 intervertebral disc disease in 6 cats.

and type II. The postmortem studies showed a high incidence of cervical disc protrusions, which were less common in clinically affected cats. It has been suggested that the cervical disc protrusions do not cause clinical signs because of the relatively larger size of the cervical vertebral canal.[38]

It is likely that the increased incidence of IVDD at certain locations of the spine is associated with the stance configuration and range of motion of the spine in the cat. A radiographic study of the cat vertebral column showed that during stance, the cat spine exhibits a mild dorsiflexion in the lower lumbar segments, a marked ventroflexion in the lower thoracic and upper lumbar segments, and a severe dorsiflexion in the cranial thoracic (above T9) and cervical segments.[55] The same study looked at the mean stance angles relative to the range of motion and found that during stance the lower lumbar joints (L4-5 to L6-7) are nearly maximally dorsiflexed and the joints from T10 to T13 are maximally ventroflexed, while the other joints are held midrange; this may explain the increased prevalence of IVDD at T12-L1 and L4-6 in clinically affected cats (see **Fig. 5**B).[55] In studies of both clinically affected and unaffected cats, IVDD is also found at unusual locations like T2-3 and T3-4 (see **Fig. 5**). These locations are unusual because discs between T1 and T10 in the dog and T1-T11 in the cats are covered by the intercapital or conjugal ligament, which extends from the head of one rib to the head of the opposite rib over the intervertebral disc and across the floor of the vertebral canal. This ligament is thought to provide additional support to the disc and protection from intervertebral disc protrusions in dogs.[37,56] However, cats owe their flexibility to their vertebral column being able to achieve a total torsion of almost 180° and that most of the torsion is seen within a small range of the lower thoracic vertebrae from about T4 to T11.[56] Another reason for their flexibility is that the scapulae do not articulate with the axial skeleton, rather, the trunk is supported by muscles (levator scapulae, serratus ventralis, and major and minor rhomboids) that originate on the medial surface of the scapula near the dorsal border and fan out to insert on the trunk in a sling-like arrangement.[56] These muscles suspend the trunk from the scapulae much like the wires on a suspension bridge and help to stabilize the trunk against rolling movements.[56] The net suspensory force vector between scapula and trunk intersects the vertebral column near the T2-3 joint.[56] Therefore, it is possible that the proximity of a very flexible area (T4-11) to a much more stable area (T2-3) of the cat spine may lead to the development of IVDD at those locations, especially during traumatic events; in fact, in 2 cases with T2-3 and T3-4 IVDD an external trauma was documented.[1]

Treatment of cats with IVDD is often successful, especially with surgical decompression of the spinal cord. Thirty cats had surgery, and 16 of them had an excellent outcome with the cat returning to normal; 5 cats had a good outcome with some residual neurologic deficits, 5 had a fair outcome, 3 were lost to follow-up, and 1 died.[1,35,39–53] Ten cats were treated conservatively, 3 cats had a good outcome, and 1 an excellent outcome after treatment with corticosteroids, acupuncture, and physical therapy. Among the cats with IVDD treated conservatively, 1 cat had a poor outcome, 1 died, and 4 were euthanized; the remaining 5 cats were euthanized immediately after the diagnosis.[1,35,39–53]

CONGENITAL DISEASES

Congenital diseases can affect the spinal cord of cats; these are listed here and discussed further in the article on congenital spinal cord diseases by Westworth and Sturges elsewhere in this issue. Sacrocaudal dysgenesis is a constellation of congenital abnormalities commonly reported in Manx and Manx-crossed cats; it may affect the lumbar, sacral, and coccygeal spine, and it is often associated with malformations of the spinal cord such as myelodysplasia, hydromyelia and/or syringomyelia, meningocele or meningomyelocele, and tethered spinal cord.[57–59] Other congenital diseases affecting the spinal cord of cats are cyst-like lesions, such as spinal arachnoid cyst,[60–65] spinal intradural epithelial cyst,[66] spinal dermoid cyst and sinus,[67,68] or vertebral malformations causing compression of the spinal cord, such as hypoplasia of the odontoid process with secondary atlantoaxial luxation, and multiple cartilaginous exostosis.[57]

VASCULAR DISEASES

Vascular diseases affecting the spinal cord represented 9% in a postmortem retrospective study of 205 cats with spinal cord disease, and ischemic myelopathy was suspected in 6.5% of the cases in a study on MRI findings in 92 cats with clinical signs of spinal cord disease.[1,4] In the first study, 15 of 19 older cats (median age 9 years) presented vascular lesions affecting multiple segments of the spinal cord (11/15) and brain (5/15). The most common lesion was spinal cord malacia, in some cases vasculopathy

(5/15); hemorrhage (5/15) or thrombosis (4/15) were also found.[1] In 4 cases, history and histopathologic findings of severe necrosis involving the ventrolateral gray and white matter of thoracolumbar spinal segments were suggestive of ischemic poliomyelomalacia associated with severe abdominal compression and prolonged vasospams of lumbar arteries.[69] Focal malacia was described in 4 cases of vascular myelopathy in the author's study; the cause of the lesion could not be determined though trauma, intervertebral disc disease, or fibrocartilaginous embolism were suspected.[1]

Fibrocartilaginous Embolism

Fibrocartilaginous embolism (FCE) is not commonly reported in cats; however, publications on suspected or confirmed cases of FCE are appearing with more frequency, probably because the advent of MRI increases one's index of suspicion for the surviving cats and provides a better lesion localization for the histopathologic examination. FCE is caused by a small fragment of degenerated disc that occludes the blood supply to the spinal cord, leading to ischemic necrotizing myelopathy.[70] The exact pathophysiology of FCE is not known. It has been suggested that herniated nucleus pulposus reaches the spinal cord entering first the vertebral body vasculature, or that the disc extrudes directly within the spinal vasculature or into persistent embryonal arteries of the annulus fibrosus, or anomalous vasculature, or that the disc enters vessels that reach the nucleus pulposus following chronic inflammation.[71]

Based on information from the veterinary literature, FCE tends to affect older cats, the progression of clinical signs lasts usually less than 24 hours, and the clinical signs are often lateralized and with cervicothoracic localization (**Fig. 6**).[70–77] In 14 cats with FCE (confirmed in 9 cases and suspected in 5) that had a mean age of 9 years (median 10 years, range 4–12 years), there was no breed or gender predisposition. The mean and median progression of clinical signs was 19 and 16 hours; however, progression of clinical signs lasted for more than 24 hours in 2 cases and in 1 case there was a recurrence of clinical signs 24 hours after the onset and initial recovery. The most common clinical signs were tetra- or hemiparesis or hemiplegia (9/14), followed by posterior paresis/paraplegia and Horner syndrome, reported in 5 cases each. Spinal tap was performed in 9 cases; in 5 cases spinal fluid analysis revealed neutrophilic pleocytosis, in 2 cases it was normal, in 1 case there was albuminocytological dissociation, and in 1 case blood contamination. Myelography was performed in 3 cases and showed spinal cord swelling in all of these cases. MRI was performed in 9 cases, characterized by intramedullary lesions hypo- or isointense to normal gray matter on T1-weighted images, and hyperintense on T2-weighted images, with mild or absent uptake of contrast. MacKay and colleagues[76] reported that timing of infarct enhancement is variable; MRI performed within hours from the onset of an infarct may not enhance, whereas 5 to 6 days later the gadolinium enhancement should be more evident. The cervicothoracic intumescence was the spinal cord region with the highest prevalence of suspected or confirmed FCE (50%), followed by the lumbosacral intumescence affected in 21% of the cases; in the dog, a study suggested that the lumbosacral intumescence has the highest incidence of confirmed FCE (47%) followed by the cervicothoracic intumescence with 31%.[78] Nine cats were euthanized, and FCE was confirmed by histologic examination of the spinal cord and findings of extensive malacia and intravascular fibrocartilaginous emboli (see **Fig. 6**B). Three cats made a complete recovery within 2 to 6 weeks and 2 cats showed a significant improvement with only mild conscious proprioceptive deficits within 3 to 7 weeks.[71,74,77]

Even with only 14 cases of FCE, it is possible to observe that the MRI findings of FCE were consistent, that FCE in cats seemed to predominate in the cervicothoracic

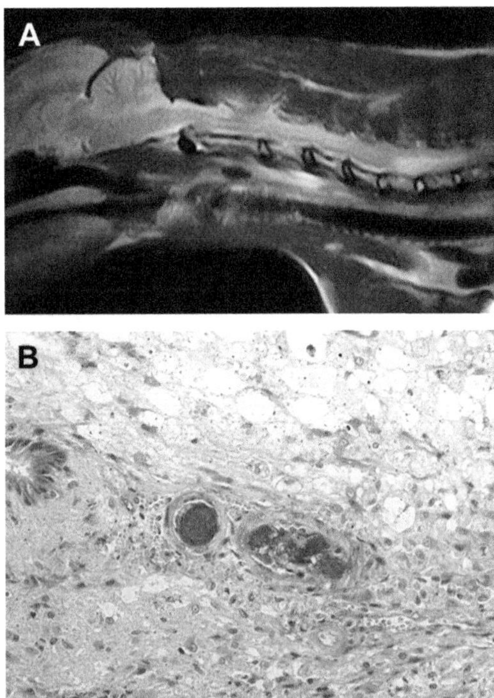

Fig. 6. Fibrocartilaginous embolism in a 9-year-old DSH cat. (*A*) Sagittal T2-weighted image of the caudal cervical spinal cord. There is a hyperintense intramedullary lesion extending from the sixth cervical to the first thoracic vertebra, and 2 degenerated intervertebral discs between the third and fifth cervical vertebrae. (*B*) Histopathological section of the caudal cervical spinal cord of the same cat in **Fig. 6**A. The toluidine blue–stained image reveals fibrocartilaginous emboli (stained purple) filling a vessel lumen within a necrotic section of the spinal cord (original magnification ×50 µm). (*Courtesy of* Sergio Rodenas, Sonia Anor, and Marti Pumarola, Neurology and Pathology Service, Veterinary College, University of Barcelona.)

intumescence, and clinical signs are markedly lateralized, especially when the cervical region is affected. The high incidence of FCE at the cervicothoracic intumescence is probably explained by the high prevalence of degenerated protruding disc in this region in the cat.[36,37] Also, the cervicothoracic junction is essential for head and neck movements in quadrupedal animals, especially for lowering the head.[79] One possible explanation for the marked lateralization of clinical signs may be associated with the arterial supply to the spinal cord of cats and dogs. Approximately half of the central arteries in the feline spinal cord alternate between branching to the right and left side, while the other central arteries have a common stem and supply both sides; the cervical region has a slightly higher frequency of unilateral central arteries (55%) compared with the thoracic (49%) and lumbar spinal cord (47%).[80]

Intraosseus Vascular Malformations

Intraosseus vascular malformations (IVM) causing spinal cord compression have been described in 3 young cats between the ages of 15 and 20 months with a history of 3 to 12 months of chronic progressive posterior paresis partially responsive to corticosteroid therapy.[81] In some cases, the presentation of IVM can be similar to a neoplastic disease; plain radiographs showed focal decreased bone density or lysis of thoracic vertebrae, T2, T4, and T10-11, respectively; and myelography showed obstruction of the contrast column or extradural compression in all cases.[81] The lesion was described as vessels of varying size with endothelial cells, prominent pericytes, and variable amount of smooth muscles among a loose connective stroma separated by lamellar bony trabeculae, with osteoblasts and infrequent osteoclasts.[81] The bony and vascular proliferations caused severe spinal cord compression. Despite the aggressiveness of vascular proliferations, Wells and Weisbrode[81] considered these lesions as developmental anomalies based on the young age of the cats and the well-differentiated appearance of the vessels including endothelial, perithelial, smooth muscle, and fibrous cells.

Myelopathy Secondary to Aortocaval Fistula

A recent report described myelopathy secondary to aortocaval fistula in a 15-month-old male DSH with history of progressive paraparesis of 3 months' duration.[82] A large aneurysmal dilation of the caudal vena cava and an anomalous vessel arising from the vena cava were identified on abdominal ultrasound. Myelography, nonselective angiography, and contrast-enhanced CT confirmed an aortocaval fistula and vena caval aneurysm, with an engorged vertebral venous plexus causing a bilateral ventrolateral spinal compression from T12 to L4. An attempt to surgically occlude the anomalous vessel was unsuccessful; on necropsy, the ventral and lateral portions of the spinal cord from T7 to L4 showed Wallerian degeneration, which was more severe from T11 to L1 spinal cord segments. Vascular malformations of the CNS such as the one reported are often developmental anomalies, but they can also be acquired secondary to trauma, rupture of an arterial aneurysm, or surgical ligation of blood vessels.[82]

DEGENERATIVE/INHERITED DISEASES

Storage diseases, spinal muscular atrophy, and neuroaxonal or neuronal dystrophy are degenerative and inherited diseases of the spinal cord of cats.[83] Other degenerative myelopathies may have an infectious or nutritional etiology, such as the FeLV or cobalamin deficiency associated myelopathies described below.[84,85] The storage diseases affecting the feline spinal cord are: gangliosidosis GM1/GM2 reported in Siamese, Korat, and domestic cats; glycogenosis type IV reported in Norwegian Forest and domestic cats; sphingomyelinosis (Niemann-Pick disease) in Siamese, Balinese, and domestic cats; and mucopolysaccharidosis type VI in Siamese and domestic cats.[83,86]

Neuroaxonal Dystrophy

Neuroaxonal dystrophy (ND) is a degenerative condition characterized by swelling of the distal segment of axons (spheroids) within the CNS.[87] ND is thought to be hereditary and transmitted by an autosomal recessive gene.[88] The clinical signs are hind limb ataxia progressing to paresis and paralysis, head tremors, and hypermetria.[87] ND was initially described in 6 litters of tricolored DSH cats; the most prominent histopathologic findings were presence of spheroids in the brainstem, atrophy of the cerebellar vermis, and depletion of neuron within the spiral ganglia.[88] Affected kittens developed the first clinical signs at 5 to 6 weeks of age and had a diluted coat color.[88] More recently, ND was reported in 3 DSH cats with onset of clinical signs between 7 and 9 months of age and in 2 Siamese cats with first clinical signs at 2 weeks of age; the 2 Siamese cats and 2 of the DSH had a normal coat color, and no signs of inner ear involvement was found in the 3 DSH.[87,89]

FeLV-Associated Degenerative Myelopathy

Chronically FeLV-infected cats may present with various neurologic signs including lethargy, abnormal behavior, vocalization, hyperesthesia, urinary incontinence, and posterior paresis progressing to paralysis.[84] In a retrospective study of 16 cats with chronic FeLV infection, the most common clinical signs were posterior paresis progressing to paralysis within 1 year.[84] The average age for cats with known birth dates was 9 years. All cats were FeLV seropositive for 2 to 4 years, only 4 of 12 cats had the typical hematological abnormalities associated with FeLV infection, such as anemia, macrocytosis, neutropenia, macrothrombocytes, and thrombocytopenia; 10 cats had lymphopenia, and CSF was analyzed in 7 cats and was unremarkable. On histopathology there were widespread lesions in the spinal cord and brainstem characterized by white matter degeneration with dilation of myelin sheaths; some of the dilated myelin sheaths were devoid of axons and others had intact or swollen axons. Positive FeLV p27 immunostaining was present in glial cells, neurons, and endothelial cells of the sections of all spinal cords examined. FeLV proviral DNA was extracted from spinal cord alone in 5 cats and from spinal cord, brain, spleen, and intestine in another 5 cats; CSF was positive only in 1 cat.[84]

METABOLIC/NUTRITIONAL DISEASES

Hypervitaminosis A

Hypervitaminosis A causes a metabolic osteopathy in cats fed a liver-based diet for months to year.[90] This metabolic osteodystrophy is characterized by bony osteophytes and exostosis around joints, and tendon, ligament, and joint capsule attachments, with the occipital bone and cervical and thoracic vertebrae the most commonly affected sites.[91] Initially, the osseous hyperplasia involves the cranial cervical vertebrae, then with progression of the disease the joints of the cervical and cranial thoracic vertebrae may coalesce and cause complete bony ankylosis. The pathophysiology of vitamin A toxicity is not well understood. It has been hypothesized that vitamin A increases lability of cytomembranes and renders them prone to mechanical injury, leading to the formation of exostosis.[92] Vitamin A toxicity causes also an inhibition of the collagen synthesis and breakdown of musculotendinous insertions in the periosteum during muscular activity, therefore in cats the excessive muscular activity during grooming could explain the predisposition of the cervicothoracic spine to be more commonly affected.[91] Pain, reduced mobility of the neck, and forelimb lameness due to bony ankylosis and nerve root compression are the early clinical signs of vitamin A toxicity in cats. In some cases the lesions may progress to induce paralysis. Radiographic evidence of vitamin A toxicity may be detected after 15 weeks in kittens on an induction diet.[92] It is usual for chronically and severely affected cats to have a poor prognosis for functional recovery, and correction of the diet merely stops progression of the clinical signs; however, in some cases some neurologic deficits seemed to be reversed by correction of the diet.[91]

Nutritional Secondary Hyperparathyroidism

Nutritional secondary hyperparathyroidism (NSH) due to chronic dietary calcium deficiency, which leads to increased serum levels of parathormone and accelerated bone resorption, has become rare since the advent of balanced commercial pet food. In the past this disorder was commonly reported in puppies and kittens fed an all-meat diet.[93] A diet low in calcium will especially affect young growing animals that have an increased demand of calcium for bone growth and minimal calcium reserves. In response to a decrease in serum calcium concentration there is an increase in secretion and synthesis of parathyroid hormone, which leads to increased bone resorption, renal calcium reabsorption/phosphorus excretion, and renal synthesis of active vitamin D. The clinical signs will reflect the effects of severe osteopenia and hypocalcemia. In a report of 6 cats with NSH, 2 cats presenting with spinal fractures associated with severe osteopenia were euthanized due to severe neurologic deficits; the other 4 cats improved after a change in diet.[93]

Myelopathy Associated with Cobalamin Deficiency

A 9-year-old cat with history of chronic pancreatitis associated with deficiency of serum cobalamin and folate concentrations presented with a progressive history of ataxia affecting all 4 limbs and tetraparesis.[85] Spinal reflexes were within normal limits. At the postmortem examination, the spinal cord presented bilateral and symmetric degeneration of the white matter. The most severe lesions affected the center of the dorsal columns of the caudal cervical and cervicothoracic segments with severe loss of fibers, marked astrocytosis, fibrosis, and proliferation of blood vessels. The cat had low serum concentration of cobalamin and folates, and clinical signs consistent with exocrine pancreatic insufficiency (EPI), confirmed by the histologic examination of the pancreas. Serum cobalamin concentrations are markedly decreased in most cats with exocrine pancreatic disease, because the intrinsic factor, which allows cobalamin absorption in the liver, is produced only by the pancreas in the cat. It is likely that chronic EPI and cobalamin deficiency caused the severe myelopathy in this cat as has been described in humans.[85]

REFERENCES

1. Marioni-Henry K, Vite C, Newton A, et al. Prevalence of diseases of the spinal cord of cats. J Vet Intern Med 2004;18:851–8.
2. Marioni-Henry K, Van Winkle TJ, Smith SH, et al. Tumors affecting the spinal cord of cats: 85 cases (1980-2005). J Am Vet Med Assoc 2008;232:237–43.
3. Bradshaw JM, Pearson GR, Gruffydd-Jones TJ. A retrospective study of 286 cases of neurological disorders of the cat. J Comp Pathol 2004;131:112–20.
4. Goncalves R, Platt S, Llabres-Diaz, et al. Clinical and magnetic imaging findings in 92 cats with clinical signs of spinal cord disease. J Feline Med Surg 2009; 11(2):53–9.
5. Simons AF, Vennema H, Rofina JE, et al. A mRNA PCR for the diagnosis of feline infectious peritonitis. J Virol Methods 2005;124:111–6.
6. Kornegay JN. Feline infectious peritonitis: the central nervous system form. J Am Anim Hosp Assoc 1978;14:580–4.
7. Baroni M, Heinhold Y. A review of the clinical diagnosis of feline infectious peritonitis viral meningoencephalomyelitis. Prog Vet Neurol 1995;6:88–94.
8. Kline KL, Joseph RJ, Averill DR. Feline infectious peritonitis with neurologic involvement: clinical and pathological findings in 24 cats. J Am Anim Hosp Assoc 1994;30:111–8.
9. Pedersen NC. A review of feline infectious peritonitis virus infection: 1963-2008. J Feline Med Surg 2009;11:225–58.
10. Hartmann K, Binder C, Hirschberger J, et al. Comparison of different tests to diagnose feline infectious peritonitis. J Vet Intern Med 2003;17:781–90.
11. Addie D, Belák S, Boucrat-Baralon C, et al. Feline infectious peritonitis. ABCD guidelines on prevention and management. J Feline Med Surg 2009;11: 594–604.
12. Hirschberger J, Hartmann K, Wilhelm N, et al. [Clinical symptoms and diagnosis or feline infectious peritonitis]. Tierarztl Prax 1995;23:92–9 [in German].

13. Foley JE, Lapointe JM, Koblik P, et al. Diagnostic features of clinical neurologic feline infectious peritonitis. J Vet Intern Med 1998;12:415–23.
14. Kitagawa M, Okada M, Kanayama K, et al. A feline case of isolated fourth ventricle with syringomyelia suspected to be related with feline infectious peritonitis. J Vet Med Sci 2007;69:759–62.
15. Okada M, Kitagawa M, Ito D, et al. MRI of secondary cervical syringomyelia in four cats. J Vet Med Sci 2009;71:1069–73.
16. Hartmann K, Ritz S. Treatment of cats with feline infectious peritonitis. Vet Immunol Immunopathol 2008;123:172–5.
17. Legendre AM, Bartges JW. Effect of polyprenyl immunostimulant on the survival time of three cats with the dry form of feline infectious peritonitis. J Feline Med Surg 2009;11:624–8.
18. Levy MS, Mauldin G, Kapatkin AS, et al. Nonlymphoid vertebral canal tumors in cats: 11 cases (1987-1995). J Am Vet Med Assoc 1997;210:663–4.
19. Rossmeisl J, Lanz O, Waldron D, et al. Surgical cytoreduction for the treatment of non-lymphoid vertebral and spinal cord neoplasms in cats: retrospective evaluation of 26 cases (1990-2005). Vet Comp Oncol 2006;4:41–50.
20. Lane SB, Kornegay JN, Duncan JR, et al. Feline spinal lymphosarcoma: a retrospective evaluation of 23 cats. J Vet Intern Med 1994;8:99–104.
21. Zaki FA, Hurvitz AI. Spontaneous neoplasms of the central nervous system of the cat. J Small Anim Pract 1976;17:773–82.
22. Spodnick GJ, Berg J, Moore FM, et al. Spinal lymphoma in cats: 21 cases (1976–1989). J Am Vet Med Assoc 1992;200:373–6.
23. Engle GC, Brodey RS. A retrospective study of 395 feline neoplasms. J Am Anim Hosp Assoc 1969;5:21–31.
24. Bitetto WV, Patnaik AK, Schrader SC, et al. Osteosarcoma in cats: 22 cases (1974-1984). J Am Vet Med Assoc 1987;190:91–3.
25. Liu SK, Dorfman HD, Patnaik AK. Primary and secondary bone tumors in the cat. J Small Anim Pract 1975;15:141–56.
26. O'Brien D. Osteosarcoma of the vertebra causing compression of the thoracic spinal cord in a cat. J Am Anim Hosp Assoc 1980;16:497–9.
27. Wheeler SJ. Spinal tumors in cats. Vet Annu 1989;29:270–7.
28. Radaelli ST, Platt SR, McDonnell JJ. What is your diagnosis? J Small Anim Pract 2000;41:84–6.
29. Troxel MT, Vite CH, Van Winkle TJ, et al. Feline intracranial neoplasia: retrospective review of 160 cases (1985-2001). J Vet Intern Med 2003;17:850–9.
30. Ross J, Wybrun RS. A report on the clinical investigation of a paraplegic cat. N Z Vet J 1969;17:251–3.
31. Jones BR. Spinal meningioma in a cat. Aust Vet J 1974;50:229–31.
32. Wheeler SJ, Clayton Jones DG, Wright JA. Myelography in the cat. J Small Anim Pract 1985;26:143–52.
33. Yoshioka MM. Meningioma of the spinal cord in a cat. Compend Contin Educ Pract Vet 1987;9:34–8.
34. Asperio RM, Marzola P, Zibellini E, et al. Use of magnetic resonance imaging for diagnosis of a spinal tumor in a cat. Vet Radiol Ultrasound 1999;40:267–70.
35. Munana KR, Olby NJ, Sharp NJH, et al. Intervertebral disc disease in 10 cats. J Am Anim Hosp Assoc 2001;37:384–9.
36. King AS, Smith RN, Kon VM. Protrusion of the intervertebral disc in the cat. Vet Rec 1958;70:509–15.
37. King AS, Smith RN. Disc protrusion in the cat: distribution of dorsal protrusion along the vertebral column. Vet Rec 1960;72:335–7.

38. Rayward R. Feline intervertebral disc disease: a review of the literature. Vet Comp Orthop Traumatol 2002;15:137–44.
39. Seim HB III, Nafe LA. Spontaneous intervertebral disk extrusion with associated myelopathy in a cat. J Am Anim Hosp Assoc 1981;17:201–4.
40. Gilmore DR. Extrusion of a feline intervertebral disk. Vet Med Small Anim Clin 1983;78:207–9.
41. Littlewood JD, Herrtage ME, Palmer AC. Intervertebral disc protrusion in a cat. J Small Anim Pract 1984;25:119–27.
42. Sparkes AH, Skerry TM. Successful management of a prolapsed intervertebral disc in a Siamese cat. Feline Pract 1990;18:7–9.
43. Bagley RS, Tucker RL, Moore MP, et al. Intervertebral disk extrusion in a cat. Vet Radiol Ultrasound 1995;36:380–2.
44. Kathman AS, Cizinauskas S, Rytz U, et al. Spontaneous lumbar intervertebral disc protrusion in cats: literature review and case presentations. J Feline Med Surg 2000;2:207–12.
45. Knipe MF, Vernau KM, Hornof WJ, et al. Intervertebral disc extrusion in six cats. J Feline Med Surg 2001;3:161–8.
46. Lu D, Lamb CR, Wesselingh K, et al. Acute intervertebral disc extrusion in a cat and MRI findings. J Feline Med Surg 2002;4:65–8.
47. McConnell JF, Garosi LS. Intramedullary intervertebral disc extrusion in a cat. Vet Radiol Ultrasound 2004;45:327–30.
48. Jaeger G, Early P, Munana K, et al. Lumbosacral disc disease in a cat. Vet Comp Orthop Traumatol 2004;17:104–6.
49. Smith PM, Jeffery ND. What is your diagnosis? A case of intervertebral disc protrusion in a cat. J Small Anim Pract 2006;47:104–6.
50. Maritato KC, Colon JA, Mauterer JV. Acute non-ambulatory tetraparesis attributable to cranial cervical intervertebral disc disease in a cat. J Feline Med Surg 2007;9:494–8.
51. Böttcher P, Flegel T, Böttcher IC, et al. Partial lateral corpectomy, for ventral extradural thoracic spinal cord compression in a cat. J Feline Med Surg 2008;10:291–5.
52. Harris J, Dhupa S. Lumbosacral intervertebral disk disease in six cats. J Am Anim Hosp Assoc 2008;44:109–15.
53. Choi KH, Hill SA. Acupuncture treatment for feline multifocal intervertebral disc disease. J Feline Med Surg 2009;11:706–10.
54. Heavner JE. Intervertebral disc syndrome in the cat. J Am Vet Med Assoc 1971;159:425–7.
55. Mcpherson JM, Ye Y. The cat vertebral column: stance configuration and range of motion. Exp Brain Res 1998;119:324–32.
56. Evans HE. Arthrology. In: Evans HE, editor. Miller's anatomy of the dog. Philadelphia: WB Saunders; 1993. p. 219–57.
57. Shell LG. Spinal cord diseases in cats. Vet Med 1998;6:553–64.
58. Leipold HW, Huston K, Blauch B, et al. Congenital defects of the caudal vertebral column and spinal cord in Manx cats. J Am Vet Med Assoc 1974;164:520–3.
59. Plummer SB, Bunch SE, Khoo LH, et al. Tethered spinal cord and intradural lipoma associated with a meningocele in a Manx-type cat. J Am Vet Med Assoc 1993;203:1159–61.
60. Grevel V, Schmidt-Oechtering GU, Harms N. Eine arachnoidalzyste bei der Katze. Kleintierpraxis 1989;34:55–62.

61. Shamir MH, Shahar R, Aizenberg I. Subarachnoid cyst in a cat. J Am Anim Hosp Assoc 1997;33:123–5.
62. Galloway AM, Curtis NC, Sommerland SF, et al. Correlative imaging findings in seven dogs and one cat with spinal arachnoid cysts. Vet Radiol Ultrasound 1999;4:445–52.
63. Vignoli M, Rossi F, Sarli G. Spinal subarachnoid cyst in a cat. Vet Radiol Ultrasound 1999;40:116–9.
64. Schmidt MJ, Schachenmayr W, Thiel C, et al. Recurrent spinal arachnoid cyst in a cat. J Feline Med Surg 2007;9:509–13.
65. Sugiyama T, Simpson DJ. Acquired arachnoid cyst in a cat. Aust Vet J 2009; 87:296–300.
66. Lujan A, Philbey AW, Anderson TJ. Intradural epithelial cyst in a cat. Vet Rec 2003;153:363–4.
67. Henderson JP, Pearson GR, Smerdon TN. Dermoid cyst of the spinal cord associated with ataxia in a cat. J Small Anim Pract 1993;34:402–4.
68. Tong T, Simpson DJ. Spinal dermoid sinus in a Burmese cat with paraparesis. Aust Vet J 2009;87:450–4.
69. Summers BA, Cummings JF, de Lahunta A. Degenerative diseases of the central nervous system. In: Summers BA, Cummings JF, de Lahunta A, editors. Veterinary neuropathology. St. Louis (MO): Mosby-Year Book; 1995. p. 208–350.
70. Zaki FA, Prata RG, Werner LL. Necrotizing myelopathy in a cat. J Am Vet Med Assoc 1976;169:228–9.
71. Coradini M, Johnstone I, Filippich, et al. Suspected fibrocartilaginous embolism in a cat. Aust Vet J 2005;83:550–1.
72. Bichsel P, Vandevelde M, Lang J. L'infarctus de la moelle épinière à la suite d'embolies fibrocartilagineuses chez le chien and le chat. Schweiz Arch Tierheilkd 1984;126:387–97.
73. Turner PV, Percy DH, Allyson K. Fibrocartilaginous embolic myelopathy in a cat. Can Vet J 1995;36:712–3.
74. Scott HW, O'Leary MT. Fibro-cartilaginous embolism in a cat. J Small Anim Pract 1996;37:228–31.
75. Abramson CJ, Platt SR, Stedman NL. Tetraparesis in a cat with fibrocartilaginous emboli. J Am Anim Hosp Assoc 2002;38:153–6.
76. MacKay AD, Rusbridge C, Sparkes AH, et al. MRI characteristics of suspected acute spinal cord infarction in two cats, and a review of the literature. J Feline Med Surg 2005;7:101–7.
77. Mikszewski JS, Van Winkle TJ, Troxel MT. Fibrocartilaginous embolic myelopathy in five cats. J Am Anim Hosp Assoc 2006;42:226–33.
78. Cauzinille L. Fibrocartilagineous embolism in dogs. Vet Clin North Am Small Anim Pract 2000;30:155–67.
79. Graf W, de Weale C, Vidal PP, et al. The orientation of the cervical vertebral column in unrestrained awake animals. Brain Behav Evol 1995;45: 209–31.
80. Culkin SE, Purinton PT, Oliver JE. Arterial supply to the spinal cord of dogs and cats. Am J Vet Res 1989;50:425–30.
81. Wells MY, Weisbrode SE. Vascular malformations in the thoracic vertebrae of three cats. Vet Pathol 1987;24:360–1.
82. Kube SA, Vernau KM, Wisner ER, et al. Myelopathy secondary to aortocaval fistula in a cat. Vet Radiol Ultrasound 2004;45:528–31.

83. Marioni-Henry K. Myelopathy, paresis/paralysis, cats. In: Tilley LP, Smith FW, editors. Blackwell's five-minute veterinary consult: canine and feline. Ames (IA): Blackwell Publishing; 2007. p. 920–3.
84. Carmichael KP, Bienzle D, McDonnell JJ. Feline leukemia virus-associated myelopathy in cats. Vet Pathol 2002;39:536–45.
85. Salvadori C, Cantile C, De Ambrogi G, et al. Degenerative myelopathy associated with cobalamin deficiency in a cat. J Vet Med A Physiol Pathol Clin Med 2003;50:292–6.
86. de Lahunta A, Glass E. Visual system. In: de Lahunta A, Glass E, editors. Veterinary neuroanatomy and clinical neurology. St. Louis (MO): Saunders Elsevier; 2009. p. 389–440.
87. Carmichael KP, Howerth EW, Oliver JE, et al. Neuroaxonal dystrophy in a group of related cats. J Vet Diagn Invest 1993;5:585–90.
88. Woodard JC, Collins GH, Hessier JR. Feline hereditary neuroaxonal dystrophy. Am J Pathol 1974;74:551–66.
89. Rodriguez F, Espinosa de los Monteros A, Morales M, et al. Neuroaxonal dystrophy in two Siamese kitten littermates. Vet Rec 1996;138:548–9.
90. Goldman AL. Hypervitaminosis A in a cat. J Am Vet Med Assoc 1992;200:1970–2.
91. Polizopoulou ZS, Kazakos G, Patsikas MN, et al. Hypervitaminosis A in the cat: a case report and review of the literature. J Feline Med Surg 2005;7:363–8.
92. Seawright AA, English PB. Hypervitaminosis A and deforming cervical spondylosis of the cat. J Comp Pathol 1967;77:29–39.
93. Tomsa K, Glaus T, Hauser M, et al. Nutritional secondary hyperparathyroidism in six cats. J Small Anim Pract 1999;40:533–9.

Index

Note: Page numbers of article titles are in **boldface** type.

Vet Clin Small Anim 40 (2010) 1029–1040
doi:10.1016/S0195-5616(10)00108-7 vetsmall.theclinics.com
0195-5616/10/$ – see front matter

D

E

F

G

H

I

N

O

P

W

Printed and bound by CPI Group (UK) Ltd, Croydon, CR0 4YY

03/10/2024

01040458-0010